About The Author...

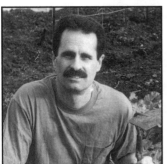

Photo taken August '96

When John Thomas began his pursuit of agelessness, his *calendar age* was only 27, while his *real* age—that is, his **bio-electric age**—was 39. Today 2006, John is 61 years by the calendar; yet his bio-electric age is is only 19 years **"young!"** Thomas is living proof that aging and aging reversal are matters of "choice."

John was heavily influenced by the exemplary lives of Paul C. Bragg, and Jack LaLanne.

At age 61, John can personally attest "I've *been there and done it!"* He has **reversed** all of the signs of aging in his body by following a *"model"* that is based on the way the body *actually* works—rather than relying on **"experts"** and their **faulty** "medical model" which does **NOT** deliver the desired results!

Except for emergency procedures and "parts" replacement, Thomas says medical "science" is a mess of *confusion* and *failure.* The "alternative" approach is based on a similar *faulty* model—offering people safer band-aids, but little "meaningful" progress. The **"PROOF"** says Thomas is *"All the sick and dying healers!"* Young Again! is an **indictment** of a faulty medical "model"—and the "sick care" system it seeded and perpetuates!

Thomas uncovered the **mysteries** behind the aging process; then **developed** and **tested** the *Young Again Model*™— a model based on thinking and living **outside the box!** The results are **undeniable** and **available** to anyone seeking a better life—free of dependence on the "sick-care" system. *Young Again!* is **meaningful** because the author has **personally** lived the subject matter—and is **living** proof that aging reversal is within people's reach if they want it. [See author's photo on back cover.]

Writing a book like *Young Again!* requires "keen" observation skills and a broad background in life-sciences, philosophy, politics, history, nutrition and agriculture. John Thomas thinks *"outside the box"* and *write "low tech"*—using a writing style that ensures *"communication"* with the reader rather than "conversation!" [See *Chicken or Duck,* Chapter 39.]

Young Again! is a practical *"How To!"* book that tells **exactly** what must be done to **recapture** youth, **reverse** disease and **extend** life. The book was **NOT** written for pretentious **"experts"** who *cannot* demonstrate *living proof* in their lives or in that of their patients. Critics of the *Young Again Protocol*™ argue "theory" because they don't have a viable working model.

Young Again! is a **living testimony** that encourages everyone to **walk the talk** through personal responsibility!

Thoughts From Patricia Bragg

What a masterpiece! *Young Again!* is the best of the best! It will help millions of people.

We are a nation of half-dead people! Cancer, heart trouble, high blood pressure, osteoporosis, etc. The health of our people is slipping fast. The question is why?

Good health is something that cannot be purchased from a doctor or in a bottle of pills. Good health is the product of a healthy lifestyle. America needs to know more about how to achieve health and vitality. Staying youthful, no matter what your age, is central to the health message and to the message of this book.

My father, Dr. Paul C. Bragg N.D., Ph.D., was a teenager dying of tuberculosis when he *chose* a life of health. Dad was ninety-seven years "young" when he died of a surfboard accident. During his life, he helped thousands of people find the path to agelessness. One of those people was Jack LaLanne.

Jack was a sickly boy. His health was so poor he was forced to drop out of school. Dad's message changed his life. Today, Jack LaLanne is a legend. He is living proof that the health message really works.

Dad said the world was lacking strong, courageous men and women who were not afraid to buck the trend of commercialism in the food industry and in the healing arts—people who could stand tall.

Here we have a strong crusader who *believes* in the health message and who *lives* what he preaches. John Thomas' wonderful book is his gift of love to the world.

Now, dear reader, it is your turn to experience a life of boundless energy and health. The keys are in your hand. Read and follow this book and it will change your life. *Young Again!* is the most thorough and concise message ever written on the subject of healthy living.

No excuses. You know right from wrong. Remember, what you eat and drink you become. It's either sickness or it's health. It's time to choose. Now! Today!

Young Again! is truly a personal guide to ageless living. I am honored to be a part of it.

Author's Introductory Comments
To The 6ᵗʰ Edition Of *Young Again!*

The 6ᵗʰ edition marks a major **"SHIFT"** from earlier editions. **Five new chapters** have been added; the book has been **TOTALLY** rewritten to provide a smooth flow of information and throught. Significant content changes have been made and all pertinent information has been retained.

Readers of earlier editions will benefit by **"reading"** this 6ᵗʰ edition in the **"order written"**—and in its **ENTIRETY**. New information is presented on nearly every page of the book.

"Window box" pages following each chapter direct the reader's attention to specific subjects and protocols for better understanding of "fundamental" concepts—and to provide the reader with ideas that are useful in everyday life.

"Links" have been added to the original "first" 35 chapters—referencing the reader to related subject matter located throughout the book and in "new" chapters.

"New" chapters are: 35, 36, 37, 38 and 39. Topics are discussed in multiple places throughout the book in "context" of related subjects to insure "continuity of thought" and to cause the reader to recognize that body physiology and health issues are "interconnected"—and never "isolated" issues.

The Glossary and Index have been substancially expanded to accommodate new **words** and **concepts** for clarification and understanding by the reader and to assist the reader in locating subjects and points of interest quickly and easily. Also, significant cross-indexing has been added within the body of each chapter for quick reference.

Your author is taking **"personal"** responsibility for a grammatically correct and hopefully error-free 6ᵗʰ edition. Typographical errors are the territory of the "proof reader!" Context and continuity issues are the author's responsibility. Clarity of thought is "unique" to the author and cannot be "farmed-out!" The reader should enjoy the improvements.

Writing of the 6ᵗʰ edition of *Young Again!* absorbed thousands of hours due to the volume of new information and the difficulties encountered when **"weaving"** new information into the fabric of concepts and protocols from earlier editions.

Your author hopes the reader will come to know the wonderful feeling that comes with *aging reversal* and being "in-control" of one's life and health.

May "you" dear reader become *Young Again!*

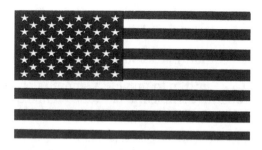

Authored and published under the jurisdiction of the
Title 4 U.S.C. 1 Flag of Peace of the united States of America
as confirmed by the flag on front cover.
Young Again! is a "common law" offering into the public domain.
Printed in the united States of America

Young Again!
How To Reverse The Aging Process
By John Thomas

Plexus Press P.O. Box 1240 Mead, WA 99021
Phone (509) 465-4154   Fax: (509) 466-8103
(800) 659-1882
(Sorry, no email. Please use above contacts.)

Cataloging-In-Publication Data
Thomas, John
Young Again! How to Reverse The Aging Process / by John
Thomas. (1st edition April, 1994)
p. cm. • References: p. • Includes index and glossary.
ISBN 1-884757-80-4 (6th edition, April, 2006)
1. Aging. 2. Rejuvenation. 3. Longevity. 4. Health. I. Title
RA776.75.T56   2006
613.04—dc20   94-65131

Printings: 20 19 18 17 16 15 14 13 12 11 10 9 8

LEGAL NOTICE

Aging reversal requires the investment of time, energy, and money by the reader/Citizen desiring the experience, knowing that aging reversal is "personal and unique" to the indivdual. The **"intent of mind"** of the author and publisher in making *Young Again!* available in the public domain is limited to the dissemination of health-related information for causing THINKING among Citizens and QUESTIONING of medical modalities and advice. Neither the publisher nor author offer "medical" advice, and the book *Young Again!* is not to be used for medical diagnosis. The author and publisher believe the information provided is complete and accurate, but mistakes both typographical and in content may be discovered after printing; and therefore, the reader should use *Young Again!* as a general guide only and not as the ultimate source of information. Neither author nor publisher have liability or responsibility for any reader/Citizen respecting loss or damage caused or alleged for reliance on information in *Young Again!*

➡ **THE READER IS PERSONALLY RESPONSIBLE FOR SEEKING "PROFESSIONAL" MEDICAL CARE BY THE READER'S OWN CHOICE.**

vi

DEDICATED TO...

Robert McLeod—You will meet Bob in Chapter One. He became my mentor, a living example, and a good friend.

Dr. Paul C. Bragg N.D., Ph.D.—Paul Bragg was the point man of the health movement in the United States. Millions of people owe their lives to him. He served his fellow man well, and his Creator to the fullest. Paul Bragg saved my life!

Charles Walters—Charlie is the editor of *Acres USA*. He taught me to winnow the wheat from the chaff. He helped me establish the link between "live food and live soil." His editorial pen is the harbinger of TRUTH in matters of agriculture and national economics. He is another Thomas Paine!

Diane DeFelice M.S., R.D.—Diane was my upper level college nutrition instructor. She is unselfish in her effort to help students make the connection between diet, lifestyle and good health. She helped me realize that *Young Again!* simply had to be written in order to set the record straight.

Patricia Bragg N.D., Ph.D.—Patricia *challenged* me to write this book. She also challenged me to pick up the baton her father handed to her and to Jack LaLanne. Patricia is the daughter of the great Wizard—"Paul Bragg." Patricia is a mighty force in the health movement worldwide. She is a voice crying in the wilderness!

Jack LaLanne—Beginning in the 1950's, Jack LaLanne became "Mr. Fitness." He is a living example of the benefits that accrue from a healthy lifestyle and regular exercise. Jack has been the point man in the fitness industry for over 40 years! He deserves our applause and thanks. Many people have been blessed by his work.

Leonard Ridzon—Of all the people I've known in 61 years, this farmer makes me think more than any other. Leonard is a simple man, but he isn't simple. He sees the Creator's handiwork and asks questions to whoever will listen. His questions can hold a pack of doctors at bay; they seldom risk an answer. And when Leonard talks, you had best be listening. He says as much *between* the lines as he does in words. Thank you Leonard for teaching me to observe, think and question!

TABLE OF CONTENTS

Chapters...

Acknowledgements

The author would like to take this opportunity to acknowledge and thank the following people who were involved, directly and indirectly, in bringing this book to fruition and to the attention of the public.

Robert Stephan D.D.S., Dr. John Briggs D.C., Linus Pauling M.D., Edward Arana D.D.S., Hal Huggins D.D.S., Joseph Kramer M.D., Ignaz Semmelweis M.D., Thomas Gerber M.D., Arnold Lorand M.D., Max Gerson M.D., Dr. Carey Reams, Drs. Paul C. and Patricia Bragg, Dr. Bernard Jensen, Guenther Enderlein M.D, and Robert F. Hofman M.D.

Also, Bob Mcleod, Jack LaLanne, Charles Walters, Christopher Bird, Roger Lent, Ellen Rosbach, Merlyn Anderberg, Diane DeFelice, Ray and Carolyn Teagarden, Dan Poynter, Tom Mahoney, Pat and Kay Lee, Cathy Cameron, Keith Ries and to the family into which I was blessed to have been born.

Special thanks to Marjorie Fisher and Douglas E. Wells.

Cover Design by:　　　John Thomas

Cover Preparation by:　　Dunn + Associates
P.O. Box 870
Hayward WI 54843
(715) 634-4857

CREDITS:
Credit hereby given for Progressive *Spinal Deformation In Osteoporosis* medical illustration shown on page 100, per:

Introduction by Robert B. Stephan D.D.S.

Man's ways are the antithesis of Nature's ways. They have little resemblance to the natural healing process. Nature provides the basis of life and the potential to help man correct his tendency towards disease, but drug-based medicine has chosen to increase health care productivity rather than identify the constraints which inhibit good health.

Allopathic medicine seems to be infatuated with technology, powerful drugs, and the suppression of symptoms. It prefers to *cut, poison,* and *burn,* when less would do. Medicine's world is physical and chemical.

We are moving away from this physical and chemical-based system of disease care and into the realm of energy and spirit. This is not a new movement, but a rediscovery of ancient wisdom. It is a mix of "proven" wisdom combined with technology.

As we move away from a *disease* care system and into a *health* care system, we will need a compass and a road map to navigate by if we hope to find our way through the maze of exploding knowledge and rediscovered tradition that is fast approaching us.

Young Again! serves the dual purpose of a navigation tool and a survival manual. It is easy to read and it is a very complete gathering of information. It will guide you to a healthy, vibrant life; *and* it will take you where Western Allopathic doctors fear to tread.

It is a divine privilege to be involved in the march to a preferred future, and it is a great pleasure to have John Thomas' wonderful book to use as a fount of information in my position as a Holistic Biological Dentist. Discover in this book the joy and path of good health!

Dr. Robert B. Stephan, D.D.S., B.S., F.A.P.D.
731 Indiana, Spokane WA 99205   (509) 325-2051
Holistic Dental Association, Board of Directors
International Academy of Oral Medicine and Toxicology
American Academy of Biological Dentistry
Occidental Institute, Research Faculty
Environmental Dental Association

Introduction by Dr. John A. Briggs

Our body is an incredible work of art. Unfortunately, it does not come with an owner's manual—as does a car—that tells us *how* to care for our body.

Consider the master mechanic. He has knowledge of the workings of his car. He knows how to protect his investment. His world is a world of regular maintenance and mechanical details. He avoids the pitfalls of ownership through individual responsibility. He knows *how* to maintain his car's youthfulness and vigor.

The medical world is not like the world of the master mechanic. In my practice, I have seen people with the full range of health-related problems—problems directly related to modern living—problems that could be avoided if people only had an owner's manual.

These people come to me willing to spend their fortunes. They have tasted the bitterness of disease and old age—they cry out for good health. They also DREAM of regaining the health of their youth.

I help them as best I can. I point the way, but my time is limited as is their money. What these people really need is an owner's manual for the care and maintenance of their body. I have wished for such a manual.

My wish was fulfilled when John Thomas wrote *Young Again!* It contains all the information my patients need to maintain their youth and vigor.

Young Again! arms the reader with practical, valuable information. This book is correctly aligned with the concepts of Naturopathic medicine. It will help the reader to stay young no matter what their age.

Thomas' research is exhaustive. He has a thorough working knowledge of the healing arts. Most importantly, he drives home his points with simple examples designed to help the reader understand.

Read this book and follow the information it contains. If you do, you too can achieve the radiant health I observed when John Thomas first introduced himself.

Dr. John A. Briggs
Naturopathic Physician
Clatskanie, Oregon

Foreword by Charles Walters

"People can be 'fed' to live peacefully or fight, to think or dream, to work or sleep, to be virile or pathologic, physically, mentally, and spiritually developed or retarded, and for any possible degree of advance or variation within the mechanical limits of the organism."

This was the late Albert Carter Savage speaking during the early years of WW II, and Winston Churchill took him seriously. After all, the health of England's fighting men was all that stood between the freedom of Englishmen and Hitler's thirst for world domination.

It was realized that food had to carry a fair complement of minerals in order to confer health, and the idea that vitamins could function without minerals was at least as strange as the concept that coal-tar drugs—capable of making a healthy person ill—could make a sick person well.

These few thoughts came to mind when John Thomas' manual *Young Again!* arrived on my editorial desk.

Individual health is too important to be left in the hands of physicians. How can a person make informed decisions to preserve health and conquer sickness as well? Most books deal with individual problems—single factor analysis, we call it—but leave unanswered the silent killer in our lives, namely *shelf life.* For it is shelf life in the grocery store that annihilates the quality of life for the consumer.

When most of today's senior citizens were still youngsters, strange words in type too small to read became an indispensable part of almost every label. First came the emulsifiers and stabilizers—carrageenan in cheese spreads, chocolate products, evaporated milk, ice cream and dairy products. All evidence of mutagenicity, carcinogenicity, and teratogenicity remained neatly tucked away in the scientific literature.

Dioctyl sodium sulfosuccinate became the wetting agent of choice, even though infants suffered gastrointestinal irritation and reduced growth rates as a consequence of its use. There were also dozens of flavorings and colors other than Red Nos. 2 & 4, all inimical to sustained human health. Aspartame (Nutrasweet™) is a sweetener with approximately 160 times the sweetness of sugar. The problem is that people with phenylketonuria can't handle it. It accumulates in the system and causes mental retardation and even death. Cereals, chewing gum, and gelatins are loaded with it.

As shelf life for foods improved, strange anomalies in the population multiplied. The public prints became filled with reports of bizarre crimes (youths dumping gasoline on old ladies and setting them on fire, for instance); and asylums for the insane became a growth industry, finally to emerge with credentialed practitioners and a new nomenclature—mental health!

Did shellac—a food grade version of furniture finish—used as a confectioner's glaze have anything to do with this? Or xylitol, a sugar substitute that is a diuretic and causes tumors and organ damage in test animals? Or propylene glycol alginate or oxystearin (a modified glyceride) or glycerol ester of wood resin, or guar gum? All annihilate lesser life and whittle away at human health a bit at a time!

John Thomas' message in his manual on health is clear and to the point. Witless science has worked its mischief, but we are not helpless. We have only to take command of our own health and make sensible judgements without reference to higher approved authority.

Young Again! has little to do with mirror image vanity and everything to do with the "mechanical limits of the organism," as Albert Carter Savage put it, meaning the human body.

Young Again! has to be read with a box of marker pens handy. It is a matchless narrative and an encyclopedia of health. It covers the secrets of the ancients and projects forward to encompass the range of the electromagnetic spectrum. The advice—page by page, chapter by chapter—may not entirely reverse aging, but it is certain to put the process on hold.

Charles Walters
Editor, Acres USA
Kansas City, Missouri

Aim High!

The "purpose" of this book is to provide the reader with **ANSWERS** and a **REALISTIC** "model" for dealing with health issues—and to improve the quality of the reader's life. Hopefully, these are the reasons you are reading *Young Again!*

Your author's approach to health and longevity is **TOTAL** and **BASIC!** He does **NOT** believe in band-aids or magic bullets. He wants readers to understand how loss of control over the body's **terrain** occurs—and exactly what must be done to reverse the process.

It is not the author's *intent* to be absolute or overzealous. Few people will be able to comply 100% with all of the suggestions contained in these pages. The reader is encouraged to advance in personal knowledge at his/her own pace. Do not feel doomed because you are unable to follow all suggestions at once. Please realize, the material presented represents the BEST you can shoot for—the goal—the ideal!

The ideal world of health is a lifestyle that includes wholesome food, pure water, moderate exercise, adequate rest, low stress, a clean body and a strong mind. These things are worth striving for even though the *perfect* lifestyle is very difficult to "live" in a world where disease and human suffering are the norm.

Hopefully, this book will help the reader find a middle ground where enjoyment of good health can be realized and perpetually maintained, consistent with one's circumstances.

We live in an imperfect world and we fall short of the ideal. Sometimes we are subject to events and circumstances beyond our control. Yet, each day, we **DO** have the opportunity to make "choices" that affect our lives and health—and the lives of those around us—for good and bad. We must strive to make the **BEST** choices we can each and every day.

The reader is reminded that health and disease are **cumulative** states of being, and the *alternative* to good health is a sorry existence indeed. Poor health cheats people of the opportunity to fully experience "life" at its best. True happiness can only be experienced when we are emotionally, spiritually and physically "healthy!"

Aim high—and do the very best you can. Good health is worth **whatever it takes** to get it and keep it!

Think About It!

"In the health arena, there are only two classes of people. Those who are young and healthy and those who are old or sick. The former want to hold onto their youth and the latter desperately want to reclaim what they have lost."

John Thomas

1

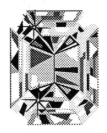

Something Of Value

*"If you want to look and feel as I do when
you are my age, you must begin now!"*
Robert McLeod

It was a strange place for me to meet the person who
would become my mentor. Stranger still were the circumstances—a restaurant meeting room in San Bernardino, California in 1971. The event: A district sales meeting for ARCO
(Atlantic Richfield Company), formerly Richfield Oil Company.

Having graduated from college the previous September,
I stood in awe of the grandeur of it all. The Company, the oil
industry and all that.

We had instinctively corralled ourselves into groups
based on our position on the corporate ladder. Barnyard
pecking order they call it.

And as a few of us were talking, I overheard my
immediate superior and his cronies laughing and poking fun in
a rather contemptuous way at one of their peers—a man named
Bob McLeod.

McLeod was somewhat ostracized by others of his own
level. "Status inconsistent" the sociologists call it! His peers
mocked him in "ignorance!" As I listened to their gossip,
something caught my attention.

"You know," one of them said, *"McLeod is a vegetarian.
He doesn't eat meat. He's...real strange!" "Yah! He's into health,
whatever that is,"* said another.

It was difficult to compare McLeod to this arrogant,
egocentric bunch of executives. I could NOT account for the
differences between the *group* and the stranger, McLeod.

McLeod looked young. His smile, his eyes, his laugh—
nothing squared with someone of 49 years. His hair was
vibrant! His waistline was trim and slim. I liked what I beheld!

The "other" executives, well, they all looked 20 years

older than McLeod. Paunchy stomachs, grayed hair, bald heads, fat, cigarettes blazing—and booze! Many were ready for their gold watches, but by this time in history gold watches had been replaced by the old glass hand, a slap on the back and the epitaph on the grave stone *"He was a good old boy!"*

McLeod Knew

McLeod knew something they did not, for he was 49 years "young" and the others who were in their late thirties and early forties were well,...older!

I took my first step into the world of ageless living as I navigated in McLeod's direction. Life would never again be the same for me. I was destined to be there on that day, at that moment, and Bob McLeod was destined to become my mentor. God works in strange ways!

I introduced myself to this 49 years *young* enigma, and as we talked it became crystal clear that he was a very special human being. Immediately, my mind was made-up! "When I reach 49 years of age, I am going to *LOOK* and *FEEL* like Bob McLeod!" [I was 27 years of age then.]

"It's a long story and you are going to have to search it out for yourself, but I would consider it a privilege if I can assist you," he said.

Instant friends we were! Fellow travelers for sure! Our paths only crossed a few times in the months that followed. When they did, he would take me under his wing and talk with me and point the way.

"If you want to understand how I have managed to look and feel 20 years younger than I am, you will have to study. I recommend you begin by reading a book by Dr. Paul C. Bragg entitled The Miracle of Fasting.

"You will not find all the answers there, but this book is a good place to start," he said.

Six months after meeting Bob, I left the company and lost ALL contact with him until August of 1993. At that time, he still looked *young and vibrant!* If you saw him on the street you would guess him to be in his late forties. Not too bad for someone 69 years **"YOUNG!"**

Thirty-one years have passed and now it is my turn. At 61 years of age, I am here to tell you that you **CAN** stop the clock and you **CAN** reverse the aging process—that is, if you will follow my lead and stay the course.

Fear

People are reluctant to venture out, to break new ground, to sail uncharted waters—particularly when it involves being *different.* Perhaps it is social pressure. Perhaps people think they are giving up *something of value.* Regardless, pride, fear and ignorance are the primary stumbling blocks that keep people from following the path of good health. Instead, people hang onto destructive habits—habits that become the glue by which they seal their coffins.

Most of my peers at that fortuitous meeting are well on their way into old age. All of them were past their anabolic **PEAK** at that time. Today, most of them suffer from degenerative disease—and many of them are dead. **All** of them are old beyond their years—each the product of poor choices. There is no room for blame. We are responsible for our **CHOICES!**

People do not think "they" are going to get old. They know they have to die, but it is the other guy who gets old, never them. One day they wake up and look in the mirror, and their mind says, *"Heh! Better enjoy it while you can! Time is short!"* As friends grow old and die, the image in the mirror is confirmed—disease and old age have arrived.

It's important to understand the difference between disease and a "condition!" A disease is a condition that has "officially" been given a name. Diseases and conditions **BOTH** alter lifestyle and prevent us from enjoying life as we would if we were in a healthy state of being.

We do **NOT** *catch* disease! We *develop* conditions! Disease should be "hyphenated" and spelled **"dis-ease"**—and I will do so for the remainder of this book to drive home the point. We die of "conditions" **NOT** dis-ease!

How we define our health issues greatly influences our **attitude** about aging and our ability or inability to take control of our lives and redirect those energy forces that cause the *bioelectric body* to grow **"OLD!"**

It's Your Decision

Would YOU like to become *Young Again?* All that is required is that you complete this book and apply its lessons in your life. If you want to experience the **miracle** of reversing the aging process, you **MUST** *visualize* the end result in your mind's eye. The miracle is available to *anyone* who wants it, but it is **NOT** free! The reader will become fully acquainted with the price as each chapter unfolds.

Once you understand **HOW** you *"grow"* old, you will understand **HOW** to become *Young Again!*

PREVIEW: *In the next chapter, you will discover that you have four different classifications of age. You will also determine your anabolic PEAK and learn of its significance in your life.*

The "Terrain!"

This book is **NOT** about "curing" anything. It is about **altering** and **restoring** the "terrain"—so disease will **"disappear!"**

Vorago™ SunRise & "Breast" Protection

"Protecting" breast tissue is of *primary* concern to women. Chapter 35—a new chapter—teaches women how to **protect** their breasts and keep their breast tissue "healthy"—and how to avoid "trouble!" Read about the **Vorago™ Effect** and it's link to female—and male—health and longevity in *Vorago™ SunRise.*

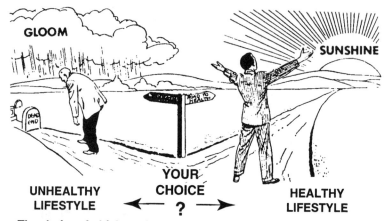

The choice of which road to take is up to the individual. He alone can decide whether he wants to reach a dead end or live a healthy lifestyle for a long, happy, active life.   – Paul C. Bragg

Reality Self-Check

When you look down the street, do you see a STOP sign instead of the horizon? Young people see only the horizon because their entire life is in FRONT of them.

Don't lose sleep over the doctor's diagnosis—for it is nothing but a confirmation of yesterday's poor choices. Instead, focus on today and tomorrow will be yours.

When you look in the mirror and the image looking back at you *isn't the image you remember,* you better believe the image looking back at you!

"In this book [Young Again!], the author goes a long way to provide hope that, in a world beset by health-threatening pollution of all kinds, we are afforded some tools with which to build healthier, longer and perhaps happier lives."
Christopher Bird, *The Secret Life of Plants*

2

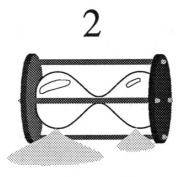

Young Again!

*"Youth is a wonderful thing. What
a crime to waste it on children."*
George Bernard Shaw

Old age follows days filled with new hopes and new dreams of good times to come—good times that go "unfulfilled" because our body fails to keep up with our mind.

An **old body** with a **young mind** is a phenomenon where conflict and misunderstanding abound. It is a condition where the body we once knew becomes *lost* in **TIME** and unable to communicate with the mind. Flip sides of the same coin: a young mind, an old body—each expressing itself in a different language with no interpreter to translate.

Aging occurs through ignorance—and by **CHOICE!** People grow old because they do not know **HOW** to stay young. They are becoming old much faster than they once did. This is particularly true among the young—and particularly women between ages 25-35. The young now experience ONSET of old age by year 24. **Dis-ease** that once belonged to the "old" now belongs to the "young!" **CHOICE** of lifestyle is the single biggest factor controlling **"degenerative"** transformation.

Despite the statistical claims of the *experts*, life expectancy is *not* greater today than it was yesterday. The statistics used to support this claim of greater life expectancy have been skewed by the number of children reaching adulthood. At one time, **half** the population of the United States died prior to reaching age twenty—holding down "life expectancy!" The *statistical* rise over the last fifty years has caused a gullible public to buy into the "sick-care" system's false claim to fame. The public has fallen for a **"Kabuchi Dance!"** [See Chapter 38.]

We are NOT better off today than yesterday. "Degenerative" **conditions** have replaced "infectious" **dis-ease.** Moreover, contagious conditions are rising and returning with a vengeance. Their resurgence bodes ill for those who are unprepared and unwilling to change their lifestyle "choices!" A long, **HEALTHY** life is what we were **meant** to enjoy during our days on Mother Earth. This book focuses on that goal.

Dividing Line

At my initiation into the study of aging in 1971, it was considered difficult to turn the body's biological clock backward if someone had *survived* 35 years of **NORMAL** living. If we made the same statement today, we would have to reduce age **"35"** down to age **"24."** The dividing line between youth and the **ONSET** of old age has fallen!

When we are young, our health is at its peak and the body is able to repair itself quickly and easily. The word *anabolism* best describes this "state-of-being." Anabolism is the "absence" of slowdown and loss of function in body tissues and vital organs. It implies **ongoing** repair and the ability to **restore** organ function. Anabolism is a *building up* process!

As we age, vital organ function slows. When we are under "stress"—we become "fragile" and injuries do not heal as quickly. *Catabolism* best describes this negative "state-of-being." Catabolism is the opposite of anabolism. Both **conditions** are central themes of the *Young Again Protocol*™.

Catabolism is a kind of *self-digestion* where the body lives off the energy released from the digestion of its own tissues. This "bare-bones" energy helps meet the body's *minimum* energy needs. Energy produced through catabolic activity is *starvation energy.* Catabolic activity can keep us alive—but it should **NOT** be equated with health and longevity. Death has its roots in catabolism.

When we are young, we are **anabolic!** When we are old, we are **catabolic!** Of course, there are degrees within these categories. In this book, *anabolism* and *catabolism* refer to the **OVERALL** condition or trend direction of the *bio-electric* body—and the implications that go with it.

The age **"24"** dividing line we spoke of earlier is our **anabolic PEAK.** [More on this in a few pages!] The **"peak"** is that point in **TIME** when young people begin their *slide* into old age. Some people reach their anabolic peak earlier than age 24; for others, it comes a little later. The **point** is that "onset" of old age is arriving much too soon!

Once Upon A Time

There was a time when it was uncommon to see the first **SIGNS** of old age until the fortieth or forty-fifth year—unless one was subject to hardships beyond the norm. Obesity, gray hair, balding, slowing of sexual function, wrinkled skin, diminished vitality, etc. are all classic **SIGNS** of old age.

Before we can erase the **SIGNS** of old age, we must come to understand *why* they occur. We also need to understand *how* they express themselves. When we become **AWARE** of the passing of **TIME**, we also become aware of the invisible forces of aging—forces that cause the young to wake up old.

When we reach our *anabolic peak,* we are at the crossroads of **TIME**. We are caught between the wonder of youth and the approach of old age.

Aging occurs quietly and without notice. It is a **self-ordained** process that speeds the passing of **TIME** and hastens our date with death.

Change The Script
Life Should NOT be miserable and end poorly! We can change the script if we *choose*—no matter what our age! We can *reverse* our course if we are willing to learn and act upon new-found knowledge.

It is **NOT** the idea of growing old that people fear. Rather, it is the idea that old age will *cheat* them of the enjoyment of the things they once took for granted. For most, the thought of old age gives rise to visions of a dead-end street, loneliness, pain, suffering and finally death.

When your author chose the title for this book, he wrestled between *Forever Young!* and *Young Again!* The former title did not fit those people who are on the *anabolic* side of the pyramid. They will not read this book because they cannot grasp the meaning of the word *old*. Their world is *young*. They are never going to get old—or so they think.

Only those who **recognize** that they have *passed* their anabolic peak understand the **implications** of the word **OLD***!* To them, the idea of becoming *Young Again* is but a dream!

Hosea proclaims, *"My people are destroyed for lack of knowledge!"* However, it is not knowledge that mankind lacks,

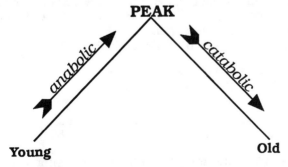

Anabolic Peak—That point in TIME when youth is spent and the onset of old age has begun. [Also see pages 22 and 198.]

but the wisdom to discern the difference between false knowledge and truth. *Old age* and *old* are not necessarily synonymous. They do not have to mean the same thing.

The Doctor

When we are dying, we hear the pronouncements of medical science, *"Nothing can be done!" "Accept that which cannot be changed!"*—and other expressions designed to worm their way into our consciousness and numb our wits as our will to live is "excised!" ***"Oral pacifiers these pronouncements!"*** Empty words designed to help us accept and rationalize the phenomena we call *"life"* and *"death!"*

In the beginning—when poor health first manifests itself—the medical folks talk of recovery. In time, recovery gives way to high-tech jargon and **"HOPE!"**

For the terminal patient who has cast himself or herself before the altar of science, medical science quickly exhausts its mumbo-jumbo, turning instead to steely words that chisel our name on the tombstone.

The doctor announces death's call. The patient answers that call with forced preparation and frustration along the nagging questions *"Why?"* and *"How?"* The "mystery" of health and happiness, life and death goes unanswered.

The Clergy

Religious training convinces us that we have an "appointed time" and to "accept what God has foreordained"—soothing words that placate our emotions and numb the reality of the moment. Few people dare to question religion's pronouncements. There is little quarter for rationality here.

Instead, we elevate to dogma that which we do **NOT** understand. We blindly follow our beliefs, never pausing to question "Why?" and "How?" as life slips away.

We give up. We grow old. We accept what we have been taught and we die decades ahead of **TIME** because medical science said *"Sorry!"* and our religious leaders offered us little consolation—except a *"hereafter!"*

Society attempts to buffer the *"Why?"* and *"How?"*

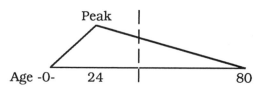

Aging Pyramid—note how far left of the center line the anabolic peak of "age 24" is located.

with cynicism set to music in songs like Peggy Lee's *Is That All There Is!* Because we do not know the answers, we keep dancing—pausing only to *"Break out the booze!"*

Our inability to winnow truth from falsehood is *not* totally our fault. We have been schooled to accept the flood of distortions emanating from societal organs—government, newspapers, schools and universities. Together, they are nothing but a "Kabuchi Dance" [See Chapter 38.] wired to the halls of "science"—the god of our civilization. Science has become a national religion—but it fails to answer *"Why?"* and *"How?"*

Pilgrimage

Daily, we *voluntarily* make the pilgrimage to Science's cultic altar, paying homage to the idea that cause and effect can be explained using single factor analysis. We accept the *theory* that there is a **bug** responsible for every dis-ease, a **pill** to cure every ailment.

We are told we have a built-in alarm clock that signals our time to die, when longer days—good days—filled with health and happiness are within our reach if we will only act and accept our greatest gift of all—good health!

Medical science blames the bacteria and viruses for our dilemma and health problems—while Christianity blames Eve for bringing the curse of **sickness** and **death** upon Adam and his progeny. We need to **STOP** the *"blame-game!"*

Instead of taking responsibility for ourselves, we *blame* events and other people for our shortcomings. We prostrate ourselves before the "altar" of science and pay homage with the fruits of our labor—trading hard earned money for pharmaceuticals that treat **symptoms**—but leave the **causes** untouched—and more importantly **"unidentified!"**

Palliation is a term that comes to mind. It says much about medical science in a few syllables. It means: relief of **SIGNS** and **symptoms** "without" addressing underlying cause(s). Drugs alter organ function! Supposedly, they are prescribed to **prevent, diagnose or cure** dis-ease. "Palliation" is the **fourth** reason used to **justify** drug usage and "standard of care" guidelines that hamstring good doctors. Palliation tricks the patient and leads the physician astray!

How different life would be if people possessed a valid medical "model" of dis-ease and aging—and acted upon that knowledge. Sadly, mankind lives in a medically induced **stupor** where the *"Why?"* and *"How?"* of life and death, health and dis-ease goes unanswered.

Make no mistake, 99% of "aging" comes down to the "choices" we make each and every day of our lives. This book was written to answer the *"Why?"* and *"How?"*—and to point the way to the **path** of agelessness!

What Is Your Age?

How we define age makes a big difference in our *attitude* toward life because **attitude** dictates the choices we make and "drafts" our physiologic future and our *bio-electric age.*

Age can be defined on the basis of **calendar** age (chronological age), **mental** age, **functional** age and most importantly, *bio-electric* age. Please review them, carefully!

Calendar age is how old we are in years upon this earth. We celebrate our calendar age each year with a birthday party. Unfortunately, we celebrate in *past tense* and in the *negative* by defining age in years *old,* instead of years *young!*

Mental age is defined by the way we "think!" It is our perspective on life. If we "feel" physically **OLD,** our mental perspective is "old!" We suffer a mental "disconnect" when the physical body breaks-down. If we "feel" physically **YOUNG,** our mental perspective is "young!" Body and mind are connected. The dividing line between being physically young and physically old is our anabolic peak. **RESTORE** your body "terrain" and you automatically restore your "mental" terrain as well as your anabolic peak. Old body = old mind; young body = young mind. It behooves us to stay physically and mental young!

Functional age is based on our ability to function. *Nursing* and bogus *holistic* medicine define functional health as our ability to experience normal, everyday desired activities. Wellness is defined as the way we "perceive" ourselves. These definitions "allow" for one or more degenerative **"conditions!"** Plastic definitions like these bother your author because they mislead and dodge the issues and causes of aging and dis-ease! They are **dead-end** definitions that ignore mental and physical limitations that deprive us of a truly youthful existence.

Bio-electric age is the "real" age of the physical body Reversing your *bio-electric* **age** is **"THE"** issue. Your *bio-electric* age is **measurable**—and it is infinitely **malleable!** In future chapters, the reader will learn how to "manipulate" and "control" the forces of aging that influence *bio-electric* **TIME.**

We experience **peak** health in the **ABSENCE** of disease. This book teaches you **HOW** to achieve that goal .

When you look young, think young and feel young—you truly *are Young Again!*

PREVIEW: *In the next chapter, you will determine your REAL age and identify those things that are causing you to become old before your time. The information you provide will become YOUR foundation for the balance of this book. Are you ready?*

| Fast Asleep |

If you want to go to sleep and your hands and feet are cold, soak your hands and feet in a basin of hot water, put on some warm wool socks, and you will go to sleep "fast!"

The Stress Cycle

Stress has "physical" consequences! All it takes is a stressful "event" to ruin your day and weaken your "health!" Stress of any kind causes the **adrenal glands** to go into **OVERDRIVE** "triggering" a cascade of reactions in the vital organs of the body. Next, stress hits the **liver** causing "reduced" bile-flow with **HUGE** implications for female and male hormone levels, the bowels and digestion of food. Ultimately, stress causes the body to turn "acid"—and the more acid your body the poorer your health. **"HOW"** your emotions and your "physical" body deals with stress is the issue. [More later!]

Congestion & Mucous

Colds and flu, pneumonia and sinus issues, allergies and ear aches involve mucous congestion. Cystic Fibrosis is a worst-case example! Heavy mucous is confirmation of waste overload of **both** soluble acid waste and structural amyloid plaque. Mucous and amyloid wastes provide a "perfect" breeding ground for viruses, bacteria and yeast. **Nano-dosed** DNA—**called MX**™—is used to **breaks up** mucous and cause it to "flow"—so the head, chest and ears "clear!" [See pages 121, 127 and 344.] Clear Head™ is used to destroy microbial infection and breeding grounds in the sinus cavities, and to break up congestion with the help an irrigator tool called the Neti Pot.™

Brown Eyes Green

We are taught that eye color, balding, diabetes, obesity and hormonal problems are "genetic" in origin—but it's not so. Children are **born** with bluish eyes **before** they change to brown or black. Men *with* hair **become** bald *after* they *lose* it. People **become** diabetics! Women **develop** female problems. Blondes **become** brunettes. People **become** fat. People **grow** deaf. The list goes on! Your author had dark brown eyes for 48 years. **Now** the're half green. Bald men can **regrow** hair. Diabetics can **become** normal. Women can **resurrect** their "hormone cycle." Fat people can **become** thin. "Genetic" problems are solved by restoring the **TERRAIN**. Genetic problems are **symtomatic** and "past tense" in nature—**never** "causative!" Dis-ease manifests in the "terrain" **BEFORE** it manifests in the genes. Your author **regrew** his hair, **increased** his muscle mass and saw his health "blossom" **after** age 50—and so can you!

Who's In Control
Question medical authority. Get-up off your knees. It's YOUR body and YOUR life. Take control of YOUR future.

NORMAL COLON AND SICK COLONS

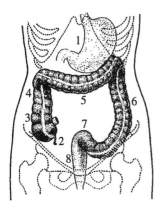

A. The Normal Colon
The normal colon in the proper position in relation to other structures: 1) stomach 2) appendix 3) cecum 4) ascending colon 5) transverse colon 6) descending colon 7) sigmoid flexure 8) rectum

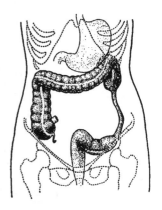

B. The Spastic Colon
The colon in spastic constipation.

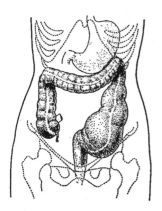

C. The Engorged Colon
The colon in engorged constipation.

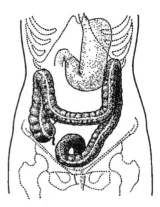

D. The Sagging Colon
Ptosis, or sagging, of the transverse colon, accompanied by displacement of the stomach.

Programmed To Die
We *program* ourselves to die by our actions, words and thoughts. And as we prepare, the *reaper* takes our friends and siblings—a signal that "our" time is approaching. We do our best to make sure we are not left behind!

3

Any Old Road

*"If you don't know where you're going,
How will you know when you get there?
If you don't know how you got there,
Any old road will NOT take you back."*
John Thomas

Aging is considered to be part of the "normal" life process when it's really the "abnormal" part of the process. Normal growth takes us from infancy to our anabolic peak at age 24—abnormal aging takes us from that "peak" to our grave.

Aging follows a procession of **TIME** related events that we identify with **SIGNS** and **symptomatic** "descriptions" like gray hair, menopause, balding, diabetes, wrinkles, cold body, loss of energy, low sex drive, dental problems, obesity, etc.— things that serve to **"document"** the passing of **TIME**.

The aging process can be *slowed, stopped* and *reversed.* But doing so is **ONLY** possible when we have correct knowledge and understanding—supported by action! Fundamental to getting "results" is **personal responsibility.**

People speed the aging process and the *passing* of **TIME** when they **ignore** the **SIGNS and symptoms!** "Tuning-out" causes us to age by default! The *Young Again Protocol*™ teaches how to *re-cycle* **TIME** itself **not** by "reliving" old experiences— but by "exchanging" **TIME** already spent for "new" **TIME** and "new" experiences. [See Chapter 31.]

Aging and **TIME** are related—but they are **not** the same! Aging is the result of **TIME** poorly lived, whereas **TIME** is the *vehicle* of aging. For example, cancer is the product of **TIME** *poorly* lived. Cancer causes the passing of **TIME** to accelerate. When this occurs, the body experiences a slump in its *bio-electric* balance and we grow OLD—fast! Dis-ease is **TIME** in motion—and it warps our concept of **TIME**! Aging is **TIME'S** trail—a confirmation of biologic deterioration.

Rate Yourself
Shortly, the reader will be asked to **"personalize"** the *types of aging* discussed in Chapter 2. This simple project will

provide tangible "meaning" to new and different concepts of **aging** and **TIME!**

Use an erasable pen or pencil. *Estimate* and place *your* age on each line. Leave the last line **blank** until *after* you have scored your *bio-electric* age at the **END** of this chapter.

Mental Age   0_____ 80 yrs

Calendar Age   0_____ 80 yrs

Functional Age   0_____ 80 yrs

Age You Feel   0_____ 80 yrs

Bio-electric Age   **0_____ 80 yrs ++**

"SIGNS" & Symptoms

TIME poorly lived produces **SIGNS** and **symptoms** of *bio-electric* aging and dis-ease that results in diminished activity in the **vital organs** and **glands**.

Symptoms of dis-ease are *subjective* changes in body function that are **NOT** apparent to an outside observer—like nausea, anxiety, low-level pain, dryness of mouth, poor appetite and low sex drive. Symptoms often go unnoticed by the host in the early stages because alterations in the body "terrain" are subtle. Symptoms eventually "morph" into **SIGNS** ! Aging is a "polite" word for *slow-down! Slow-down* eventually leads to **shut-down!** Aging is "falling-apart" *one day at a time!*

Aging first occurs in the "invisible" realm where the "electric" body resides. Eventually, aging is seen in the mirror and/or confirmed by the doctor's diagnosis.

TIME Made Visible

SIGNS are different from **symptoms. SIGNS** are *external* in nature; they are "observable"—and they can be "measured!" **SIGNS** support a doctor's diagnosis of a morbid condition. They also cause the "individual" to become acutely **aware** of alteration of body function! Hence, **SIGNS** are *confirmation* of aging and the passing of **TIME**. Think of **SIGNS** as yesterday's time capsules in "visible" form.

SIGNS speak of an **abnormal** "condition" in the aging process called dis-ease and pathology! When viewed as "normal and expected," the impact of **SIGNS** on our consciousness is greatly lessened—and by "default" their effect on the *bio-electric* body goes unnoticed until one day we are **"OLD!"**

Dis-ease is like the unwelcome guest who drops-by "unannounced!" Unlike the guest, however, dis-ease doesn't go away. Instead, it "steals away" our very life, and we can no longer do the things we could once do. Eventually, we find ourselves in serious trouble. Only then does dis-ease *remove its "cloak"* and the passing of **TIME** "accelerates" before our very eyes! *Too soon old, too late smart!* ***Damage to the vital organs is dis-ease's shadow. Slow-down and loss of vital organ function should be our cue to change our lifestyles immediately!***

Charting Your *Bio-electric* Age

The remainder of this chapter is your **key** to managing "your" bio-electric age. The "checklist" is your brush and canvas for determining *"How?"* and *"Why?"* your *bio-electric* age is what it is. The list is **your** *personal* **road map** to ageless living that points the way back in *bio-electric* **TIME**—that is, if the reader absorbs and learns the lessons contained in this book. Each "listed" item will be **"fleshed-out"** as the *Young Again* story unfolds chapter by chapter.

Each item reflects an assigned point value based on its long-term **cumulative effect**. Most items are unisex and apply to both sexes, while the male/female lists apply to the respective sex only. *Contributing factors* that accelerate aging are included and carry heavy score values. This list is **NOT** a diagnosis of a particular dis-ease condition—but it is a list of markers! "Scoring" provides a close approximation of true *bio-electric age*—providing you are honest with yourself.

Check the boxes that apply. Serious **past** health conditions **should** be counted if they have left their mark or are of recent vintage. If under medical care or taking medications, do "count" it. Complete this exercise **"NOW"** and **"AGAIN"** after you have completed the book when you better understand the significance of each listed item. Each listed item provides direction and meaning in the quest for agelessness.

Please **do not** diminish or pass judgement on the items listed. The list is comprised of **SIGNS, symptoms** and **contributing factors** that affect your life—for good and for bad.

Let your author assure the reader that "every" item deserves *attention!* Please think "cumulative!"

Brave New World - 2006

In Huxley's book, *Brave New World,* everyone **"appears"** happy and healthy with **NO SIGNS** of aging or ill health—up until the moment they *"drop dead!"*

Today 2006, the **SIGNS** are "visible" everywhere. We are **beyond** the *Brave New World!* We live in a world totally removed from reality—an *Alice in Wonderland* world that only "appears" real! We are actors in the "kabuchi dance" called the "health care" system—as described in Chapter 38.

SIGNS & Symptoms Of Bio-Electric Aging

Height: Loss of physical height:
- •1/4" shorter   50 ❑
- •1/2" or more   200 ❑

Facial: •Crow's feet around eyes/upper lip lines   30 ❑
- •Cheeks sunken, hollow   35 ❑
- •Cheeks sagging/puffy   65 ❑
- •Cheeks/nose have spider capillaries   50 ❑
- •Face losing "tone"   40 ❑

Skeletal: Muscle deterioration/loss of muscle mass   60 ❑
- •Flabby body; no muscle tone   40 ❑
- •Leg cramps/charleyhorse   18 ❑
- •Stature mildly hunched-back   80 ❑
- •Stature severely hunched-back   120 ❑

Belly: •Paunchy/pot   20 ❑
- •Grossly distended   200 ❑

Eyebrows: thick, bushy   25 ❑

Nose & Ear hair (external)   25 ❑

Body Odor: •Needs deodorant   50 ❑
- •Overpowers deodorant   80 ❑

Bad Breath: Chronic   30 ❑

Teeth: •Decayed   40 ❑
- •Cleaning required once a year   25 ❑
- •Cleaning every 6 months   40 ❑
- •Mercury amalgam fillings   150 ❑
- •Root canal(s) present in mouth   40 ❑
- •Gingivitis, bleeding gums   70 ❑

Nails: •Fungus/yeast growth under toe/finger nails   80 ❑
- •Slow growth   30 ❑
- •Thickening of toe nails   40 ❑

Hearing: Progregressively worse with age   60 ❑
- •Tinnitis   60 ❑

Skin: •Dry, scaly (includes dandruff)   20 ❑
- •Psoriasis/seborrhea/eczema   50 ❑
- •Wrinkled/leathery   40 ❑
- •Fat bumps on upper arms ; back   10 ❑
- •Pimples/acne/skin blemishes   30 ❑
- •Do not sweat easily   20 ❑
- •Brown *liver* spots on hands/body   40 ❑
- •Bruise easily; painful to touch   60 ❑
- •Heavy oil secretion   15 ❑

Hair, Mustache, & Beard:
- •Predominantly gray/white   50 ❑
- •Bald head   50 ❑
- •Loss of body hair (legs, chest, groin)   80 ❑
- •Slow hair growth   30 ❑
- •Head hair (once wavy, now straight)   40 ❑
- •Gray or white pubic, axillary, or leg hair   40 ❑

Physical Activity:
- •Inability to perform hard physical work   30 ❑
- •Joint pain/inflammation after hard work   20 ❑
- •1-3 days required to recover from hard work   30 ❑

Weight:
- •Easily gain pounds   30 ❑
- •Unexplained large weight loss   40 ❑

Mental:
- •Depression   50 ❑

	•Confusion/can't face day	45 ❏
	•Need coffee to get/keep going	30 ❏
Stools:	•Lack of medium dark brown color	30 ❏
	•Formed/hard or dry	50 ❏
	•Defecation requires effort	20 ❏
	•Food transit time over 24 hours	40 ❏
	•Overly foul gas/odor	40 ❏
	•Bright red blood on stool	15 ❏
	•Less than "complete" bowel evacuation	20 ❏
Illness:	•Often feel sick, but no fever	30 ❏
	•Colds more than once a year	25 ❏
	•Succumb to flu most years	30 ❏
Eyes:	•Require reading glasses	20 ❏
	•Sensitive to sunlight	40 ❏
	•Poor night vision (car lights bother)	20 ❏
	•Brown spots in iris (colored portion)	30 ❏
	•Racoon shadows under eyes	90 ❏
	•Macular degeneration/glaucoma	50 ❏
	•"Floaters" in eyes	30 ❏
Joints:	•Joint pain (general)	40 ❏
	•Osteo arthritis, bursitis	100 ❏
	•Rheumatiod arthritis	200 ❏

Minor Wounds:
- •Scab drop-time requires over 1 week   20 ❏
- •Subject to secondary infections   50 ❏
- •Scars form easily   40 ❏

Capillary Blood:
- •Does not form a "pearl" when finger is pricked (blood flows instead)   75 ❏
- •Color is dark red; not bright red   60 ❏
- •Non-instant color return when nail beds are squeezed and released   40 ❏
- •Blood full of "debris" (Rouleau effect)   80 ❏
- •Use of blood thinners/aspirin required   50 ❏

Respiratory (lungs):
- •Heavy breather/can't catch breath   90 ❏
- •Prone to pneumonia/bronchial trouble   80 ❏
- •Angina-tightness of breath   150 ❏
- •Asthma   80 ❏

Gut & Bowel/gastro-intestinal:
- •Constipation (less than 2 BM's/day)   90 ❏
- •Irregular bowel habits   60 ❏
- •Alternating diarrhea/constipation   30 ❏
- •History of appendix problems   50 ❏
- •Appendix removed   60 ❏
- •Colitis /diverticulitis/Crohn's   75 ❏
- •Removal of any part of small intestine   90 ❏
- •Colostomy   90 ❏
- •Untreated for intestinal/organ parasites   90 ❏
- •Gas, indigestion, cramping after meals   30 ❏
- •Acid reflux syndrome   50 ❏
- •Abundant/ongoing foul gas   40 ❏
- •Diagnosed with Leaky-Gut Syndrome   90 ❏
- •Bloated abdomen after meals   50 ❏

Blood Circulatory System:
- •Heart Attack   80 ❏
- •Anemia (low "iron")   40 ❏

- •Diagnosed arterio/atherosclerosis — 100 ☐
- •Poor circulation — 50 ☐

Lymphatic System:
- •Lymph nodes swollen/painful groin, armpits, breasts — 50 ☐
- •Lymph nodes surgically removed — 50 ☐
- •Cancer of lymph system (lymphoma) — 200 ☐
- •Spleen surgically removed — 60 ☐
- •Tonsils have been removed — 70 ☐

Fat: Body & Dietary:
- •10-20 lbs overweight — 20 ☐
- •30-75 lbs overweight — 90 ☐
- •75-200 lbs overweight — 200 ☐
- •Fatty tumors beneath skin covering body — 50 ☐
- •Dietary fat intake (butter/olive oil) less than 20% of diet — 50 ☐
- •Use of ANY type margarine — 50 ☐
- •Use of soy/canola oils or products — 70 ☐
- •Fat-free diet — 100 ☐

Urinary:
- •High albumin in urine — 50 ☐
- •High urea level in urine — 40 ☐
- •A/G ratio 1.6 (need blood test; see page 113) — 90 ☐
- •Prone to kidney stones — 40 ☐
- •Generally **dark** urine color — 25 ☐
- •Foul urine odor — 30 ☐
- •Sweet urine odor — 50 ☐
- •Bladder infections (female) — 75 ☐
- •Urine volume small (less than 4 oz) — 35 ☐

General Metabolic:
- •Drink less than 1/2 gal water/day — 100 ☐
- •Drink water/liquids with meals — 80 ☐
- •Drink chlorinated/fluoridated water — 60 ☐
- •Substitute soft drinks/juice for water — 95 ☐
- •Failure to drink 1 qt. of mineralized water with fresh lemon immediately upon rising — 50 ☐
- •Failure to drink 12-24 oz. of mineralized water per hour in heat, during hard work, when flying — 30 ☐
- •Use fluoridated toothpaste — 50 ☐
- •Use common deodorants — 30 ☐
- •Drinking water comes from city "tap" — 80 ☐
- •Regularly drink over-counter store "bottled" water — 30 ☐
- •Use any medications for headaches — 40 ☐
- •Regularly take Rx drugs — 80 ☐

Liver/Gallbladder:
- •Diagnosed/prone to gallbladder problems — 60 ☐
- •Surgical removal of gallbladder — 60 ☐
- •Diagnosed for hepatitis A, B, C, D, E, mononucleosis, Epstein-Barr, malaria, Chronic Fatigue, or "lime" disease — 95 ☐
- •Diagnosed with Herpes (genital) — 60 ☐
- •Suffer with "shingles" (past/present) — 80 ☐

Saliva: •Dry mouth — 30 ☐
- •Require liquids to swallow food — 30 ☐

Body Temperature:
- •Below normal body temperature — 60 ☐
- •Cold hands and feet — 60 ☐
- •Sensitive to cold temperatures — 30 ☐

•Suffer in hot weather 30 ❏
Connective Tissue & General Energy:
  •Diagnosed with lupus, MS, fibromyalgia,
  peripheral neuropathy, restless legs syn. 200 ❏
  •Suffer from gout (use medication for) 80 ❏
  •Stiff joints/loss of flexibility 50 ❏
  •Must eat often to have energy 30 ❏
  •Subject to mood swings/energy drops 30 ❏
  •Knee, shoulder or hip problems (cartilage) 80 ❏
  •Poor energy; energy "drops" 40 ❏
  •Sleepy/listless after lunch meal 35 ❏
Stress and Headaches:
  •Inability to function under stress 30 ❏
  •Regularly stressed-out 40 ❏
  •Chronic headaches 70 ❏
Cancer:
  •Diagnosis of any type of cancer 200 ❏
  •Received chemo/radiation therapy 300 ❏
  •Cysts or tumors of any kind 50 ❏
Tobacco: •Smoke or chew 95 ❏
Tongue: •Coated, pasty white-daytime 40 ❏
  •Coated upon rising in morning 20 ❏
  •Heavily grooved 40 ❏
Sleep: •Sleep less than 7 hours per night 20 ❏
  •Sleep less than 6 hours per night 80 ❏
  •Sleep broken; usually interrupted 20 ❏
  •Sleep with windows closed 30 ❏
  •Sleep under electric blanket 50 ❏
  •Insomnia (can't sleep) 70 ❏
  •Hypersomnia (sleep all time) 40 ❏
  •Narcolepsy (involuntary daytime
    sleep lasting about 15 minutes) 40 ❏
Dietary:
  •Use "non-food-based" vitamins/minerals 20 ❏
  •Take calcium supplements 30 ❏
  •Lump in throat (difficulty swallowing) 50 ❏
  •Use insulin for diabetes 80 ❏
  •Vomit after meals (bulimia) 95 ❏
  •Eat when nervous 30 ❏
  •Increased appetite w/o weight gain 30 ❏
  •Acid foods upset stomach 30 ❏
  •Nervous stomach 20 ❏
  •Always hungry 60 ❏
  •Poor appetite 25 ❏
  •Milk causes indigestion/bloating 50 ❏
  •Spicy foods a problem 20 ❏
  •Greasy foods cause indigestion 50 ❏
  •Eat or snack more often than every 4 hrs 55 ❏
  •Devour food...fast eater 30 ❏
  •Salt food 30 ❏
  •Eat alfalfa sprouts 20 ❏
  •Food not "organic" or home grown 80 ❏
  •Eat restaurant food often 90 ❏
  •Eat junk, packaged or preserved foods 100 ❏
  •Prepare food in a microwave oven 200 ❏
Computer & Cell phone:
  •Use computer more than 1 hour daily 50 ❏
  •Computer closer than 30 inches 50 ❏
  •Use cell phone daily 100 ❏

Fluorescent, Mercury, Sodium Vapor lights:
- •Use for work light — 30 ❑
- •Receive under 1 hour sunshine daily — 50 ❑

Exposure to electrical interference devices:
- •Radar (police/military) — 40 ❑
- •Electronic Equipment — 30 ❑
- •Smoke Detector — 20 ❑

Exercise: Lack of aerobic activity 3 times a week — 80 ❑
Wake-Up: Slow; require hours to get going — 40 ❑

Blood Pressure:
- •Resting pressure above 70/120 — 50 ❑
- •Working pressure above 90/140 — 90 ❑

Emotions:
- •Keyed-up, can't relax — 30 ❑
- •Melancholy/unhappy — 40 ❑
- •"Snap" personality — 50 ❑

Vegetable Juicing:
- •Failure to drink 1 glass of fresh beet, carrot and ginger juice daily — 50 ❑

Eat according to rules for blood type/food combining — 30 ❑

Colon Therapy:
- •Do not do colon therapy weekly — 100 ❑
- •Do not do colon therapy at all — 200 ❑

Females Only

Menstruation & Menopause:
- •Over age 40; & no vitamin B-12 shots — 70 ❑
- •Over age 40; WITH vitamin B-12 shots — 50 ❑
- •Exposure to mammograms — 60 ❑
- •Premenstrual tension (PMS) — 50 ❑
- •Painful/difficult menses — 40 ❑
- •Depression before menstruation — 20 ❑
- •Painful intercourse — 60 ❑
- •Vaginal dryness; itching — 50 ❑
- •Ovaries/uterus removed — 80 ❑
- •Thinning hair — 40 ❑
- •Vegetarian/vegan — 70 ❑
- •Menses irregular/skip often — 40 ❑
- •Acne worse during menses — 30 ❑
- •Painful breasts — 60 ❑
- •Body painful to touch — 60 ❑
- •Ovarian cysts/uterine fibroid tumors — 95 ❑
- •Hot flashes — 95 ❑
- •Can detect active ovary each month — 40 ❑
- •Used birth control pills (ever) — 150 ❑
- •Used any form of estrogen replacement — 150 ❑
- •Thyroid condition/thyroid medication — 90 ❑
- •Yeast/bladder infections; vaginal itching — 80 ❑
- •Endometriosis — 200 ❑
- •Food binges/cravings before menses — 40 ❑
- •Brain fog, poor memory, confusion — 90 ❑
- •Lack of sexual interest — 90 ❑
- •Cellulite formation (hips or thighs) — 100 ❑
- •Vertigo (dizziness) — 70 ❑

Male Only

- •Impotence — 90 ❑
- •Prostate problems — 90 ❑

•PSA count elevated	60	❏
•Painful ejaculation	60	❏
•Urination dribble, can't release	90	❏
•Frequent night urination	80	❏
•Pain inside leg or heels	30	❏
•Leg spasms, cramps at night	20	❏
•Vegetarian/vegan	50	❏
•Over age 40; & no vitamin B-12 shots	50	❏
•Lack of sexual interest	100	❏

Total Score... _____

Divide: (men divide by 226; women by 243) ⌐_____

Your *bio-electric* "reference score" is........... _____

Add points together and divide score by 226 for men or 243 for women to obtain your **bio-electric reference score.** **Example:** If you are man and your score is 1790, divide by 226 to obtain a **reference score** of 7.92, and so on.

Next, use the conversion scale to convert your reference score to your *bio-electric* age of 70 years. This is your **"real"** age!

Bio-electric Score Conversion Scale
The number on the left is your reference score. The number on the right is your *bio-electric age.*

.18 = 18	.22 = 20	.30 = 22	.33 = 24
.66 = 28	1.10= 30	2.42 = 35	2.86 = 40
3.30 = 45	3.96 = 50	4.40 = 55	5.28 = 60
6.60 = 65	7.92 = 70	8.81 = 75	11.00 = 80+ etc.

Your *bio-electric age should* **MOTIVATE** you to evaluate your life. **Please do NOT panic or feel hopeless if your *bio-electric* age is older than you think it should be. It is only a reference age.** Remember, it took your entire life to reach your present *bio-electric* age. Allow yourself a little time to undo the damage. *Circle* your *bio-electric* age and *transfer* your score to the chart on page 28. Please "re-calculate" your *bio-electric age* **every year** to see your progress. Your **reference score** is a very important number.

Think About It!
If your *calendar age* is 27 years and your bio-electric age is 39 years—as was your author's age in the old days—you are **"losing"** the battle! The younger you are, the less effect a few extra years will have. But if you are already "older," those extra years are more "meaningful!" Aging must not be ignored or written-off or casually dismissed just because you don't have any **symptoms** or see any **SIGNS**—yet!

The older you are, the faster **TIME** flies and the faster you become old! You "know" you are in trouble when the **SIGNS** appear. Aging **SIGNS** and **symptoms** appear after age 25, except for acne, cellulite, obesity and dental problems. Later, its menstrual problems, obesity, arthritis, diabetes, connective tissue disorders, digestion and bowel problems, heart attack. The wise person deals with these issues in the formative stages **before** the doctor is asked to provide a diagnosis. It's a matter of **CHOICE!** Don't waste **TIME**—looking back! Finish reading this book and apply it! The answers you SEEK are here!

TIME is not on your side if your bio-electric age is equal to or greater than your calendar age.

[Your author's present calendar age is 61—and his bio-electric age is holding at 19 years *young!* **TIME** is standing still for John Thomas—and **TIME** will "reverse" and "stand-still" for you, too—if you will take responsibility for your life!]

Action Steps For Ageless Living
1. Evaluate your score and review items checked.
2. Complete the reading and study of this book.
3. Recalculate your score at least once a year.
4. Accept responsibility for your life.
5. Implement the truths contained herein.

Each and every step taken to improve health—no matter how small—produces big benefits. The combined effect of several small steps can be *astounding!*

No one's situation is hopeless! The *bio-electric* body has AMAZING resiliency! Follow the lessons contained herein, and your body will heal itself. Let your body prove to you that you can become *Young Again!*

PREVIEW: *In our next chapter, you will meet a few great people of science, get a glimpse of the "behind-the-scenes" maneuvering within medical science—and you will be offered an explanation of mankind's present environmental dilemma.*

| Sauerkraut |

Non-pasturized "raw" saurkraut is extremely good for the digestive tract and a wonderful help to women with yeast and bladder issues. Sauerkraut is a "must" food for anyone fighting cancer because it improves and restores the "terrain!" It is easy to make—and better, too! Use all of your garden produce to make it—red or green tomatoes, green beans, peppers, broccoli, summer squash, whatever!

Life is simpler when you plow around the stumps!

Shedding "Your" Skin!

Humans and snakes have something in common. Both shed their skin. Snakes shed their skin from the "outside" as often as necessary as they grow. Humans, on the other hand, shed their skin from the "inside" during old-time "cleansing" procedures. Everyone acquainted with alternative healing has been taught that cleansing of the body can cause it to "shed" a rubber-like mucoid-matter from the colon wall. Victor Irons and Bernard Jensen often referenced the phenomenon in their writings.

Your author has had many discussions with gastro-enterologists, surgeons, etc. about the "mythical" mucoid matter that is supposed to inhabit the bowel and coat the colon wall. They tell me they have **NEVER** seen it when they look inside someone's colon during a colonoscopy. They see either healthy or unhealthy tissue—but no mucoid lining. So as far as they are concerned, us "health" folks are *"nuts!"*

The answer to the riddle goes something like this. When people go on fasts, do major cleansing and drink fresh vegetable juices, the body dumps "acidic" waste from the tissues into the blood and lymphatic systems. The waste is then filtered by the liver and stored in the gallbladder as "bile." Bile empties into the 15 foot-long small intestine known as the "gut" before traveling through the colon (large intestine) on its way to the toilet. [Bile and waste are easily "re-absorbed" in a sluggish intestinal tract.]

Traditional "fasts and cleanses" allow waste **to COLLECT** on a "sluggish" colon wall and people often "shed" the "mucoid-matter" lining from the colon wall like a snake sheds its skin. Humans shed their skin from the "inside" via the bowel.

The reason the medical folks never see the mucoid matter is because prior to doing their procedure, they give the patient some rather caustic stuff to drink in order to empty the colon. So who is correct? BOTH parties are correct, they are simply out of time and sequence with each other.

The "stuff" that comprises our intestinal "skin" is best described as "cancer that hasn't happened yet!"

The *Young Again (Tissue and Liver) Protocol*™ is a full-body **"deacidification"**—and is one of the **MOST** valuable processes available to people who want to avoid the medical system and enjoy good health for the balance of their lives.

Dr. Jensen's colon book contains forty colored slides of people's "skins!" They aren't very pretty to look at, but they are real as real can be! Your author has pulled this "stuff" from his body many times in the old days. [The *Young Again Protocol*™ avoids the need for this unpleasant experience because the waste moves out of the system in "liquid" state and does not accumulate!]

So what's it going to be, dear reader? Rid your body of the horrible burden it is laboring under—or continue to suffer, grow old and die early?

Readers who follow the *Young Again Protocol(s)*™ and "deacidify" their **"terrains"** now—on their own terms—can **AVOID** the doctor's terms later. [High Enema Therapy™ is very much a part of the deacidification process—and it is very easy to do!]

It's more fun to be healthy and young every day of your life, than sick and old—for the rest of your life! You decide!

Yeast

Here are a few of the symptomatic health complaints associated with Candida Albicans or "yeast!" Eye floaters, bad breath, depression, constipation, foul and excessive gas, low energy, bloated abdomen, aching joints, arthritis, moodiness, low blood-sugar, acne, skin dryness, hearing problems, ear aches, colic in babies, hair loss, sinus and lung mucous etc. Yeast is associated with all dis-ease, but yeast is **NOT** the cause. Rather, yeast "feeds" and "lives" in a highly **"ACID"** body terrain. Non pasteurized sauerkraut eaten 2-3 times daily is a wonderful, old-time remedy for yeast outbreaks—especially in women. [The *Young Again (Tissue & Liver) Protocol*™ deacidifies the "terrain" so the system can restore.]

Vitamin B-12

Common vitamin B-12 related "symptoms" are: memory loss, sleeplessness, nervousness, irritability, spinal problems, constipation, poor motor function, shingles, heart palpitations, ringing in ears, chronic fatigue—the list is "500" long!

Central to the vitamin B-12 molecule is cobalt, hence, *cyan-o-cobal-o-min.* Oral intake of B-12 from food or oral supplements requires the mucoprotein "intrinsic factor" [Secreted from the stomach wall!]—or B-12 is not absorbed. Sublinguals don't work after about age 30. The only place in the small intestine that B-12 can be absorbed is in the ileum.

Vitamin B-12 injections are commonly given to women after age "40"—but it's synthetic B-12 and it leaves a lot to be desired. [The *Young Again Protocol*™ calls for Cobo-12™ transdermal B-12 skin creme that is absorbed easily. [Women deplete their B-12 supply about 20 years ahead of men. Menopausal complaints always involve vitamin B-12 issues.]

Osteoporosis

Contrary to popular belief, calcium intake is **NOT** the issue behind loss of bone density in women over 35 years of age. Osteoporosis has "three" common denominators—and "calcium" is **NOT** one of them. The denominators are: 1) an acid terrain; 2) poor hormonal activity; 3) inability to lay down collagen. All three issues are discussed in future chapters.

All Played Out

Life is like a an old-time record player that plays in three speeds: 33, 45 and 78. At 33 life is great. At 45 you're not so sure. At 78, you're all played out. To avoid being a 78 at 45, all you have to do is "reduce" your *bio-electric* age to decimal **.33!** See pages 24 and 28-29 to better understand *bio-electric age.*

Foaming Urine

In the mid 1950's, Ajax cleanser was a popular household product. The advertisements sang a little song that went like this: *"Ajax, the foaming cleanser, baba baba ba ba, sends stains, right down the drain!"*

It is a **very good SIGN** if your urine produces massive amounts of foam. The more waste that is excreted, the more the urine foams! As the aging process reversed itself, your author's urine became more and more *foamy!* Just thought you might like to know one of the **SIGNS!**

Medical Grade Ionized Water™ (MGIW™) produces foamy urine in large quantities. Your author drinks this high "ORP" therapeutic water daily!

Diabetes

Diabetes is an "auto-immune" condition. Adult Onset Diabetes, Type-II is "linked" to a leaky-gut. This form of diabetes was once the domain of people over age 40 and overweight, but the age threshold is dropping—especially in females. **Diet** is an important diabetes management tool. **Stress** causes the adrenal glands to boost cortisol production, upsetting female hormone balance. **Poor bile-flow and a sluggish bowel make matters worse!** A "acid" body *terrain* goes **WITH** diabetes. Insulin is a "bad" crutch—and certainly not a "cure!" Better to avoid the need to use it!

The *Young Again Protocol™* for diabetics calls for closing a "leaky gut," High Enema Therapy™ and the Tissue and Liver Protocol.™ CWD™ is very useful—as is R/C™ and MZ.™ Fresh vegetable juices require *CAUTION!* Green beans—steamed, raw, canned —all you can eat— work wonders! Non-pasturized saurkraut is very helpful.

Diabetes is one of the "BIG 4" dis-eases—cancer, arthritis and heart attack/stroke are the other three. All four are "terrain" and "auto-immune" conditions!

Food & Light

After food is digested, circulating blood moves the food energy into the capillaries beds behind the eyes—where "light" activates it. Hence, the phrase *"Let there be light!"* takes on new meaning. [See Vorago™ SunRise, Chapter 35.]

West Nile Fever

Like malaria and AIDS, West Nile Fever is transmitted by mosquitoes. People with weak "terrains" are "at risk" Terrain issues always involve a "weak" liver. [Use L_sP_cC™, VZ™, PAC™ and OX™ with the *High Enema Therapy™* and the *Young Again Protocol™* to restore and manage your *terrain!*]

A System Of Experts!

When a system becomes overly *complex*, a cadre of *experts* soon appear with their agenda, codes and private vocabulary. And in the people, this spawns resentment followed by skepticism as to the system's fairness.

Most of what we're taught and much of what we believe either isn't true or doesn't work. The experts understand this fact—and so should you! We are in uncharted waters in world history—and the ability to "truly" understand what is going on is absolutely crucial. The Uncle Eric Book Series is perhaps the **very best** book series to come along in the last hundred years! They are equally useful for adults and children alike. [Call 800-509-5400.] Other good books to read are: *If You Want To be Rich & Happy, Don't Go To School; Trust Us, We're Experts* and *The Crazy Makers.* [See Source Page 400.]

"Perception is reality! What counts is the way things are, NOT the way things are perceived!"

Puberty & The "Middle Years" Window

Hormones DRIVE the changes that occur as children enter adulthood. When the hormones kick-in, baby fat turns to lean muscle mass. Boys become as strong as mules; girls become shapely. Physical height manifests on a daily basis.

Most teens enjoy good health—in spite of the abuse they deal themselves. By age 24, the hormone miracle "peaks" and growth levels out. The middle years begin at puberty and end around age 45. The "unravelling" process known as *aging* begins by age 24, as **vital** organ function slows and acidification of the "terrain" accelerates. Women age faster and more harshly than do men. There is a lesson here, ladies!

Early **SIGNS** and **symptoms** of aging are: cellulite, cold body, thinning hair, fatigue, loss of muscle mass, digestion and bowel issues, teeth and gum problems, overweight, use of drugs and alcohol, depression and diagnosed dis-ease.

Central to these things is the closing of the "puberty window" and acidification of the "terrain." By age 45, the process is complete and the middle years are **over!** Use the *Young Again Protocol™* to **reopen** your middle-years "window." [See pages 72, 164, 178, 212, 374 and 378.]

Young Again Protocol™

The *Young Again Protocol™* deals with **restoration** of the "terrain" and **stimulation** of vital organ function over months and years. It takes about 1 year for every 10 years of age to completely awaken the *bio-electric* body. It's worth the effort!

4

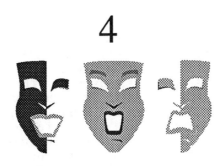

See What You Look At

Said Dorothy to the Wizard:

"You're a very bad man!"
"Oh no!" responded the Wizard.
"I'm just a very bad Wizard!"

It's difficult to comprehend the human dilemma without some understanding of the forces within science and medicine that blur our vision and confuse our thought processes. Once understood, however, the reader will more fully grasp why he or she is discovering the path of agelessness in the pages of this book versus the media or medical system literature.

The truly GREAT wizards of science and medicine are a breed of their own. They are often light years ahead of their time. They are also a problem for those who want to control and manipulate society. There have been many of these great people in science and medicine. Many of them lived out their lives on the fringe—away from mainstream medicine and science. We hear little about them, but the impact of their vision is all around us—often with another's name on their discoveries! A few of these hardy souls chose to function *within* the system. Their insight usually created craters that could neither be denied nor erased by the powers that be.

I refer to these people as WIZARDS. Wizards understand medical science's loss of direction—and the dilemma of TRUTH vs. THEORY.

Medical science's tragic loss of direction did **NOT** occur by accident. Rather, it was foreordained—and it is a tale of *manipulation* and ***behind the scene*** control!

Let us paint the historical landscape of a few great men and women of **"REAL"** science so we can better understand the politics of "medicine" today—and why we **MUST** accept responsibility for our own lives by **"unplugging"** from the medical system. Here's a brief history of a few medical Wizards.

The Great Wizards

Dr. Carey Reams was a Wizard. Reams had a sixth sense about nature and the energy forces of life at the subatomic level. Most of Ream's focus work was in the agricultural arena. Reams *dared* to expose the connection between diet, lifestyle and dis-ease. He used simple, inexpensive testing procedures to determine the "state" of people health; procedures that only called for the pH of the urine and saliva plus the mapping of the blood capillaries in the white of the eye. He suffered professional ridicule and legal abuse for his efforts.

Dr. Linus Pauling was a Wizard! He gave us his monumental discoveries about vitamin C. He also suffered professional ridicule for the **TRUTH** he heralded. Dr. Pauling was the harbinger of the fantastic DNA molecule discovery in 1954. Your author spoke with Dr. Pauling many times in the years before his death at age 94. At age 92, he was still teaching at Stanford. Pauling was a wonderful scientist and a monument to **TRUTH**. Truth separates good scientists from a poor ones. Pauling won TWO nobel prizes. [See *MoonShine*, Chapter 37, for the "rest of" the vitamin-C story.]

Dr. Guenther Enderlein was a Wizard. He proved that the blood is NOT a sterile medium. He heralded the **pleomorphic** nature of microbial life forms that are always present in the blood of healthy people. He explained "why" and "how" life forms—from viruses and bacteria to yeast and fungi—*appear* in the blood as people lose control of their "terrain." Enderlein was the first person to use body fluid pH to detect the presence of cancer. His final exam question to test his understanding of life before becoming a doctor in 1898 was: *"What is the difference between plant and animal?"* Enderlein responded, *"There is NO difference!"* He was correct and his discoveries proved it.

[When your author returned to school at age 45 to become "enlightened" in the ways of science, he took a sound understanding of plant and soil physiology with him. This background provided greater understanding and helped him make "connections" than were NOT "taught" in classroom. Soil and plants became the foundation of the Young Again Protocol™—and the basis of this book.]

Rene M. Caisse, R.N. was a Wizard. Rene was Canada's "cancer nurse." She was a keen observer of nature's ways and understood life at the subtle energy level. She developed "Essiac Tea" and was hounded by health officials unmercifully.

Dr. Max Gerson was a Wizard. His discoveries are of tremendous importance to the aging process. He was an excellent example of "low-tech" medical brilliance. What made Gerson unique was that his therapies worked. He cared about people and he was an astute observer. He *cured* cancer with simple, inexpensive modalities—and therein was the rub! Gerson was hounded mercilessly by established medical authorities because he threatened their dogmatic position on the nature of cancer. He died in 1959 tired and overworked.

Rachel Carson was a Wizard. She was the scientist who took on the military-industrial complex by herself. In 1959, she wrote the book *Silent Spring*. Rachel was the beginning of the *legitimate* environmental movement. Her findings shattered Science's litany of lies and brought the evils of pesticides into focus. She was proclaimed a *witch* and was verbally burned at the stake before and after she died in 1964. Her epitaph reads: **TRUTH!**

Theo Colborn is a Wizard. She is the author of *Our Stolen Future* and the woman who took on the entire medical and scientific world in the grand style of Rachel Carson, author of *Silent Spring*. Colborn's book defines the hormonal dilemma we face. [The *Young Again Protocol*™ offers a solution to it.]

Dr. Ignaz Semmelweis was a Wizard. He has particular significance to medical science and our story. He was a physician in Budapest during the middle 1800's. Semmelweis made the mistake of confronting a thoroughly entrenched male-dominated profession that had only recently wrestled away control of the healing arts from female midwife "healers." His contribution to medical science was a simple one, but it involved the use of uncommon good sense—a dangerous commodity in the face of arrogance. Semmelweis said *"Doctors, wash your hands between patients!"*

[There had been unrelenting outbreaks of childbirth fever (Puerperal Fever) among women and hundreds of deaths in area hospitals. The year was 1840. His detractors laughed good Dr. Semmelweis from the scene. They destroyed his reputation by character assassination—a ploy that leaves neither trail nor record of those in bloody gowns. They also used professional ostracism—a time-tested tool of the trade. Today, they resort to revocation of a physician's license to practice—putting a doctor out of his trade. Ostracism, licenses and belittling are common maneuvers used to this day to CONTROL physicians who dare to step out of line.]

Norman Walker was a Wizard. Walker was a health researcher and reporter who *practiced what he preached* and lived well past age 100. His primary contribution to the alternative health arena was his ability to piece together seemingly unrelated pieces of medical facts into a cohesive fabric of usable information. His life was a tribute to **TRUTH!**

Bernard Jensen was a Wizard. Jensen expanded the fields of colon therapy and iridology and helped thousands of people. Jensen served his fellow man well.

Victor Irons was a Wizard. It was Irons who first

brought colon hydrotherapy to the fore as a viable, health modality. We owe him our utmost gratitude for his "gift!"

Comments

A doctor's status derives from the State. When the State grants permission, the professional is created by way of a license. The doctor is a "political being" that exists at the whim of the State. Licenses are **supposed** to protect the public. More often than not, licenses are a mockery—a Kabuchi Dance of sorts—as described in Chapter 38. Behind the scenes, State licensing boards, insurance companies and "peer review" organizations badger and control doctors who discover **TRUTH** and dare to question scientific and medical "dogma!"

History provides a long list of good Wizards—Galileo and Copernicus, for example. who were hounded and destroyed. **"Control"** is the name of the game. Control is ALWAYS carefully maintained despite political "staging" provided for its theatrical effect. In history, nothing happens by accident!

The history books tell us *nothing* of the political maneuvering by Dr. Semmelweis' peers, nor of the women who died, nor of the money siphoned-away from people who prostrated themselves at science's "altar!" Today, some arrogant doctors still "fail" to wash their hands between patients. The more things change, the more they are the same.

How It Happened

To understand how science and medicine lost their way and why mankind is at war with Mother Earth, let us go to the roots of Christianity, for it is there that we will find our clue.

And God said to Adam *"Take dominion over the Earth and every living thing thereon."*

This one command, credited to Deity, has done more to pillage the Earth and its inhabitants—plant, animal and man—than any words ever put to print. The problem isn't the command, but its **interpretation** and **implementation.**

Misunderstood and certainly **misapplied**, this biblical edict set the course and destiny of history from Christ to Isaac Newton and the present-day order. By **blaming** *sin* and the *fall* in the garden on Eve—instead of acknowledging that **BOTH** male and female made their own choices—*man* **dogmatized** jurisdiction over woman and proclaimed **WAR** against Nature and the Earth. Done in the "name" of GOD, mankind's present "health" dilemma appears to be the result of misapplied "blame"—instead of respect for life!

Adam & Eve

"Power and dominion over nature" shaped science and its tributary, medicine, into the **CULT** it is today. Man over God.

Man over the Earth. Man over Woman. For it says, *"Eve caused Adam to sin!"*

Interwoven in this tragic story was the shift from mankind's original primeval state as a *matriarchal* society to that of a *patriarchal* one. No longer would the **blood line** flow through the woman. Instead it would flow through the man. No more would Woman be exalted and recognized as the *giver* of life. Instead, she would be looked upon as the "ONE" who caused Adam (man) to sin in the garden.

"And from this day forward, you will experience pain in childbirth as a REMINDER of your transgression." And so, Woman became the villain. A commodity to be controlled, bought, sold and *"blamed"* for Adam's transgression—which was by Adam's own **CHOICE!**

It was into this arena that Dr. Semmelweis wandered. Little did he realize that the **powers behind the scene** did not care about Puerperal Fever. It was profitable business. *"So what if some women die as long as WE control access to choice in medical care, access to God—and, of course, control over the creation of a nation's money supply."*

"Control" is the name of the game! Reader's who wish to enjoy some semblance of control over their "life" must come to the realization that in matters of health, finance, religion and law—things are **NOT** what they appear. Thinking and acting outside the box are "crucial" if you wish to avoid the "matrix!"

TRUTH in medicine causes problems—and the greater medical science's **backlash** to a Wizard's message, the greater the probability that **TRUTH** is on the loose.

In medicine and science, **TRUTH** prospers **outside** the mainstream—out on the fringe. The "fringe" is where the reader will learn how to reverse the aging process. Only on the fringe can the reader become *Young Again!*

PREVIEW: *Our next chapter is where you will become acquainted with the "energy forces" that CONTROL the aging process, and you will learn HOW to identify them.*

The *Young Again!* Idea

Young Again! is about **"why?"** and **"how?"** people age. It is about enjoying and maintaining superb health by living and practicing concepts and habits that produce long-term results for those who are willing to do their part. Implied here is the need for a realistic "model." Faulty models go nowhere!

Just because you can't see it and you don't understand it, doesn't mean it came from the devil!

Hormones! Lots of Noise! Little Said!

In 2004, Suzanne Sommers—and a few practitioners—talked about "bio-identical" hormones for women. They **failed** to mention that the liver "orchestrates" women's hormones—and unless the **LIVER** and **"terrain"** are addressed—"bio-identical" doesn't mean much! They also **failed** to mention that "stress" is a **HUGE** hormonal "wild card" for women. Stress puts the adrenal glands into overdrive—spiking cortisol levels and "skewing" hormonal balance. [See pages 72, 76-7 and 362.]

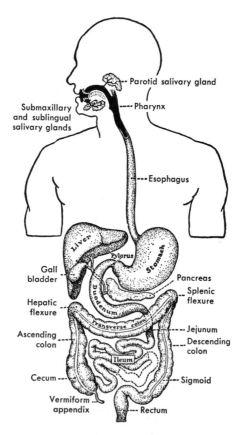

Submaxillary and sublingual salivary glands
Parotid salivary gland
Pharynx
Esophagus
Liver
Pylorus
Stomach
Gall bladder
Pancreas
Splenic flexure
Hepatic flexure
Duodenum
Ascending colon
Transverse colon
Jejunum
Descending colon
Ileum
Cecum
Sigmoid
Vermiform appendix
Rectum

Visceral Organs Of The Abdominal Cavity

Raccoon Eyes!

Circles under the eyes are a **SIGN** of "liver" overload, **not** kidney stress. Under-hydration, lymphatic congestion and bowel issues makes things worse. Follow the *Young Again Protocol*™ and you will be a *happy camper*—without raccoon eyes!

5

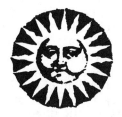

Energy & Matter

"Reason, of course, is weak when measured against its never-ending task. Weak, indeed, compared with the follies and passions of mankind, which, we must admit, almost entirely control our human destinies, in great things and small."

Albert Einstein

Little in life is seen in concrete terms of black and white. This is particularly true in the healing arts. For example, consider just a few of the differences in the following modalities (therapies) of healing presently in use.

Allopathic medicine (allopathy) attempts to heal using **"chemotherapy"**—which is "chemically" induced manipulation of **SIGNS** and **symptoms**. Included here is surgical intervention, emergency medicine and *palliation*. Allopathy is the predominant medical modality practiced in the West. It uses "drugs" to **OVERPOWER** body systems to **FORCE** change. Allopathy believes that "opposite cures opposite."

Homeopathic medicine (homeopathy) is the exact opposite of allopathic medicine. It is called the medicine of "similars." Homeopathy focuses on *unfriendly energy fields* in the body that vibrate at *anti-life* frequencies—frequencies that stress the vital organs and create imbalances in the system. Homeopathy uses **vibrational** *remedies* instead of chemical drugs. These remedies are potent substances *"tuned"* to cancel renegade energy forces in the body—as represented by drugs, vaccines, toxins, etc. Remedies **erase the footprint** of offending energy fields, clears the body of their "signature" and returns the patient to "homeostasis" (*homeo*-resembling; *stasis*-a state of equilibrium; balance within the system).

Chiropractic views dis-ease, in general, to be the byproduct of incorrect spinal alignment affecting the nerve plexus issuing therefrom. Poor alignment negatively influences the vital organs served by the central and peripheral nervous systems. Chiropractic has much in common with other vibrational modalities. Chiropractors often wear several hats at once—and are at best "tolerated" by M.D.'s. The reason: a good chiropractor is trained to be results and patient oriented—and they are generally open to alternative healing modalities.

Network Spinal Analysis (NSA) is a new form of chiropractic that integrates various "levels" of care in such a way as to *unfold* and *awaken* spinal energy flow. Healing occurs as a by-product of the freedom of the *body-mind* to utilize its natural, self-regulatory and self-expressive capabilities. In other words, healing is not the direct product of chiropractic, but of the "forces" of life itself at the "subtle" energy level.

The purpose of NSA is to determine the appropriate *timing* and *application* of mechanical forces to the tissues **before** chiropractic adjustment. NSA enables patients to release *non*-productive, neurological patterns that block healing. NSA allows the *whole* person to express and experience their body's own self-intelligence and vital-energy force.

NSA speeds healing and helps the patient become aware of and "erase" negative energy *memory* patterns *at* and *below* the cellular level. [A "whiplash" is a memory of physical truama. See Gua Sha below.]

Network Spinal Analysis produces significant improvement in patient self-awareness and ability to make life changes. This promising new healing modality was developed by Donald Epstein, D.C., and is offered to the public by highly trained healers under the trade name Network Chiropractic™.

Yoga & Pilates are not exactly new to the health scene, but they are wonderful and **proven** modalities for people who practice them. Your author was taught some yoga techniques by his daughter and saw wonderful progress in the sacrum and low back from an injury 25 years earlier. Yoga is very ancient. Classes are taught at local schools, YMCA and on video.

"Pilates" [pronounced *pee-lot-ees*] was developed by Joseph Pilates about 90 years ago. Pilates rejuvenatory and unique body conditioning "moves" to tone muscles, increase flexibility and lengthen and align the body.

Your author can testify to the wonderful anti-aging effects that yoga and Pilates' have on **"older"** women who practice them. "Yoga ladies" are way ahead of their peers! They are "easily" 20 years younger than their girlfriends.

Acupuncture came from Asia and promotes healing and numbs pain using tiny needles to *manipulate* energy meridians similar to reflexology and High Enema Therapy™.

Gua Sha [pronounced *gwa saw*] is a 3000 year old modality that is easy to learn and is very effective and is used to relieve pain, promote healing and *free* bound **"chi"** energy. [A teaching video and kit are available for "in-home" use. The technique is very effective on whiplash, joint and neck problems. [See page 370.]

Bio-Magnetics uses magnetic energy flowing from *therapeutic* magnets. This promising modality has broad application for people desiring *personal* control over their health. It is an effective, inexpensive in-home modality. "Medical grade" mattress pads and pendants are the primary applications.

[Therapeutic magnets are specific in nature and application. They are useful for tissue trauma; they nullify the effects of 110v, 60-cycle alternating electrical current, and they protect and stimulate the immune system. Therapeutic magnets are DC (direct current) energy fields that "awaken" energy meridians and manipulate pain. Healing follows "repolarization" of cellular organelles, increased production of ATP, and increased flow of blood and lymphatic fluids. Therapeutic magnets restore energy "flow" in and around injured or inflamed tissue. Millions of people get drug-free relief and improved health through magnetic therapy. It is widely used in Japan. Allopathic medicine considers magnetic therapy "quackery"—but patients who experience "results" think otherwise. See pages 82, 144 and 233.]

Vibrational Medicine is a composite description that includes dozens of healing modalities that rely on the manipulation of the body's *energy* fields to induce healing. Vibrational medicine teaches that health and sickness are "manifestations" of **"ERRANT"** energy at the subtle energy level. Healing requires establishment of energy "balance" **before** the body can become "whole."

Vibrational medicine is a **blend** of Western and Eastern thought and produces wonderful results. Its roots **ante**date allopathic medicine by many thousands of years.There is no question that this form of medicine **is** replacing the Frankenstein called "allopathy."

[A few examples of vibrational medicine are cold laser, photo-luminescence, aroma therapy, flower essence, High Enema Therapy™, therapeutic magnets, qi gong, tai chi, deep breathing, essential oils, chiropractic, homeopathy, yoga, Pilates, good food and BFRV™ and MGIW™ water(s). These modalities promote energy flow within the bio-electric body.]

Compare The Difference

Allopathic medicine is based on the *Newtonian* view of reality. Sir Isaac Newton saw the world as an elaborate mechanism. Newton so influenced allopathic medicine that for the past 300 years, the body has been **viewed** as a grand machine that takes its orders from the brain and central and peripheral nervous systems. This view was replaced by a newer "model" that sees the body as a flesh-and-blood biological computer. Nuts and bolts gave way to circuit boards and DNA. Both approaches **fall short** of the reality of life at the **"subtle"** energy level of our existence.

The Newtonian approach fails to account for "Fourth Dimensional" energy forces like spirit, intuition, subconscious mental activity, biofeedback, dowsing, etc. which are subtle energy manifestations composing the metaphysical **"sixth" sense** (*meta*-**beyond** physical). **"Sunlight"** is Fourth Dimensional. All things "physical" are nothing but "frozen" sunlight energy. Fourth Dimentional energy **CANNOT** be measured by length, width and height—the First, Second and Third Dimensions. [See Chapters 31 and 35 for expansion of these ideas.]

Paradigm Shift

Vibrational Medicine (VM) sees the physical body as the *signature* or *footprint* of the invisible **"electric"** body. VM is based on Einstein's view of matter which says "matter will release energy when taken apart." For example, the splitting of an atom in a atomic explosion . This is a **MAJOR** *paradigm shift* from Western medicine's archaic approach to healing. The word **paradigm** means *para*-beside, *digm*-an example that serves as a model.

The Einstein model sees the human being as a network of energy fields that co-exist and coalesce; that is, **condensed** energy resonating at a healthy or sick frequency. [Mother Earth frequency is between 7.8-8.1 Hertz.]

Vibrational healing *manipulates* energy, where allopathic medicine uses negative energy inputs (drugs, surgery) to **over-power** and **force** the body into submission—*bypassing* the body's innate intelligence. Homeopathy uses "similar"—but opposite—frequencies to neutralize offending energy force fields. Vibrational medicine does **NOT** endorse the Germ Theory of Disease—but it **does** recognize that the **"TERRAIN"** controls the microbes (bacteria, viruses, yeasts, fungi, parasites, etc.).

Present day drug therapy is a mixture of *hoped for* therapeutic effects and **KNOWN** adverse effects—the good *hopefully* outweighing the bad! A better translation is *"Acceptable collateral damage!"* or *"Acceptable body count!"* or *"The one for the many!"*—as Spock would say!

Drugs are drugs! They alter body function in negative ways. They do violence to the body and to the liver in particular. At best, they ease patient suffering through *palliation* (relief of signs and symptoms **WITHOUT** cure of underlying causes)—while "killing" the patient. Collateral damage!

Health Through "Manipulation"

An example of energy manipulation would be running a magnet over a computer disc or a DVD. The magnet **neutralizes** *energy* stored on the disc by cancelling the "signature" or "footprint" of the energy message. If the energy message on the disc were a dis-ease "condition," a positive change in health would occur when the "signature" is **neutralized!** Whenever positive energy gains the upper hand, the body returns to a state of "homeostasis." Because life is energy and energy is matter, we must conclude that life and energy are manifestations of the same phenomenon. Vibrational medicine's focus is "energy."

Magneto Hydro Dynamics (MHD) focus is the field of dentistry at the "consumer" level through **prevention** of periodontal issues and reduced accumulation of dental plaque. Plaque formation results in cavities and gum problems. MHD utilizes a small counter appliance that produces electromagnetically **"CHARGED"** water. When hydrogen ions are "freed" from the H_2O [water] molecule, the ions carry a positive (+) charge that causes them to "bond" to bacteria and plaque deposits—**neutralizing** them! [The device is an inexpensive way to care for teeth and gums. It works on pets, too! [See pages 79, 117-8-9, 149, 187, 204 (photo), 233 and 329.]

[The Young Again Protocol™ calls for Oral Advantage™ (O/A)—a product that is mixed with a small amount of water and held in the mouth immediately prior to bed. O/A "pulls-out" infection from below the gum line—reducing inflammation and causing loose teeth to "tighten-up!"]

Teeth and gum problems are some of the very earliest SIGNS of acidification of the body's "terrain."

Radionics is used by some alternative farmers. It involves "broadcasting" beneficial energy frequencies into soil and air to "feed" plants, animals and microbes. Compare this practice to a radio station that transmits a melody that is picked-up by radio for our enjoyment. Properly used, radionics enhances production of highly nutritious food by controlling the "energy" environment—and therefore weeds and insects.

Biodynamics is *homeopathic* agriculture that uses biodynamic "preparations" and techniques. Books on the subject are *Biodynamic l, ll,* and *lll +Introduction, A Biodynamic Farm* and *The Rock Dust Book.* This is valuable information for anyone seriously interested in growing vibrantly healthy food.

Your author has a one acre garden and orchard and "practices" these techniques because they work!

Medical Science Challenged

Medical science is threatened by alternative paradigm **"shifts"** because they **conflict** with their textbook "model." Paradigm shifts challenge accepted theories that medical science has elevated to the status of "law" by way of the mumbo-jumbo called the **"scientific method!"** Misuse of the so -called scientific method has gotten us into a lot of trouble. It should be abandoned because it shackles individual creativity. The **"POINT"** your author is making is: vision **MUST** "precede" inquiry rather than the other way around.

Vibrational medicine is gaining popularity because it delivers **RESULTS** with little risk and no damage to the patient. It behooves us to embrace these newer "models."

The Young Again Model involves the management and manipulation of energy fields by controlling the "terrain" of the bio-electric body.

The *Young Again Protocol*™ calls for the application of vibrational medicine at the layman's level—where people live out their daily lives. There is **NO** better *return on investment* than good health and the ability to work as long as one needs or wishes to work. Good health is the **ULTIMATE** alternative to forced "retirement!" For many people, retirement is a health disaster. This book provides the framework of knowledge needed to maintain control over one's life and health.

The Young Again Protocol(s)™ *discussed in this book—and each person's response to them—are unique to the individual and are adjusted as needed.*

New View

The universe is composed of but two things: **ENERGY** and **MATTER.** Our body is matter in the form of frozen light energy. If this is true, then drugs, which are matter, must also be energy—and they are! However, they are **NEGATIVE** energy—energy that manipulates illness in the short term at the expense of health and longevity in the long term. **No one can deny** the advances allopathic medicine has made—especially in the replacement of body parts and in emergency medicine. But there is a negative side also. We must realize that medications and surgical intervention carry **substantial** "risk" and tradeoffs—and should **ONLY** be used as last resort.

Aging is a cumulative process. The combined effect of personal neglect, dis-ease and drugs accelerates aging in the youngest of people.

Energy Shifts

When we choose to live an unhealthy lifestyle, energy **"shifts"** result in dis-ease and accelerated aging. Aging "reversal" is the **product** of manipulation of negative energy so the body can enjoy and maintain a state of "homeostasis"—indefinitely! When your author talks about having an ageless body, he is talking about a "state" of being where positive energy "dominates"—and the body that does **NOT** require perpetual jump-starts with drugs and surgery to keep going.

Everything we do, eat and drink involves "energy" and influences the "terrain!" We must learn to "decipher" what is good for us and what is not by identifying those energy forces instead of turning to drugs or invasive surgery.

Dis-ease is the manifestation of negative energy. Vibrational medicine offers the ordinary person more CONTROL over their health and life!

We *must* recognize that we are **more** than hunks of flesh and blood, **more** than biological machines—and **more** than spiritual beings *trapped* in bodies during our time on Earth. We are **energy**—and because we are energy—we are part of the cosmos. And yes, we are created in the likeness of God who is also **ENERGY**—positive, beautiful energy!

Anions & Cations

Anions and **cat**ions are usable forms of **"electron"** energy that are released when a chemical reaction takes place—as in the gut and liver when we eat and digest food. The release of energy opposites—one (+) the other (-)—produces the electrical activity that grants permission for life.

"Matter" is a combination of (+) and (-) energy forces with a particular **"footprint"** of anions and cations. For example, the metal "steel." When the energy "footprint" of matter is altered through fusion, we may get lead or alchemist gold—instead of steel. Break the bonds holding atomic structures together and energy is released—and sometimes with a big "bang." [The reader will learn more about these concepts in Chapter 18.]

Good & Bad Energy

The terms **positive** and **negative** energy mean the same as **good** and **bad** energy. *Good* energy is "right-spin" energy and *bad* energy is "left-spin" energy. We know good energy from bad energy by their *effect* on our health and the *bio-electric* body.

Positive energy has a particular *spin* of its own—it *spins to the right,* meaning clockwise. **Negative** energy *spins to the left,* meaning counter clockwise. Hurricanes spin left.

Solar energy is **an**ionic energy. It is life-giving energy. The Earth's spin is the product of **an**ionic, clockwise, right-spin energy entering the Van Allen Belt (ozone layer). As these energy particles penetrate the ozone layer, they are deflected, bombarding the Earth and causing it to spin. When Van Allen theorized this belt in 1948, he was laughed down by "experts!" Later, he was vindicated when NASA lost contact with astronaut John Glenn as he passed through this belt [ozone layer] on his return to Mother Earth.

Anionic energy passes "through" matter. It is also very comforting and soothing. Have you noticed the difference in the heat produced by a wood fire compared to the heat produced by gas or electricity? Wood heat warms *"clear to your bones!"*

Wood heat is **an**ionic energy; it comes from the Sun. Its effect is *right-spin* and it warms us because the **an**ions released by oxidation (burning) of the wood pass **through** the body, warming the cells. This is similar to how a microwave oven works—with one very important exception. Microwave energy is left-spin—and food cooked with the device is **VERY** destructive to health—and **NOT** fit for consumption!

Right-spin **positive** energy keeps you young. Left-spin **negative** energy causes you to "grow" old. The former keeps you on the *anabolic* side of the pyramid as illustrated on pages 21 and 198. The latter puts you on the *catabolic* side. One spins RIGHT; the other spins LEFT. We are interested in the way these energy forces affect living things and HOW they influence the aging process. Please check your understanding by reviewing the following drawings.

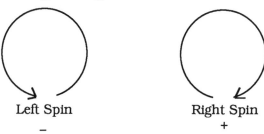

Left Spin   Right Spin

−   +

How To Determine The Spin

There are several ways to determine the spin and/or predict the effect a substance will have on living tissue.

For instance, look at a bottle of vitamin E and you will see that the word *tocopherol* is preceded by the letter(s) d or dl. "d" indicates that when infra red light is beamed through the tocopherol, the light is bent to the *right* or clockwise indicating that the vitamin E has life giving energy. "dl" tocopherol has the opposite *footprint*—an isomer—and provides nothing useful.

Please note, almost all "d" vitamin E is encapsulated in SOY or CANOLA oil—causing the positive energy to go "negative." Substances that exert a negative influence on the body must be **neutralized, disposed of or isolated** to minimize their effect on the "terrain!" This includes food and non-food substances like drugs, food additives, colorings, ALL artificial sweetners, excitotoxin type salts—like "MSG"—and other substances which we will discuss in more depth later.

Neutralize

The word **neutral** doesn't mean much to most people. It's kind of a *neutral* word. We must be more specific in its use. When we say that the body must **"neutralize"** toxic or left-spin energy substances, we mean that those substances which exert a negative influence on the body must be **de-energized** by the body. To de-energize something requires energy. Please recall our magnet and computer disc example. Both are forms of **stored** energy. The magnet's energy neutralized the disc's energy using an opposite energy force and footprint.

The body handles negative energy in similar fashion. Consider a potato—a stable form of food energy. The potato is **stored** complex carbohydrate energy put there by the plant for future needs. Depending on how the potato was grown, it may produce positive or negative effects in the body. All potatoes or carrots or peaches or apples, etc. are **NOT** equal!

Negative energy potatoes cause the body to squander "reserve" energy to *process* and **de-energize** the potato's negative energy "signature." If the body is unable to accomplish the task, the potato's negative energy circulates and diminishes vital organ function weakening the "terrain!"

Left-spin energy—when turned loose in the body—has **momentum** like a boulder rolling down a hill. Stopping it requires the body to waste **vital force**—creating an energy "deficit" that **reduces** health and vitality. The body is **FORCED** to try and remove the toxic energy from **circulation**. Isolating "noxious" energy is a damage-control tactic designed to preserve anabolic activity. Negative energy is *catabolic* in nature. [Please refer to the aging pyramid on page 198.]

Back to "spin." When you read "right-spin," think "good" for my body. When your read "left-spin," think "bad" for my body." It is **NOT** oversimplification! It's the way things work.

Kinesiology

Kinesiology, as defined here, relates to body response to "energy fields" and their affect on body physiology. In vibrational medicine, kinesiology is concerned with the energy dynamics a substance imposes on the *bio-electric* body.

Kinesthetics involves "muscle sense." It is known as Dynamic Reflex Analysis, Applied Kinesiology or plain old "muscle testing." It involves gain or loss of strength in the digits and limbs, using various testing techniques.

Some practitioners use this procedure to **diagnose** and **prescribe**. Your author does **NOT** consider "muscle testing" to be a viable, trustworthy technique. Muscle testing is a **crude** form of dowsing that is extremely **"SUBJECTIVE"** and of questionable value to the practitioner and patient. The same can be said for hair analysis, food combining, and eating for your blood type. All of these are **"questionable"** yardsticks and temporary management tools—at best! Better to restore the **"terrain"** and forget about the *hocus-pocus!*

The problem with "muscle testing" is that good, biologically active substances often produce exactly the same response as "known" bad substances. [For example, racemized™ products are **VERY** biologically active and produce **MAXIMUM** body response. That is why the *Young Again Protocol*™ is adjusted for each person.]

Analysis by a "machines" that supposedly analyse the "terrain" is no better than muscle testing because the machine relies on "programmed" inputs based on a "faulty" medical "model." Testing is **GROSSLY** influenced by the effects of systemic heavy metals on the **"autonomic"** nervous system—a "wild card" variable that is **NOT** accounted for when the machine makes its "determination!" Now for some testing techniques used by some "alternative" practitioners.

How To Test

You will need a helper and the food, drug or supplement to be tested. First, form a ring with the thumb and middle finger of your dominant hand. Next, have your friend attempt to gently, but firmly, pull your fingers apart, while noting the amount of effort required to *separate* the fingers. Then, place the substance in question in the mouth or opposite hand and repeat the process. Supposedly, if the substance is good for the body, the fingers become **STRONGER,** and visa versa. Testing by yourself is difficult. This process involves just enough "voodoo" to elevate its status above that of a "warm fuzzie."

*[Sometimes, the body gives **false results** because it instinctively **KNOWS** that the "substance" will produce a **healing crisis** and cause body to "cope, cleanse and heal!" Rejuvenation is "stressful"—and the body seeks to **minimize** stress, especially when it **knows** that the "host" does **NOT** truly desire healing and will be unwilling to "cope!" Your author sees this phenomenon all the time. Sadly, these people **never** heal.]*

The above procedure can also be done by extending the dominant arm so that it is level with the shoulder and have another person gently press down while the person being tested holds the substance in question. Do a **before** and **after** test to gauge arm resistance to movement.

Other Examples

People who drink too much alcohol have cirrhotic livers. So do people suffering from hepatitis, mononucleosis, malaria or yellow fever. You can check the condition of their liver—or its response to a product or procedure—using the arm method described above, while at the same time touching the liver area (just below rib cage on right front). Loss of strength implies a messed-up liver!

My friend bought some tomatoes at the super market—the kind that grow mold before you get them home. I tested them with a **refractometer**, pendulum and vibration chain. All three tested negative in his body, weakening his **"aura"**—which reflects the body's life force—and vitality. They were returned. Better to buy organic or from a gardener or a farmer's market in your area. Forget the grocery store!

Foucault's Pendulum

A pendulum is one way to measure right and left spin energy. A pendulum is an "antenna"—and it works just like a radio or television antenna except that here, the antenna is **"moving."** An antenna can both send and receive energy signals. Trees are antenna growing on the surface of the earth.

All substances emit energy signals—including the body. A HIGH vitality body issues "right spin" signals. The opposite is also true. The body's aura "mirrors" it energy "state"—be it right or left, healthy or sick. Rocks, drugs, food, etc. have an aura. Kirlian photography can capture a picture of an "aura."

Suspend a pendulum over something and it will "spin" left or right. Some pendulums are more sensitive than others—as are individual dowsers. Dowsing is highly subjective, hence, variations in interpretation is a problem.

The strength of the pendulum's spin reflects the "strength" of the substance being checked. Gut instinct guides the "interrogatories" and "direction" of inquiry—but only if the dowser can negate personal interference. [Remember, the pendulum is the antenna and the dowser is the interpreter!]

Learning to use a pendulum and vibration chain requires practice. The skill must be "developed." *The Pendulum Kit* and *Vibrations* are very good instructional works on the subject. [See pages 50-1, 144, 188, 210 and 283.]

Other Vibrational Therapies

Therapeutic Touch involves the **transfer** of positive energy to heal or help restore someone's health. It is used in the fields of nursing and massage therapy. Here, energy from a healthy person is used to transform the sick person's energy fields. **Laying on of hands**, a religious practice, and **Qi Gong**, an ancient Chinese modality, are similar to therapeutic touch—as is Reiki. We will develop these ideas in a future chapter.

Scar Application Technique

While having my mercury amalgam fillings removed, my dentist noticed a one inch scar under my chin and asked when and how it got there. After I told him, he asked me to do the finger exercise we just described, only instead of placing a substance into my left hand, he had me touch the scar with my left hand. BINGO! No strength!

The **effect** the scar was exerting was strong because it

was directly in the path of a major **"energy"** meridian flowing from my abdominal chakra (energy center) to the top of my head. The scar was *blocking* the flow of "chi!"

To "temporarily" *erase* the scar **memory**, the dentist injected a homeopathic *remedy* along its length, and instantly *full strength* returned to my joined fingers.

[Scar tissue is negative energy tissue. Scars and the "trauma" that usually accompanies their formation are recorded in the skin's "holographic" memory. Scars are like energy footprints on a computer disc—no difference! [Read The Holographic Universe. See Source Page 400.]

Physical trauma produces "physical" scars—internally and extrenally. A body under "stress" at the moment of injury, scars readily. The *Young Again Tissue and Liver Protocol*™ restores the "terrain" so healing can occur. [VZ™ and L_sP_cC™ and SOC™ accelerate the restoration process.]

VZ™ "eats" and "breaks down" both scar tissue and amyloid plaque. SOC™ increases blood flow and nerve activity to tramatized areas of the body.

Functionally "healthy" tissue is composed of **parenchyma** cells. Non-functional "unhealthy" tissue is composed of **stroma** cells. "Scarred" vital organs accelerate aging because their "energy profile" is poor—meaning the "vital" organs are unable to do their "vital" work—and as the reader is learning, all life processes are energy-based.

Ours is a world of *energy* phenomena and knowing how to "dowse" is a huge advantage. Humans dowse when they use "intuition" in making routine daily decisions—so **WHY NOT** follow your "gut" in medicine, healing and food choices? Learning to understand "energy"—in all its manifestations—will light the path to becoming *Young Again!*

PREVIEW: *Our next chapter is an overview of "high-tech" modern medicine and its "magic bullet" promises. It will help you see the futility of relying on medicine's quick-fix techniques and to appreciate the value of good health.*

| **Beautiful Skin** |

Repair of scarred, damaged and wrinkled skin requires that **ALL** "terrain" issues be addressed. **De**acidification, hormones and digestion of scar tissue using SOC™ caps, VZ II,™ SOC™ Lotion and R/Skin™ Creme—plus High Enema Therapy.™

| **Causes of Osteoporosis** |

Osteoporosis has "three" causes and **NONE** of them have anything to do with "calcium" intake! The reader will learn how to "reverse" this awful condition as the book unfolds.

➡️ | **Telephone "Magic!"** |

Cellular and cordless phones "use" is dangerous! The brain is an "electrical" grid—and wireless phone devices **EMIT** powerful "signals" that **interfere** with brain function. If wireless phones can "transmit" and "receive" voice signals through concrete and steel buildings—penetrating a bit of skull bone is a "no-brainer!" Young people who use these devices "24/7/365"—and whose brains are still "growing"—are facing **serious** long-term consequences in the **FUTURE!** "**Teeth**" are also "grossly" affected by these powerful "transmitters!" "**Unprotected**" use of wireless phones is "**inexcusable**" now that a practical solution is available. The device "harmonizes" and "neutralizes" dangerous electrical "signals." And as for those wireless hands-free "headsets"—they are **3 times MORE** potent than the phone itself. Go to: www.mybiopro.com/heavenlydragon or call 877-224-6422 to "**protect**" your brain and "**avoid**" damaging your **TEETH**!!

| **Acid Reflux** |

Medical "experts" talk about acid-reflux *as if* it is a disease. But, it is **not** a dis-ease—it is a "condition."

The questions "thinking" people should be asking are, "**Why** do people develop this condition?; and **Why** didn't they have it earlier in their life?; and **Why** can't the "experts" figure WHAT the "real" problem is?; and lastly "Is there a "fix?"

Lots of "Why's?"—and the experts don't have a clue—much less **ANY** answers! Here is your author's answer!

When the *flow* of bile "slows" digestion problems manifest and the bowels do not move like they should. **When** the stomach cannot empty its acid-laden contents into the small intestine, food *regurgitates* up into the esophagus, damaging the delicate mucous membrane lining. **When** people do not move their bowels 2-5 times per day, the digestive system eventually fails! **When** people fail to chew their food, digestion suffers! **When** people drink liquids with meals, they shut down digestion. **When** people fail to drink enough water throughout the day, they will not secrete enough saliva to digest their food. **Stay-away from "experts!"**

| **Scar Tissue & Stiff Joints** |

SOC™ helps blood flow and nerve activity which promotes health! SOC™ soften scars, clears acne blemishes, softens wrinkles and eases joint pain, supports hair, **promotes** bilateral movement of nutrients and waste across cell membranes, and **shuttles** heavy metals **OUT** of the body. Limber Life™ helps you feel "limber"—and is used with SOC™. VZ™ "**eats**" amyloid plaque and scar tissue. L_sP_cC™ accelerates the lay-down of collagen for restoration of connective tissues like bones, cartilage, muscles, ligaments and skin. [See pages 82, 149, 182, 247, 285, 293, 313 and Chapters 36 and 37.]

"Protect" Your Liver & Skin

"Three" Stage "oxidation/reduction" shower filters are the best filters available! There are **no** cartridges to change! They **last** 5-10 years! They are **"full-flowing"** so you can get **"wet!"** They are **easy** to install and your skin and hair—and "colon"—will LOVE the water! [See Pages 212 and 400.]

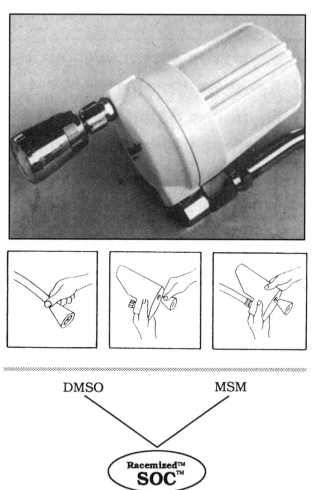

DMSO   MSM

Racemized™
SOC™

DMSO (dimethylsulfoxide) has been around for over 50 years, and except for the fact that it "stinks," it is a very useful product—especially for snake bites! [Buy DMSO in **"liquid"** at any veterinarian supply and keep it on hand. Use it "generously" on damaged tissue and you will witness a "miracle!"] Then, along came MSM which got rid of the smell! Now we have SOC™—a racemized™ and "enhanced" MSM with increased activity when used with R/A Catalyst™ to activate the SOC.™ Better results, less money and "no" odor. That's progress! [See pages 64, 82, 152, 162, 177, 184, 247, 293 and 304.]

6

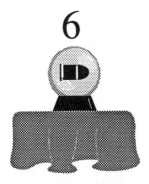

Magic Bullets

"We know life only by its symptoms."
Albert Szent-Györgyi
(Discoverer of vitamin C)

Allopathic medicine is no closer to understanding the *essence* of life today than it was a hundred years ago. It understands little about **basic** functions like sleep, growth, pain, aging and "healing." It attempts to manipulate these functions—but it does **NOT** understand them.

Today 2006, we labor under an **endless** procession of new drugs and high-tech equipment concocted for the treatment of "degenerative" conditions like heart dis-ease, cancer, diabetes and arthritis. These conditions are **technology "driven"**—requiring ever more expensive diagnostic equipment and a long line of experts to operate the "gadgets!"

We have **substituted** "high-tech" medicine for the old *"take-the-pill; solve-the-problem"* approach of yesterday. We have **substituted** dis-eases of *civilization* for the contagious maladies of the past. The problems of dis-ease and aging are **still** with us—despite medicine's passion for **"technology!"**

High-tech medicine has become an extension of our national consciousness. It is the same "magic bullet" approach used in the movies. We wrongly equate medical science's efforts with "healing!" Magic-bullet technology "blurs" our vision and sedates our mental faculties, causing us to accept life on marginal terms under the **assumption** that the wonderful body God gave us is incapable of healing itself "naturally!" Technology is **NOT** the answer. It is only a "tool!"

Yesterday & Today

Yesterday, medicine knew us as people. Today, we are "bodies" in a cattle line—stripped of our human dignity! The difference is the *system.* The system has quashed the human being on both ends of the continuum. The doctor is denied training in nutrition and vibrational medicine—and the patient gets neither. Modern medicine and the public have traded dignity for "magic bullets" and technology!

Medical science does **NOT** understand dis-ease at the subtle energy level. Yet, medicine attempts to diagnose dis-ease symptoms with tests, X-rays, CAT scans and MRI's. People take refuge in *magic bullets* and *hope*—instead of addressing the root causes of degenerative dis-ease.

Daily, newspapers gush with glowing reports of a promising new "Flash Gordon" therapy. Just as fast, people fill the stalls—like cattle in slaughter yards—waiting for a *magic bullet* that will cure their misery. Desperate people doing desperate things—ignorant as to the cause of their plight.

Poor Health • Life of Simplicity

Poor health isn't a sin, but it's awfully inconvenient and terribly expensive. There's a better way.

A life of simplicity allows you to take control of your life and health. It's the drive for money and things that stands between us and a life of simplicity. We must evaluate what is *really* important and learn to "walk away" from the rest.

If we lose our health chasing a dollar, we lose. Even if we catch lots of dollars, we still lose. When we fail to take care of our greatest treasure—our health—we give our dollars to the doctors and hospitals. When we become desperately ill, money and things mean little. They are a poor trade for good health.

We partake of magic bullet mentality because it offers us a quick, effortless "fix!" People **LIKE** smoke-and-mirror technology! But it's a **"past tense"** approach and a fancy band-aid to a health event that has already taken place.

We are confounded by high-tech magicians in white coats. We seem unable to differentiate between empty promises and empty "hope!" There is **NO** difference! Magic bullets are a distraction and a salve for an old body. Just because you enjoy good health today does **NOT** mean you will enjoy it tomorrow—an erroneous assumption people make over and over again. Your author prefers a simpler, more realistic approach.

"Keeping" your health is a lot easier than getting it back after you lose it!

Why experience the hell of old age when you can enjoy **perpetual** good health? **TIME** stands still when you are truly healthy. Do "whatever" you need to do to get your *bio-electric* reference score under "0.33." When you are *Young Again* **YOU** are in control and you won't need medicine's "magic bullets!"

PREVIEW: *In our next chapter you will learn WHY food—by itself—fails to supply the ENERGY needed to stay young and WHAT you can do to remedy the dilemma.*

The "Amyloid" Connection

Alzheimers is a **HUGE** problem—and the "experts" don't have a clue what is "driving" it. Alzheimers favors women over men 3:1! There is a hormonal "disconnect" going on here! As brain tissue **"deteriorates"** for lack of hormonal protection, it fills with "amyloid" plaque. [See pages 58, 111, 157, 259, 265, 277, 285, 293, 368-9 and Chapters 36 and 37 to learn more about "Alzheimers"—and how to **"AVOID"** it!

The 65% Watery Human Being

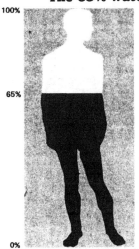

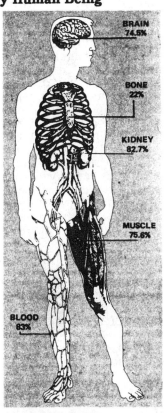

100%

65%

0%

BRAIN
74.5%

BONE
22%

KIDNEY
82.7%

MUSCLE
75.6%

BLOOD
83%

THE 65% WATERY HUMAN
The amount of water in the human body, averaging 65 per cent, varies considerably from person to person and even from one part of the body to another (right). A lean man may have as much as 70 per cent of his weight in the form of body water, while a woman, because of her larger proportion of water-poor fatty tissues, may be only 52 per cent water. The lowering of the water content in the blood is what triggers the hypothalamus, the brain's thirst center to send out its familiar demand for a drink.

Multiple Chemical Sensitivity

Environmental illness is a **BIG** issue for children and adults. Perfumes and building material off-gassing can push one's "liver" over the edge. The "liver" is the controlling factor.

The "COBALT" Connection

Cobalt is central to vitamin B-12 and formation of hemoglobin, strong connective tissues—and vibrant energy. The simplest and best way to get cobalt into the blood is with Cobo-12™ transdermal skin creme. [Women **"deplete"** their B-12 levels 20 years before men, due to menstruation.]

Spider Bites • Insect Bites & Stings

Spider and insect bites and stings are "energy" reactions of the body to "foreign" proteins. Some people experience severe reactions; others suffer loss of body parts. We must come to understand the nature of errant "energy fields" that produce these serious, so-called "allergic" reactions.

In front of me is a story of a lady in California who was bitten by a Brown Recluse spider, then slipped into a coma only to awake six-months later missing her arms, legs, nose and ear. The medical folks don't have any magic bullets for spider bites. Better to learn how to care for yourself. Better yet, **"restore"** your "terrain" and you won't have a "crisis" reaction!

Here is **"my"** story. I awoke at 2 a.m. with my hand throbbing and swollen and in *severe* pain. My hand looked like a balloon and was "throbbing!" So I shredded a potato, added some Epsom salts, and made a poultice using plastic sandwich wrap to cover and hold the mix in place. The **poultice** "drew" the venom into two boils. [An improved poultice formula uses crushed charcoal tablets, OX,™ R/C,™ caster oil, racemized™ clay, SOC,™ liquid DMSO, liquid aloe and water.]

I visited my "biological" dentist. He identified the energy "footprint" of the venom, then located a homeopathic remedy with a **"similar"** energy footprint, put the remedy in his MORA frequency generator and **electronically injected** the "invisible" energy into my hand and body—cancelling the spider's venom at the *subtle energy level* of my being. Instantly, the pain was gone. I regained full use of my hand.

Stop the Pain!

Regardless if it's a mosquito bite, a honey bee, yellow jacket or hornet sting—or *any other bite* from an insect of unknown origin—**STOP** what you are doing and **immediately** apply **EITHER** a "drop" of ammonia **OR** laundry bleach [**NEVER MIX THESE—DANGEROUS!**] to the sting. These simple chemicals neutralize most foreign proteins by dissolving the peptide-bonds that join amino acids into "proteins." It's the "foreign" protein your body is reacting to—just like when a child is "vaccinated!" This procedure eases "itching" that follows insect stings and bites, too! Use extreme caution to avoid eye exposure to both chemicals—and wash everyone's hands afterwards.

"Acid" Body & Wavy Hair

Cancer chemotherapy causes hair loss because it overloads the skin's waste processing capability and destroys the liver. When hair regrows, it usually comes in wavy—even where the person previously had straight hair. "Systemic" toxicity and poor liver function are behind wavy hair, as well as blue and green eyes that dull or turn dark with age or illness. Eye color is "symptomatic," **NOT** genetic. Vision problems only seem like "eye" problems. The "terrain" controls all of these things.

7

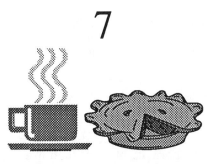

Death By Chocolate Pie

*"Chew your liquids and chew your
solids until they are liquid."*
Dr. Paul C. Bragg N. D.

"Death by Chocolate Pie," read the sign. It reminded me
that all food is **NOT** equal. Some food is *alive* and promotes
health; some food is *dead* and promotes death. We are concerned with the differences and food's influence on aging. We
are specifically concerned with food's energy **"footprint."**

Water has a similar story to tell, but there is a fundamental difference between food and water. Foods are listed in
tables and are rated, one against another based on their
nutrients, caloric content, carbohydrates, fats and proteins.
Water is **NOT** classified as a food because it does not contain
these things—but water **does** have an energy **"footprint."**

We are told that water is water, but there is **MUCH** more
to the story. Water is more than just "wet." Water's *signature*
powerfully influences life and health. Its *signature* is reflected
in its spin and measured by its ORP potential. [See page 104.]

Water is a *necessity* of life because we cannot live
without it. Oddly, the experts tell us to limit *food* intake. Then
in the same breath, they tell us to drink as much water as we
desire "without regard" to **type** of water or its *vibrational*
memory or energy **footprint**—or ORP **potential**. Water is
food—and like solid food, all water is **not** equal!

We pick and choose food on the basis of taste, appearance, color and aroma. Yet, we are not concerned about the
water we drink because we do **NOT** consider water as "food."

Water **IS** food! It certainly has foold-like qualities!
Water is **THE MOST IMPORTANT** food we put into our bodies.
Water is not important for the nutrients it contains—it contains
none. Water is important for the energy that it *should* contain.
Water with a zero contaminant load, clean vibrational memory,
therapeutic bond structure and high ORP potential is loaded
with energy and promotes health and healing of sick bodies.

BFRV™ water is pure **FOOD** and more. It has right-spin

characteristics that people can feel and taste. It is *body friendly* because it energizes, hydrates and detoxifies. People who drink it will tell you that it is *"different!"*

Live Food

Traditional food that is biologically active has a right-spin **signature** and produces right-spin **effects** in the body because it contains enzymes, charged ionic minerals, vitamins and positive "chi" energy that are absolutely necessary for good health. These components of "live" food are the foundation of life itself. Let's discuss enzymes.

Enzymes are biochemical proteins. Enzymes are also *catalysts.* A catalyst accelerates a reaction or causes a reaction to take place that either would not occur at all or would occur at a much slower rate if the enzyme were not present.

Enzymes can be compared to oxygen's affect on a fire. No oxygen, no fire. Without oxygen, fire can neither start nor continue. "True" catalysts are used over and over. They are neither altered nor destroyed in the reaction. An example is the platinum and palladium used in catalytic converters on cars. These *noble* metals convert toxic gases like carbon monoxide to carbon dioxide and water. They do it through a series of oxidation and reduction (redox) reactions. [In future chapters, you will learn how to use redox reactions to your benefit.]

In the body, most biochemical catalysts are consumed, altered or destroyed in the reactions they fuel and must be continually *manufactured* by the body or gotten from food. The liver is our **PRIMARY** enzyme and catalyst manufacturing organ—and therefore is a **MAJOR** health concern.

The constant creation of new enzymes requires tremendous amounts of right-spin energy that **MUST** come from substances that are "live" and "friendly" to the *bio-electric* body. Dead food and dead water have negative energy **signatures** and are left-spin energy fields that not only **FAIL** to contribute to health—but actually BLOCK the benefits of healthy substances with a right-spin energy *footprint.*

Biocatalysts

Biological catalysts cause reactions to occur millions of times faster than what would occur if they were not present. Without biocatalysts, life as we know it could not exist.

Vitamins do not work unless **all** needed major *and* minor (trace) minerals are present in the body in balanced form. In biochemistry, vitamins are called *cofactors* because they work **WITH** minerals and enzymes. Synthesized, man-made, vitamin "isomers" are "mirror" images that are useless and damaging to the vital organs—creating secondary problems. Many mineral supplements are **useless** because they are in "elemental" form and should be avoided. [This subject will be addressed later in Chapter 28.]

Your **BEST** source of biologically active vitamins and minerals is garden fresh food and fresh vegetable juices. The **ideal** juice is fresh **raw** beet root because of the *extreme* purple-violet "pigment." This color belongs to the ultraviolet part of the light spectrum. Other vegetables juices—and their pigments—are also fine, but not nearly as effective. Juice should **NOT** be taken unless "fully" hydrated—**NEVER** when "dry!" Juice should be "sipped" and "chewed"—**NEVER** "gulped" or drunk! Even a whiskey shot-glass of juice can be quite effective. Take juice in the morning, 30 minutes after 2 glasses of water with minerals.

"**Excess**" waste and acids in the system slow biochemical reactions as well as blood and lymph circulation. They also diminish vital organ function and hormonal balance. Acid waste accumulation speeds "systemic" degeneration and rapid aging. That is why *deacidification* of the "terrain" is absolutely crucial to good health and longevity.

The Young Again Protocol™ provides DAMAGE CONTROL while the body terrain is being restored.

Cooked Food vs Raw Food

"**Cooking**" denatures enzymes. Denatured enzymes can't do their job because they **LOSE** the characteristics that cause them to work. **Improper cooking** totally destroys food value and enzymes. "Gently" cooked food is not a problem as long as you eat plenty of fresh, raw—and preferably, home grown—green, leafy vegetables and fresh fruit.

Avoid high heat and cook no longer than necessary. Steam instead of boiling. Use stir-fry methods. Avoid microwave ovens, flavor enhancers like "MSG"—and all synthetic so-called "food." These substances *zap* the body's energy fields and block crucial biochemical pathways. Eating them **diminishes** health—causing "loss" of vital organ function!

Metabolism

Metabolism is a term that comes to mind. It means "bio-trans-formation" and refers to the way food molecules are transformed into energy molecules in the body's energy pathways. The term is often used to refer to the speed or slowness, rhythm and responsiveness of the body to both internal and external factors! Metabolism involves *fusion* reactions that join individual atoms into right-spin *energy* molecules—the exact opposite of the kind of energy reactions produced by cellular ionizing radiation as used in cancer "therapy!" Fusion reactions are right-spin and **anabolic**—they build up! Fission reactions are left-spin and **catabolic**—they tear down!

Metabolites are **by**products of biochemical reactions. Dissected the word means: *meta*-beyond; *bol*-tranformation; *ite*-product of. Hence, a substance that is **beyond** transformation. Metabolic waste is "acid" in nature. Waste is the "baggage" that **drives** old age. Oddly, chemicals of organic synthesis—like pesticides, herbicides and food additives—end up as "metabolic" waste in body tissues. Worse, many of these molecules are "zeno" estrogen analogs that confuse and gridlock the body's hormonal receptor sites and grossly affect the nervous system. **"Soluble"** metabolic waste that the liver cannot "filter" from the blood is stored in the "fatty" tissues beneath the skin. Liver "filtered" waste is stored in the gallbladder as "bile." Bile is released when we eat; bile aids digestion and activates bowel activity. ["Safe" release and transportation of highly **"acid"** tissue waste is the **"CORE"** issue of the *Young Again (Tissue and Liver) Protocol.*™

Animal Protein

Industrialized man eats high on the hog. He eats too much animal protein and not enough fruits and vegetables. Animal proteins are at the top of the food chain. **"Healthy"** animal proteins have a right-spin *signature* and these proteins sustain us. Sick animals store their wastes in the tissues and these proteins negatively influence human health and longevity. [Choose to eat healthy meat and healthy eggs!]

Food energy derived from sick animals brings on dis-ease in man a thousand times faster than does food energy from sick fruits or vegetables.

Animal proteins can be an excellent source of *energy* and nutrients—but they are a two-edged sword and must be used wisely. The "issue" with animal protein is: **quantity** eaten, **chewing** of food, body **hydration level**, liver **efficiency** and **bowel transit time** from the mouth to the toilet. [These points will be developed later.]

In his wonderful book *Fatu Hiva*, Thor Heyerdahl tells how in 1937 he and his wife lived with the last surviving cannibal of the Marquesa islands northwest of Tahiti. The cannibal told them *"Human flesh is different from other animal flesh. It is sweet!"* Interestingly, **both** healthy and sick animal flesh can be sweet and tasty. The **"terrain"** of the animals and their dietary intake and "treatment" determines whether their proteins are acceptable "sustenance" for human consumption.

The Food Chain

Here is an example of what is meant by the statement, *"animal protein is at the top of the food chain."* Crops and weeds are treated with poisons. A rabbit comes along and eats the plants, absorbs the poisonous residues and stores them in its flesh and fatty tissues. Thus, the poisons moved **UP** the food chain, from plant to animal. When we eat unhealthy meat, fish and fowl—we become the rabbit and the poisons and metabolites concentrate in us. [Eat animal proteins from healthy animals—and that includes eggs. Eat lots of eggs!]

Negative energy food from any source—animal or plant—is sick food. Sick food must be dismantled and **neutralized** by the liver. Left-spin energy food squanders vital "chi" energy—causing us to lose more than we gain!

Animal Proteins & The Bowel

Animal proteins **MUST** be eliminated from the intestines within 18 hours **"maximum!"** If they remain in the gut longer than this, they putrefy and release extremely toxic, organic molecules and metabolites—substances like indoles, skatoles and phenols. These are **WHOLE** molecules that are absorbed directly into the blood stream through a "leaky" intestinal wall. The condition is called **"Leaky Gut Syndrome"**—and it affects all people—regardless of age. The sicker, weaker or older you are, the worse the condition of your "gut wall!" Food molecules should be broken down before they are absorbed and sent to the liver for further processing. Molecules that invade the blood via a **leaky-gut** automatically "trigger" an **AUTO IMMUNE** response. With very few exceptions, **every** dis-ease you can name is an auto-immune "condition!" [Think, cancer, arthritis, lupus, fibromyalgia, diabetes, etc. The product R/C™ is used to restore gut-wall integrity.]

Food crops—like potatoes—absorb toxic compounds when grown with raw, non-composted manure. These compounds pass **whole** and **intact** into the potatoes. When potatoes are boiled, a sharp nose can identify the kind of manure that was used to grow them—pig, cow or chicken.

A toxic, **leaky-gut** is the perfect environment for parasitic activity, foul gas, bloating and conditions like colitis, diverticulitis, irritable bowel, appendicitis—and eventually cancer and cardiovascular problems. In the end, everything in the body is "connected"—and a sick liver, leaky-gut and poor bile-flow are fundamental to all of it!

Chewing of food and secretion of saliva are **CRITICAL** to good health, digestion and "terrain" management. [Use Disorb Aid II,™ Yucca Blend™ and R/BHCl™ to **insure** "complete" digestion and absorption of food and supplements. Poorly digested food is **BOTH** a problem and a loss!] When these concepts are applied they produce huge benefits. Readers who practice them are on their way to becoming *Young Again!*

PREVIEW: *Our next chapter illuminates the connection between diet, stress and accelerated aging.*

Fatty Tumors

Fatty tumors under the skin are an early warning **SIGN** that the body is "loaded" with acid waste and is "pre-cancerous!" Fatty tumors are a **TERRAIN** issue! Do not ignore them!

Portable Enema Kit

Where small bathrooms do not allow for set-up of High Enema Therapy™ equipment, provision **must** be made to learn to properly use a "fountain" style enema kit. For similar—but different reasons—people who travel need a practical way to care for themselves so they do **not** suffer from constipation, sluggish bowel, or allow their body to turn "acid!" The *Young Again!*™ Portable Enema Kit is the **perfect** answer because it is simple, inexpensive, effective, small and light weight. The process is fast and effective—and no one will *"know"* unless you tell them! [See pages 106, 123, 163, 203, 262 & 380.]

Kale & Rhubarb

Kale is easy to grow and it thrives most anywhere. You can grow it in pots, flower beds or the garden. Kale is a sweet, tasty green—and it's a "non" hybrid vegetable. Whether eaten raw in a salads, juiced or served in leaf fashion, kale promotes a healthy colon and stretches the food budget. Kale is loaded with dietary sulphur! Olive oil and a "health" type **vinegar** dressing or lemon helps digestion of "crucifer" vegetables like kale, cabbage, collards, broccoli and cauliflower. These foods are **dynamite** against "cancer!" Rhubarb is another good and easy-to-grow food—and it is a good source of bioflavonoids. To "can" rhubarb, simply wash and cut the stalks, fill jar, cover with good water, seal and store somewhere cool—like the refrigerator, cellar, etc. Cooking is **NOT** required to preserve rhubarb. *P.S.* **Never** eat rhubarb leaves, for the same reason you do **NOT** eat carrot tops—they are poisonous!

Subclinical "Dis-ease"

Throughout this book, your author refers to health issues as **"sub**clinical" in nature—as opposed to clinical dis-ease which is identified by **"SIGNS."** **90%** of health issues facing people are **sub**clinical and are **not** diagnosable—at least not in the early stages! The doctor needs **"SIGNS"** to diagnose. The *Young Again Protocol*™ focuses on what can be done on a daily basis to maintain the **"terrain"** **BEFORE** a dis-ease "state" can manifest itself. By the time **"SIGNS"** appear, you are in **trouble!** Remember *"a problem avoided is a problem solved!"*

➡ **Please Note:** The BFRV™ "trademark" replaces the "*abandoned*" BEV acronym, *DUE TO ongoing infringement and "bootlegging"* by individual(s) offering water processing equipment under the "pretense" their equipment fulfills the "terrain" management CONCEPTS of the *Young Again Protocol™*.

Water! The *Essence* Of Life!

Water has memory! It "absorbs" the *frequencies* of the contaminants it carries—and it **continues** to *vibrate* at sick frequencies after the contaminants have been removed—unless their memory is erased. Next to the air we breathe, we consume more water than any other substance. Water is an important dietary issue!

Contaminants are *energy* fields that leave their *footprint* on water by causing the molecules to **vibrate** at frequencies **unfriendly** to the body.

Conventional approaches to water purification are *incomplete*. Methods like distillation, reverse osmosis, carbon block and ceramic cartridges work at the mechanical level only. They are good as far as they go, they just don't go far enough.

The BFRV™ protocol is a Fourth Dimension approach that makes water that tastes good and feels **"different"** in the body. People like it because it *awakens* natural harmonic frequencies *at the cellular level.*

BFRV™ water *reprograms* the *rhythm* of the body causing body cells to *dance!* Its energy *frequency* is body-friendly. Its electromagnetic *signature* is complete. **BFRV™ water is liquid *music!***

The BFRV™ process "voids" waste energy frequencies in water and alters hydrogen and molecular bond angles so water can **"dance"** and become *liquid music* and *electronic food* for body and spirit.

BFRV™ theory and application *transcends* Third Dimention testing and comparison methods. It defies Newtonian physics. BFRV™ water must be experienced for its profound significance to human health and longevity. **BFRV™ captures the *essence* of life on planet Earth in liquid form.**

The BFRV™ protocol is proprietary. A discussion of the theory and application of BFRV™ and its relationship to aging and dis-ease is available in manuscript form. [See pages 74, 79, 104, 109, 117, 126, 167, 173, 220, 244, 297, 306 and 378.]

BFRV™ water is made from "raw" tap water with BFRV™ equipment. The BFRV™ process produces biologically *friendly* **DRINKING** water. *Make sure the water you put into your body is spelled BFRV™.*

"Water Is MORE Than Wet! Water Is FOOD!"

The Hormone Cycle And The Vorago™ Effect

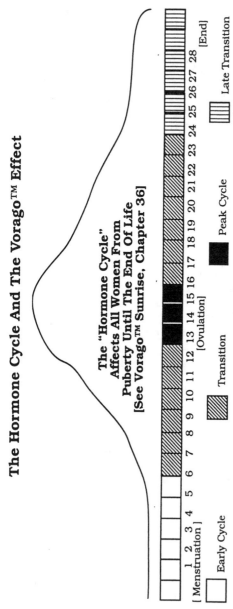

The "Hormone Cycle" Affects All Women From Puberty Until The End Of Life [See Vorago™ Sunrise, Chapter 36]

1 2 3 4 5 6 7 8 9 10 11 12 13 14 15 16 17 18 19 20 21 22 23 24 25 26 27 28
[Menstruation]   [Ovulation]   [End]

☐ Early Cycle   ▨ Transition   ■ Peak Cycle   ▤ Late Transition

Use The Female Cycle Tester™ To Measure Your Hormone Cycle!

The hormone cycle is **NOT** the same as the menstrual cycle, and having a period does **NOT** mean that you completed you hormone cycle. Management of the **hormone cycle** is crucially important for female health. Women who learn how to measure and plot their **hormone cycle** hold the keys to long term health. Women who are menstrual can use the information to regulate PMS, mood swings, conception, as well as effectively deal with conditions like lupus, fibromyalgia, MS and endometriosis. Menopausal women can use the information to deal with conditions like osteoporosis, arthritis, heart & stroke, restoration of hair and skin, and high blood pressure. Restoration of the **hormone cycle** is the key to a life free of the medical system. Racemized™ hormone precursors and the Female Cycle Tester™ allow a woman to **reopen** the **PUBERTY WINDOW**. Rebuilding of connective tissues like cartilage, bones, ligaments, muscle, tendon, hair, nails and skin is a **hormone driven** process. Hormones are a **key factor** in determining how fast women age. Hormonal health is **TOTALLY** dependent upon a healthy liver and stress management. Thyroid activity affects the hormone cycle, adrenal, liver and bowel activity. Women of puberty age and older have a hormone cycle that must "complete" **each** and **every** month of adult life—with or without a period. *The Young Again Female Protocol™* helps women make their **very own** hormones and **resurrect** and **complete** their **hormone cycle** so they can avoid premature aging and poor health. Remember, the menstrual cycle is a "dance" between the ovaries and liver. At menopause, the ovaries cease to participate and the liver is **forced** to make up for what the ovaries can no longer do. The liver is "**the**" most crucial organ affecting women's hormones. "Stress" is the ultimate "wild card" in every woman's life because stress hammers the adrenal glands skews the hormones. To further understand the riddle, see pages 46, 75-6, 152, 164, 178, 194, 212, 268, 362, 374, 378 and Chapter 36, Vorago™ Sunrise.   © 2006 John Thomas All rights reserved. Reproduction in any form prohibited.

8

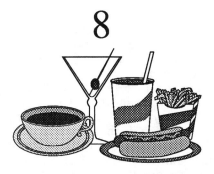

Junk Diets & Stress

"There is no such thing as 'junk food', only 'junk diets'!"
Dr. Helen A. Guthrie

All food contains energy. It is the nature of energy and its electrical **footprint** that determines what effect—good or bad—food has on the *bio-electric* body. To understand the aging process, we must concern ourselves with the "spin" or "footprint" of food energy. The direction and intensity of the spin determines food's ability to satisfy hunger and build and maintain healthy tissues and bones—or destroy health.

Nutritive tables measure nutrients. It is **assumed** that if we eat food listed on the nutrient tables, we will be nourished. It is also **assumed** that **ALL** food energy produces positive results in the body. These assumptions are both **wrong** and confusing for those seeking a healthy life.

We hear a lot about junk food because we are inundated with it. People identify junk food with quick snacks and fast food. The association is correct. But instead of calling it junk food, let's call it **"bio-junk"**—because that's what it is!

Bio-junk ("BJ") greatly accelerates the aging process. If the body cannot eliminate it from the system, it **entombs** this toxic energy in the **fat layer** beneath the skin.

*[In 1972, 6 billion dollars was spent on bio-junk diets. In year 2000, the figure was 110 billion dollars. And that is only **one** of many negative factors fueling the acceleration of the aging process. Bio-junk is NOT part of a healthy diet!]*

Dead Is Not Dead

Bio-junk ("BJ") alters biochemical reactions because of its left-spin **"signature!"** It destroys and blocks critical body pathways and cripples cellular activity. "BJ" has the ability to **multiply** its original sphere of influence by transferring its vibratory **footprint** to all of the body's tissues. This **"transference"** takes place at the **subtle energy level** of our being. Bio-junk has *radiomimetic* qualities—qualities that *mimic* the effect of ionizing *radiation* on healthy tissue. Eat enough "bio-junk" and you will eventually see the effects in the mirror.

Bio-junk has the ability to **CHANGE** its *footprint* **after** it enters the body. Its presence in the GI tract triggers **unnatural** reactions that form **"free radicals"** in the system. Free radicals cause severe damage to the vital organs and especially to the liver and kidneys—and they **continue** to interfere with normal metabolism **UNTIL** their presence is "eliminated!" In other words, free radicals have a **life of their own!**

*[It is **impossible** to keep all toxic substances out of our system because they are ubiquitous in our daily lives. And what about the "stuff" stored in the fat layer beneath the skin? The Young Again Protocol™ was developed so the body will release the "stuff" and **safely** transport it through the blood and lymph to be filtered by the liver and sent down the toilet. "**Deacidification**" of the tissues is another way of saying "**terrain management!**" Bio-junk diet causes the body to grow acid—accelerating the onset of old age.]*

Kidneys & Liver
The kidneys are crucial to good health—and it behooves us to pay attention to anything that negatively affects them. "BJ" causes tremendous long-term damage to the kidney's nephrons (blood filters). The kidneys are second to the liver in ridding the body of waste.

Restore the LIVER and you automatically lift the load from the kidneys. The kidneys were NEVER meant to do the liver's job! Kidney issues are liver issues!

Water affects the kidneys. Taoism teaches that the urinary system (kidneys and bladder) is related to the **Water Element.** Taoists believe that *Jing*—the very **essence** of life—is contained within water. They believe that careful management of the Water Element is the key to youthfulness.

Digestion & Liquids
If Pavlov's dog is an indication, digestion initiates through smell and visual and mental stimulation **BEFORE** we actually eat. In other words, the flow of digestive juices in the mouth, stomach and intestines is linked to **vision** and **thought**.

Digestion *initiates* in the mouth when we chew and mix food with saliva. The flow of saliva and digestive juices is **dependent** on fluid hydration levels in the body. When we drink plenty of water, we secrete plenty of saliva—which begins the breakdown process we call *digestion.* Saliva also lubricates food so it can be comfortably swallowed.

To maintain perfect **fluid volume** levels and electrolyte load, drink a cup of water with racemized™ sea minerals every hour of the waking day. Lots of water between meals is the "key" to **avoiding** the need to drink liquids with meals. Saliva activates and protects food enzymes so they will **not** be damaged in the stomach and GI tract. Nature designed things such that it takes 5-10 minutes to eat an apple, but only 5 seconds to drink the juice." Juices are two edged swords because they are very powerful. **Chew** your juice! Do not gulp! **Drink water throughout the day, avoiding all liquids 1/2 hour before, during and one hour after meals.**

If you take supplements at mealtime, minimize water intake and be sure to take digestive enzymes to offset the water and assist with digestion—especially after age "30."

COLD liquids are very hard on the body—and particularly on the stomach and digestive process. Cold fluids taken with a meal **retard** and **SHUT DOWN** digestion. Temperature is a **critical** "prerequisite" for chemical reactions like those involved in the digestion of food. Cold fluids with meals set the stage for **MAJOR** long-term degenerative dis-ease!

[Where indigestion, gas or bloating are a problem, DiSorb Aid ll,™ R/BHCl™ and Yucca Blend™ are very helpful! R/ BHCl™ "cleaves" the peptide bonds between the amino acids that compose proteins—including parasite proteins. DiSorb Aid ll™ is totally different than R/BHCl.™ It works in the "gut"—not in the stomach. Yucca Blend™ is an emulsifier that increases bile-flow from the liver and gallbladder.]

Women suffer with "acid reflux" more than do men—and"10" women lose their gallbladder for every man! The Young Again Protocol(s)™ solve the "riddle!"

Digestive juices are powerful "right-spin" energy fields. The liver and pancreas secrete their juices through ducts directly into the intestinal duodenum—just below the stomach. Hydrochloric acid is secreted by cells in the stomach wall as is **intrinsic factor** which "**MUST**" be present for absorption of vitamin B-12. After age 30, vitamin B-12 absorption diminishes greatly, which is **why** "oral" B-12 supplements are **useless!** [To solve this problem, Cobo-12™ transdermal skin creme was developed.]

*[Due to loss of blood from menstruation, vitamin B-12 issues become a female issue after age 30. The problem becomes **serious** by age 40 and above. The list of vitamin B-12 complaints and symptoms is in the hundreds and generally manifests as "ghost" symptoms no one can identify!]*

Hormones & Hydration

The "**ductless**" glands secrete hormones directly into the blood for distribution in the body. Low hydration (water) levels in the tissues influences hormonal secretion and response. The blood and lymph are classified as "**liquid" tissues!**

Hormones dramatically influence aging and vitality. Men and women hormonally "peak" by age 25, causing a *slowing* in metabolism. By age 30, women begin noticing subtle changes in their cycles and bodies due to their inability to effectively **"complete"** their hormone cycle. A menstrual period in and of itself is not a valid indicator. [See page 72.]

Hormones "trigger" the changes that occur at **puberty**—and again at **menopause** and **andropause**. Hormones are **CENTRAL** to aging reversal because they effect all body systems. [The *Young Again (Hormone) Protocol*™ is designed to keep the "puberty window" **OPEN** by providing the raw materials the **LIVER** needs to make your own "home-made" hormones. [See pages 46, 18, 72, 362, Chapter 35 and index.]

[Humans are "conceived" female. Male differentiation occurs later in development. Growth and development in the womb and beyond is a hormone-driven process.]

Racemized™ Hormone Precursors

A *precursor* is something that precedes the formation of something else. For example, carrots provide *beta carotene*, a natural plant food precursor to Vitamin A. The body uses racemized™ hormone precursors to make its **very own** hormones. Racemized™ hormone precursors do **NOT** carry the risks associated with conventional, synthetic, female-replacement "hormones" because your liver does the conversion!

The *Young Again Protocol*™ gives women a lot more control over their health and lives. Men are concerned with the prostate, sex drive, impotence and balding. Women **should be** concerned with **all** things "female" because they are linked to the completion of the female **hormone cycle** and **KEEPING** the "puberty window" open. [See page 72.]

In the wonderful book *Our Stolen Future,* Theo Colborn correctly defined the environmental dilemma the human race faces in relation to "zeno" estrogen analogs and their effect on hormone receptor sites in the body. "Zenos" are just **SOME** of the **"excesses"** driving aging and cancer in both sexes. And whether you are young or old, female or male, they affect your body systems. [The *Young Again Protocol*™ is designed to rid the body of "zeno" estrogens and open the receptor sites.]

Wild yam creams have been available for many years—and most are of questionable value—at best! The **only** yams worth discussion are grown on supervised farms in New Guinea between 7,000 and 9,000 feet elevation—and even then the "active" molecule in them must be isolated and purified.

"Progesterone" creme [and so-called bio-identical hormones] is useful, but most of the fanfare has to do with "minimizing" the dangerous side effects of female replacement hormones commonly prescribed by doctors. Progesterone is

ONLY one of **SIX** hormones that need tending by women—and men! The other **FIVE** hormones are DHEA, testosterone, estrogen, cortisol and thyroid. **Avoid** over-the-counter DHEA and melatonin; they have been outlawed in many countries for good reason. Anabolic steroids used by athletes and birth control pills used by women—have a lot in common! Better to let your body make your "own" hormones by following the *Young Again Protocol.*™ So-called "bio-identical" hormones from compounding pharmacies **"FAIL"** to factor in the **"state"** of a woman's liver, thyroid and stress levles—which are **"THE"** "controlling" factors. Blood tests are only "snap shots!" Relying on them is akin to chasing your tail!

Stress • Food • Pavlov's Dog

Stress and unpleasant circumstances grossly affect hormone production and digestion and absorption. Sitting down to a *quiet* meal and allowing enough time for casual, pleasant conversation is *vital* to good health. Unfortunately, few people eat this way anymore. Fast-track meals are the rule, and mealtime rarely resembles the ideal setting. People eat too fast—barely chewing—and guzzle **cold** liquids amidst noise and confusion—giving new meaning to "meals on wheels!"

The effects of "hit and run eating" on health are DEADLY—even if the very best of food is eaten.

Pavlov experimented on dogs. Dogs are known for their ability to *gobble* their food on the run. Pavlov discovered that the dog's digestive enzymes flowed the moment he rang the dinner bell. **Digestion** is "stressful" to the body, so when your dinner bell rings, prepare yourself! A meal should be a celebration. Digestion requires the body to **expend** energy—hopefully, to get more energy in return. Bio-junk creates an energy "deficit." Poorly digested food results in gas and bloating, leaky-gut, auto-immune issues, constipation and **deadly** toxic by-products that give rise to degenerative dis-ease.

Gas & Putrefication

Gas—particularly *foul* gas—is a **GOOD** indicator of an *out-of-balance* condition in the vital organs and digestive tract. The fouler the gas, the more you **should be** concerned that things are **NOT** right. Foul and excess gas are **SIGNS** of systemic overload and trouble to come. [Colon cancer and prostate trouble are two conditions that come to mine. The *Young Again Protocol*™ addresses all of these issues.]

Spoiled animal flesh (carrion) is *necrotic* flesh. Meat is flesh from dead animals, but it is **not** necrotic—or dead! In a constipated, anaerobic, leaky-gut environment, meat, fish, fowl and cheese become the equivalent of carrion, producing highly toxic by-products and foul gas. Stressful eating environments and bio-junk diets are a made-to-order cancer recipe! *The evening breeze between your knees should NOT smell like cheese!*

Otto Warburg, twice Nobel Laureate, was awarded the Nobel Prize in 1931—over 74 years ago—for documenting a vital factor behind the rise of cancer. **He said,** *"Cancer has one prime cause...and that is the replacement of oxygen [aerobic] respiration of body cells by anaerobic cellular respiration."*

Dr. Max Gerson [mentioned earlier] later determined the role of sodium [think "table salt!"] in cancer. Both Warburg and Gerson agreed that the growth of cancer cells initiates in a low-oxygen, lo-potassium, high-sodium, high free-radical, high-stress environment. That's **why** fresh vegetable juices are good. That's **why** mild aerobic exercise is good. That's **why** physical "movement" is good. That is the purpose of the L/CSF™ machine and body rollers. [See pages 38, 78 and 382.]

Table Salt

It is **impossible** to avoid sodium because it is ubiquitous. Sodium is in 99% of all prepared foods and in municipal water supplies. If you "crave" salt, your adrenal glands are severely stressed! Practical solutions are to add Racemized™ sea minerals to your drinking water and take PU™ for adrenal stress. [See page 120.] A body that "craves" salt suffers from electrolyte "imbalance" and elevated cortisol levels.

Table salt (sodium chloride) **IS** an electrolytic substance—but it should **not** be used in place of electrolytic mineral "salts" like potassium, magnesium, calcium, etc. Excess sodium is **deadly** to the body's cells and to the mitochondria that produce our ATP energy molecule. Thirst after meals indicates under hydration, over salted food, and/or adrenal stress. Use only granular salts with high levels of trace mineral electrolytes, such as Celtic,™ Redman™ or Real™ salt.

The Water Molecule

Water ifunctions as a solvent and donor of *free* electrons—as measured by oxidation/reduction potential (ORP). Water carries *energy* into the cells, and waste out! When we drink distilled, raw "tap," reverse osmosis, ozonated and common bottled waters—we fail to meet fundamental "terrain" concepts that only BFRV™ water can meet. And **failure** to use Racemized™ sea minerals in your water of choice only adds insult to injury and leads to conditions of **excess**—by "default!"

[BFRV™ water is "conception point" foundation water used to create Medical Grade Ionized Water™ (MGIW™). Racemized™ sea minerals provide the "electrons" needed to raise the ORP to therapeutic status. See pages 306 and 400.]

Below is a drawing of water molecules with their

respective bonds. Look at the shape of these "bent," "polar" water molecules—and notice how they "connect!"

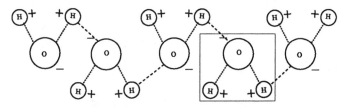

Notice that the two hydrogen atoms on each molecule are off to one side, giving each molecule a lopsided appearance. The fine dotted lines indicate a "bond" with (+) and (-) charged atoms. The box contains **one** water molecule. The oxygen atom has a (–) charge, the two hydrogens have (+) charges. The dotted line going from the hydrogen atom in the box to the oxygen to the right of the box is a **hydrogen bond** connecting one molecule to the other. The lines inside the box are **molecular** bonds "within" the water molecule itself.

The strength of bonds holding water molecules together is determined by "free" electrons. The higher the "ORP," the easier waterborne electrons enter the cells and become available for production of the ATP energy molecule. Bond angle, ORP and pH are what separates BFRV™ water and MGIW™ water(s) from other water(s). pH (alkalinity /acidity) by "itself" is a meaningless number. Drinking "alkaline" water does **NOT** make you more alkaline! **Dea**cidification and "ORP" are what we are concerned with—not pH. Conventional water testing standards are "moot" in regard to BFRV™ and MGIW™ water(s).

Why BFRV™ Water?

BFRV™ water is **biologically friendly** drinking water. It's made at home from common tap water. Equipment efficiency approaches 99.5% for removal of noxious waste and life forms, radioactivity and toxic organic chemicals. Moreover, the process manipulates bond angles while elevating the "ORP" and returning the water to the point of conception—where the egg and sperm were when they joined. [The **issue** here is **"life force"**—as diagramed on page 306.]

BFRV™ water is highly "charged" so it can carry waste **OUT** of the body. It is **"different"** from other waters—and it is very "reactive" in the body—meaning it acts like a *magnet* due its strong electrical charge and resonant frequency. People who drink it can "feel" the effect! Wonderful things happen to people who drink this strange and wonderful water. "Detractors" of the *Young Again Protocol(s)*™ poke fun at your author, but people who drink BFRV™ water "love" its Third and Fourth Dimension qualities. [See pages 104, 109, 126, 167, 220, 306 and 378.]

Real, live food is a gift from God!

Home-grown food is "ideal" and is the most fundamental and least expensive path to good health. If space is limited, grow vegetables in pots, plastic buckets and so on. It is amazing how much fresh food can be grown this way. Consider joining an organic gardening club. Many clubs rent garden space where the soil is rich and mellow from other gardeners before you. Or, hire someone to grow food for you and your family. Many older people have the time and would love to grow food for hire. These people are usually gardening pros. Pay them generously! Gardening is hard work. They deserve the money and you need the food. Drive in older neighborhoods; ask friends; make the effort to locate these people.

Gardening involves *load-bearing* work and is a good way to keep fit. Hard work is good for the body and the spirit. I suggest a spading fork instead of a tiller. Hand tools are inexpensive, they always start—and they don't burn gas. For people who **cannot** garden, fresh "live" food can be purchased at health food stores, farmers markets and co-ops. Some organic farmers deliver or have drop points in cities.

Composting • Gardening

If you are going to get into gardening, you will want to learn how to compost organic matter. Proper composting technique *controls* the break-down process so you end-up with a high-energy product. A "simpler" method is to buy composted "chicken manure" from Lowe's or Home Depot and apply to your soil 1 bag for each 100 square feet along with "flour" gypsum @ 25 lbs for same footage. Gypsum can be found at animal feed supply stores. Dig and loosen the soil 12" deep and mix these amendments into the "top" 6 inches. [If you have heavy "clay" soil, put in—1 yard of sand for above footages.]

Always use some liquified chicken or cow manure starter to get the pile going. Controlled breakdown of grass clippings, weeds, leaves, animal waste and the like will not generate foul odors **unless** the pile becomes **anaerobic.** [An anaerobic condition produces foul odors in a compost pile—and in a sluggish, human intestinal tract, too!]

Compost is MORE than old, dead things that have turned brown. It is a source of "life force" for your garden. Several wonderful books on biodynamic gardening principles are available. [See Source Page 400.]

Gardening will simplify your life and focus your energies on healthful habits. Become "hooked" on gardening and you will be a gardener forever! Besides, common store-bought food is **not** good for you—and growing food saves money!

Fresh food and biologically friendly water are *passports* to agelessness! Please do not underestimate them.

Devitalized food is so common in most people's diet that some supplementation is needed. The following "food" items are used by your author in addition to home-grown food: PAC's™, Harmonic™ pollen, racemized™ algae, predigested, organic liver capsules and VitaLight™ tablets. These products do **NOT** tax the liver. Small amounts of fresh vegetable juice provides even greater dimension and health. Beet juice in small amounts is the very best because of the purple pigments. [See Chapter 35, *Vorago™ Sunrise.*]

To become *Young Again!*

- Eat "healthy" food
- Grow a garden
- Avoid table salt & MSG
- Use racemized™ minerals
- Get some exercise
- Avoid alcohol & soft drinks
- Juice daily (breakfast)
- Eat RAW vegetables
- Avoid all processed food
- Drink BFRV™ water
- Get plenty of sleep
- Avoid liquids with meals
- Avoid soy and canola
- Do High Enema Therapy™

What you do 90% of the time is what counts! Aging reversal requires focus and commitment because the body is OLD and *SLOW* and you are not young yet! While all this takes "effort," it is well worth the effort as you will discover—especially when you see friends and loved ones sick and dying. Follow your author's lead and you will become *Young Again!*

PREVIEW: *Our next chapter explains WHY people snack and WHY they become fat and WHAT happens to the body when you eat too much or too often!*

Energy Spikes!

Light bulbs rated @ 130 v far outlast bulbs rated @ 120 v because they can take the "spike" when turned-on. A healthy body "terrain" handles energy "spikes" more easily, too!

The Big Lie!

Sadly, actor Chritopher Reeve wasted-away and died—and now his widow, "Dana" has lung cancer! This, just after newsman, Peter Jennings died of lung cancer. Dana, however, has **never** smoked! The **BIG LIE** is that "*Smoking causes lung cancer!*" The **TRUTH** is "*people need folic acid in their diet—and devitalized food does **not** contain folic acid!*" Smokers—and people who breathe other's "smoke"—and who supplement with 10 mcg. of folic acid daily will **"NEVER"** get lung cancer. Cancer is a **liver** and **terrain** issue. Cancer is **NOT** something you "catch." Ignore the experts or you will end up like them!

Angry Tissue!

Angry tissue is "traumatized" tissue—be it from injury or surgery. Angry tissue **holds** the memory of the trauma—and until the anger is released, the tissues canot fully heal. Whiplash, broken bones and sprains are good examples. The Chinese call it *"bad chi!"* [The *Young Again Protocol*™ uses a **chi gong machine** and **Gua Sha** to release and heal angry tissue. [To learn more, see "Gua Sha" page 48.]

Harmonic™ Silver Water

Few injuries equal the trauma and pain that burn patients suffer. From a medical viewpoint, the issue is infection. Socially, the issue is scar tissue. Infection and scars are both **energy** issues and they require an "energy" solution! To ease pain and prevent infection—even in the case of 3rd degree burns—use Harmonic™ Silver Water. It has a body-friendly vibrational signature and energy footprint. When "misted" onto burned tissue, gargled or drunk orally, it complements the healing process. [See photos on page 276.] "Parts per million" (PPM) of silver is **NOT** the issue! Rather, it's the "frequency" and "purity" of the silver. Scar tissue is the "end-product" of amyloid fluid that turned "structural." Digest amyloid plaque and lay down new collagen, and healing occurs much more quickly. [Use VZ II™ and L$_s$P$_c$C,™ SOC™ and liquid DMSO on burned, tramatized tissue. See index under various names and topics for a broader understanding.]

Acne, Skin Scars & SOC™

For **post** emergency and general skin damage from acne blemishes to burn scars, use SOC™ lotion and Racemized™ Skin Creme. These products help restore damaged tissue. [One man reduced 65 square feet of 20-year-old scar tissue (from burns) to less than 2 square inches.] SOC™ opens-up blood and nerve flow into damaged tissue and speeds restoration. SOC™ transports heavy metals from brain and organ tissues, cleans the arteries, restores cartilage and nerve function and helps reduce blood pressure where the arteries have become hardened. Limber Life™ and R/A™ Catalyst are used with SOC™ to restore "limberness" to an old, stiff body.

The 90/10 Rule Of Health

Strive to live your life doing things 90% correctly, and enjoy your sins [The other 10%!] to the fullest—and without guilt! The 90/10 Rule is easy to follow when your priorities are correct!

"Balance in all things is the foundation of health."

9

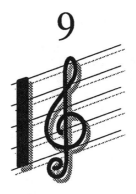

Satiety Blues

"Everything in Moderation."
Diane DeFelice

Fullness beyond desire! A primal drive fulfilled!
Who can conjure up a better feeling than a full stomach after a superb meal? Surely, food is one of the true pleasures of life. Aroma! Appearance! Taste! These are the things for which we live! Yet, in our drive to fulfill a basic physiologic need, we sow the seeds of old age and death.

Food requires a certain amount of time for complete digestion. When we eat too much food or too soon after a previous meal, the body suffers ***overload*** shock. Shock of any type puts stress on the vital organs (liver, thyroid, adrenals, kidneys, parathyroid, pancreas, pituitary and testes). **Dietary SHOCK** deserves our attention because it accelerates aging.

Snacks & Food-Related Stress

People love to snack! They snack because either they are hungry or because it is the thing to do—part habit, part social custom. The *experts* tell us it is good to eat every few hours. They tell us small meals taken more often are less stressful to the system and better for our health. They tell us small meals taken often maintain blood sugar levels and keep us on an even keel. They even tell us that multiple small meals increase productivity. ***Baloney!***

As usual, the experts are **WRONG!** These things are **NOT** true. They **NEVER** were true. Let's stop and analyze what happens to the body when we eat too much or too often, which includes snacking. Snacks are simply small meals!

Food creates stress because it involves digestion. Digestion creates stress by drawing on energy reserves to break down food and transport and reassemble it into usable energy. Substances that do not promote health must be dumped or stored. The liver is central to ALL of these functions and more.

When we eat, we borrow from our energy reserves to get the process going. If the energy generated from food does not repay the loan, we suffer an energy deficit in the form of loss of health and vitality in the vital organs.

The vital organs have *limited* capacity and resilience and require rest **BETWEEN** meals. When denied adequate rest, they become stressed. Eating too often and too much causes the organs and glands to **"stress!"**

Food "imposed" stress causes organ "burn-out" and diminished function—as the vital organs age **"together"** in chain reaction style. This scenario can occur even if food is right-spin energy—and nutritious. *Quality, quantity* and *frequency* of food intake are **some** of the controlling factors.

If dietary intake is composed of *left-spin* energy substances—organ stress is greatly increased—and when combined with meals spaced too close together, the body is left with **NO ALTERNATIVE** but to go into **OVERDRIVE** in an attempt to process, usilize, neutralize, dump or store food energy.

Food-imposed stress creates **"involuntary"** reactions because the body has **NO** choice but to process what it has been given—even to its own detriment. The body acts as much out of duty as need when fed too much, too often or when *forced* to process a bio-junk diet. Snacking **"STRESSES"** the vital organs. It upsets hormone balance by overloading the liver. It reduces vitality because food consumes energy. It creates **MAJOR** digestion and bowel issues by **slowing** the flow of waste from the body. Snacking accelerates aging by **increasing** the production of acid wastes and "rocking" blood-sugar. Dietary stress complies with the Second Law of Thermodynamics which says "energy is never lost; it merely changes "form!"

"Trophy"

Food-related stress brings about *trophy* in the vital organs. *Trophy* means change related to nutrition. If we apply the prefix *hyper* or *hypo*, we are referring to a change in physiologic activity that is above or below the norm. Both hyper and hypo conditions lead to organ burn-out and dysfunction. The terms **hypo**glycemia and **hyper**calcemia are good examples of *trophy* type blood-sugar related health conditions.

The organs are *interdependent*—and whatever affects one, affects all of them. A "condition" is **always** "multiple" in nature. The word "dis-ease" is **NEVER** singular in nature.

When "symptoms" appear—the condition is in progress; when SIGNS appear—the condition is AVANCED!

Deficiency Dis-eases & Conditions

We hear a lot about **"deficiency"** dis-eases and conditions—but there is **NO** such thing. The entire concept is but a

carry-over from the early days of allopathic medicine and the influence of Justus von Liebig's infamous agricultural theory called **The Law of the Minimum.**
Justus von Liebig developed his theory around 1830. He is regarded as the father of the synthetic fertilizer industry and the destructive practices of present day agriculture. His law says *"The nutrient that is in the* **minimum** *controls."* von Leibig viewed soil as nothing but dirt! He believed that plants only needed three elemental "salts"—nitrogen, phosphorous and potassium—commonly referred to as "NPK."
Pasteur and von Liebig were contemporaries. And like Pasteur's equally fallacious"Germ Theory of Disease," medical science also adopted von Liebig's erroneous theory. Today, clinical nutritionists **perpetuate** von Liebig's theory when they propagate the myth that **DEFICIENCIES** cause dis-ease. The experts are wrong—and so are the alternative folks who perpetuate the fallacy. [See pages 86 and 300 and Chapter 9.]
"Dis-ease" is the exact **OPPOSITE** of what is popularly believed and taught. Dis-ease is nothing but the manifestation of conditions of **"EXCESS"** within the system. Excess always manifests as deficiencies. Excesses are **"errant"** energy.
[Excess "controls!" A secular example is the stock market crash of 2001. It was* **excess** *liquidity,* **excess** *debt and* **excess** *capacity that wiped out 7 trillion dollars 2 months after 52 renouwned "experts" said everything was just "fine!"]*
In the body, "deficiencies" only appear when "excess" EXCEEDS the body's ability to cope!
Medical science teaches that the diabetic suffers from a "deficiency" of the hormone "insulin." They classify diabetics as either glucose intolerant or insulin resistant. Actually, the diabetic suffers from **excess** acid waste in the tissues and fluids—along with a "leaky-gut" and a **major** shortfall of magnesium **IN THE FACE OF** "excess" blood **CALCIUM** levels.
➡ *[Perhaps the reader can now see the "connection" between the* **dramatic** *increase in diabetes among women who are* **OVERLOADING** *on "calcium" in an effort to head-off osteoporosis. All that "excess" calcium is driving heart attacks and arthritis and cardiovascular problems in females—along with the "insane" idea that women should "reduce" or eliminate dietary fat intake. These are* **"CRITICAL"** *issues for women— and women are* **NOT** *learning of them from the "experts"—who can't even save themselves! The problem here is that the experts' medical "model" is* **defective!**]*
The diabetic keeps "carbon" sugars circulating in the blood to **BUFFER** acid wastes circulating in the system. Sugar is a carbon based molecule $(C_6H_{12}O_6)$ that "orchestrates" all life on planet Earth. [To better understand carbon's role in the life

process, see *Avogadro's Number*, Chapter 21.]

"Excess" in the diabetic creates hormonal imbalances and "leaky-gut" that makes matters worse! Leaky-gut" means the intestinal wall is overly porous, allowing overly large food and "drug" molecules **DIRECT ACCESS** to the blood stream—something that should **NEVER** occur! The result is an immune system in **TOTAL REVOLT**—and lots of **sub**clinically sick people. Asthma, allergies and sinus problems go with a "leaky-gut"—as does **EVERY** auto-immune disease known!

Type 1 *early* childhood diabetes problems are "linked" to **super antigen vaccines** "laced" with **mercury**—a "bicephalous" dilemma for parents and children alike! Low blood magnesium levels are a **MAJOR** issue here! [For further information on vaccinations, contact **New Atlantean Books** (505) 983-1856 or write P.O. Box 9638, Santa Fe, NM 87504, USA.]

Fact is, 75% of children with diabetes, autism and hearing loss suffer from **mutant** pathogenic organisms and foreign serum proteins introduced by force into healthy bodies by mad men in white coats with the support of gullible, ignorant parents! Parents should seek **"guidance"** early on **"BEFORE"** the damage is done! Parents should **"NEVER"** fight the system! Better to "play along"—and beat the "devils" at their game with a little help from someone who knows how to "buffer" the damage. **NEVER, EVER** vaccinate before 2 years of age; 4 years is even better. Avoid doctors to avoid being "pressured!"

There are ways around the vaccination problem if parents think outside the box and ask for guidance!

[Instead of worrying about "bugs" getting your children, keep their "terrain" healthy by keeping their "bile" flowing with Yucca Blend,™ PAC's,™ non pasteurized sauerkraut, Kombucha Tea, raw apple cider vinegar and enemas—especially when sick! **Control of the "terrain" is THE issue.** *The Young Again Protocol™ is about control of the "terrain!"]*

Back to diabetes! Fifty million people suffer with clinical and **sub**clincal diabetes. Science's failure to understand diabetes at the subtle energy level perpetuates needless "suffering." Independent action—**without** the blessings of higher authority—is a prerequisite to dis-ease control and return of health.

You have to THINK and ACT for yourself and your child because you are the only one who can.

Let's review. There is no such thing as deficiency disease—only conditions of **"excess"** that manifest as deficiencies! Aging is a *cumulative* condition of **"excess."** Death is *confirmation* of **"excess beyond control."**

The **vital organs** function like gyroscopes on a ship—keeping us *even-keeled* by dealing with shifts in the body's "terrain"—that is if we don't "sabotage" them with snacking, bio-junk diets, under-hydration, stress and poor bile-flow.

How we "feel" is **NOT** an accurate barometer of our true state of health. Long before **SIGNS** of dis-ease become visible, negative energy is building at the *subtle energy level.* The proof is all the **sub**clinically sick and dying people who "feel just fine"—*yesterday!* [See Kabuchi Dance, Chapter 38.] *The "lag" between symptoms and the manifestation of the clinical SIGNS of dis-ease is about 20 years!*

Mental Hype • Body Abuse

Hype is taking its toll the world over. People have become skilled in the awesome power of mind over body and drug over mind. They use both to *drive* and *whip* the *bioelectric* body. And when asked how they feel, people usually respond "great!" At the same time, over 80% of the US population suffers from **sub**clinical illness; 75% from obesity, etc.

Hype and the unbalanced person go together—as do over-excitable people and a magnesium shortfall. Hype goes with **unrealistic** mental euphoria—driving the body beyond its ability to physically respond. Coffee, drugs and "whip" type drugs and herb supplements make things much worse!

Hype DRIVES the physical body into a "twilight zone" where aging and the passing of TIME accelerates.

SIGNS of hype-driven dis-ease are are easy to spot. The doctor's diagnosis usually shatters *hype's* hold on us—but by then we are in trouble and the damage is done.

Dis-ease is the manifestation of "stress!" Dis-ease is a confirmation of aging. Dis-ease is the manifestation of Fourth Dimension **TIME** over man's Third Dimension body. Aging and dis-ease result from failure to **"square"** our energy account each day. **Death** is energy bankruptcy while **hype** is energy inflation. *Hype* is modern man's Achilles Heel because it is based on "unrealistic" thinking and "unbalanced" lifestyles.

The simple life is a life where the passing of TIME slows down. Seek simple! Boring is GOOD!

Food Digestion Requirements

Different foods require different amount of time to exit the stomach. The list below is based on the intake of "healthy" food and a "healthy" digestive system—and a meal environment "void" of stress. Note the very small amounts of food used in these examples (1/2 ounce). Large amounts of food take longer to digest. If more food is eaten **too soon** after a previous meal or snack, or if the bowel is backed-up or bile-flow is poor **"acid reflux"** and digestion-type problems manifest along with "parasite" problems! Poorly digested food putrefies in the "gut!" An anaerobic environment makes matter worse, as does a "leaky gut!" [Follow the *Young Again Protocol!* to solve these problems.]

Foods Requiring One-half To Two Hours Processing: water, wine, tea, milk, coffee, bouillon, beer and soft eggs.

Foods Requiring Two To Three Hours Processing: coffee w/cream, cocoa w/milk, asparagus (steamed), potatoes (mashed), fish (broiled), white bread, oysters (broiled), butter and eggs (scrambled, poached, fried, hard boiled).

Foods Requiring Three To Four Hours Processing: chicken (broiled), bread (whole grain), carrots (steamed), spinich (boiled), cucumber (raw), apple (raw), beef (roasted), salmon (broiled), tuna (broiled), ham, (broiled), lentils and beans (boiled), green beans (steamed) and lettuce (raw).

A Story About Satiety

Dr. Carey Reams told a story that took place during the years he and his wife were raising their large family. As the story goes, the neighbors and their children were over for dinner. When the food bowls were placed on the table, the neighbors made an effort to hide their surprise as their eyes were drawn to the modest size of the various bowls of corn, peas, mashed potatoes, gravy, meat, and desserts.

Expecting just such a response, Reams—in his characteristic style—laughed and predicted that there would be food left over. As you might guess, this is exactly what happened. Everyone had a wonderful meal, a great time, and departed with their belly "plum full!"

Your author tells this story to draw attention to the *satiety* enjoyed by all with a limited amount of food. What happened at Reams' home is exactly the **OPPOSITE** of people starving to death on FULL stomachs—as they are today!

Reams' food was "alive" and chock-full of enzymes and loaded with bio-active minerals and vitamins. Today, food is **DEAD** and **EMPTY**—providing minimal energy for the body and requiring people to "stuff" themselves in order to "feel" full because real nourishment is absent. ALL processed foods are left-spin, negative energy substances. The body cannot use negative energy and must neutralize it—or store it as FAT!

These last four words shed light on the obesity problems plaguing 75% of Americans.

We could surmise that what really took place at the Reams' dinner table was that everyone was courteous and took only small portions of food and all left the table hungry—faking-it all the way. But Reams was not a liar. He told the story to make the point that good food, bio-active food, food with a right-spin energy *footprint* is very nourishing! You can believe that everyone left the table full and gratified **BEYOND** desire which is the correct definition of the word satiety.

Few people experience real satiety these days. Instead, they know only the "other" version. *Pseudo* satiety is experienced when the stomach is full, but the body is not nourished. In other words, we quit eating because we run out of space—**NOT** because we are nutritionally satisfied. **America is full of starving people with full bellies!** It is impossible to satisfy the body's energy needs with empty calories—and left-spin energy food that is devoid of life-giving nutrients!

The Appetite

Appetite is a combination of *physical need* and *mental desire*. It is controlled by the satiety and hunger centers in the hypothalamus of the brain. It has long been established that the hunger center is **ALWAYS** active unless it is *inhibited*. The body uses two inhibitory mechanisms to regulate hunger: a **physically** full stomach and a **nutritionally** satisfied body.

The hunger center is a cluster of nerve cells that generate sensations that are a combination of physical need and mental desire. Snacking is a combination of both! Most people meet their body's need for nutritional energy—true hunger—with EMPTY calories [physical hype] and cognitive satisfaction [mental hype]—a **deadly** combination!

Real satiety is nourishment **BEYOND** desire! False satiety is a **FULL** stomach **without** adequate nourishment. When the stomach is "full"—or when nutrient energy needs are met—a message is sent to the hunger center and we lose our desire for food. This is a *negative inhibition system* because one system shuts down the other. It is a system that works flawlessly **UNLESS** we "sabotage" it!

I'm Hungry Again

Later—after the stomach partially empties—the "hungry" body **DEMANDS** more nourishment and the appetite returns with a vengeance as the cycle begins over again.

Hungry people gain weight when they **"fail"** to nourish their bodies. An "acid" terrain is another reason for weight gain. Hormonal issues are a third reason. Poor digestive capability is a fourth reason. And do **NOT** forget a stressed liver with poor bile-flow, insufficient saliva secretion and chewing of food, lack of exercise, low water intake, a "leaky-gut," insufficient load bearing activity, a sluggish thyroid—and bowels that move less than three times a day finishes the list quite nicely!

Weight control and fulfillment of nutritional and hormonal needs goes with "terrain" deacidification.

The nervous system is divided into the central and peripheral systems. The stomach is controlled by the peripheral system which is divided into the sympathetic and parasympathetic systems. We have control over the sympathetic nervous system. We control it with our *mental* thoughts. We have **NO** control over the involuntary parasympathetic nervous system. Both systems communicate with the stomach.

Load-Bearing Work

Load-bearing work is just that—load-bearing! People do not do enough of it. Society has come to view **physical work** as a curse—something to be avoided at all costs! Only poor or uneducated people do "physical" work!

Society is wrong! The body must be "worked!" Since people hate the word "work," maybe we should call "work" **load-bearing** *exercise*—which better fits the sports bent of society. Unfortunately, for many people, load-bearing activity takes place on the couch in front of the boob-tube. So let's compromise and call physical "work" **load-bearing** "activity!"

The body responds to load-bearing activity by repairing old tissue, building new tissue by circulation of lymphatic fluids and "stagnant"—but soluble—amyloid fluids. When "**worked**" on a regular basis, **anabolic** rejuvenation occurs.

We are supposed to build a "new" body every 7 years. The issues discussed in this book dictate whether your "new" body will be stronger or weaker than the one you traded in—and how long it will take to get it.

As people age, they lose their **ability** and **desire** to do physical activity. Part of this phenomenon is the physical inability to perform; part is a lack of desire; and part is a lack of energy. A sedentary lifestyle **destroys** the body and accelerates loss of bone, muscle and mobility. Circulation of amyloid fluid waste explains **why** people who exercise and work their bodies enjoy better health than those who do not "work!"

The more sedentary you are, the faster you will age. This is called the "use it or lose it" rule.

The Dowager's Hump

The dowager's hump is a classic **SIGN** of total systemic **OSTEOPOROSIS**—which is **demineralization** and **degeneration** of the bones. The humped-back, bent-over appearance—as seen among older people, particularly in women—is a **SIGN** that is becoming all too common among younger people, too. Osteoporosis is prevalent in females because of **low or unbalanced** hormones; **low** thyroid activity; **early** acidification of the tissues; the **"inability"** to lay down more collagen than is being lost; and **loss** of vitamin B-12 via menstruation.

Osteoporosis is a SERIOUS but reversible condition. Reversing the condition takes lots of work and time. Understanding WHY it occurs is the important thing!

Please turn to page 100 where you will see that the spinal column and related connective tissues of the "osteoporotic" person have *shrunk*. Notice that the person has lost *inches* from their maximum height—which was achieved

at their ***anabolic peak!*** [Also see pages 21, 22 and 198.] Lost inches occur mostly in the spinal column through deterioration of the vertebrae, tendons, ligaments—and the discs **between** the vertebrae. Eventually, the rib cage *settles* and rests on the pelvis (hip). The process takes about 40 years to occur! Settling of the spine and rib cage **distorts** the visceral cavity, prolapses the colon, and contributes to "bladder drop"—causing the belly to protrude. Sluggish bowels and the *humped* appearance goes with the territory!

Osteoporosis begins at about age 25 and greatly accelerates after age 30 and again in the forties with the onset of menopause. This condition is seldom diagnosed before age 45. Bone "density" tests identify the problem but offer women no solution.

By the time **"menopause"** manifests, osteoporosis is a reality. Please do **NOT** dismiss osteoporosis. It is a 100% guaranteed "issue" for women—just as prostate is a 100% guaranteed issue for men. These conditions are "fixable!"

*[A "dower" is a deceased man's estate. Dowager is an old English term for the man's widow who holds property from her deceased husband's estate. These women had the imposing appearance of a "humped" back and shoulders. Hence—a "dowager's hump." The condition was predominately seen among wealthy, older women. The poor usually died too soon in life to get the hump. The wealthy dowager did **NOT** do load-bearing work because physical work belonged to the domain of the poor. The dowager's hump is confirmation of advanced osteoporosis—and a VERY acid body "terrain!"]*

The story of the dowager provides an **IMPORTANT** lesson. Here are a few things every woman—and man—can do to **STOP** and **REVERSE** osteoporosis and degeneration:

• Reopen the "puberty window" (see pages 72,164,212).
• Use B.T. racemized™ thyroid creme.
• Drink fresh beet and carrot juice every day.
• Do High Enema Therapy 2-3 times each week.
• Deacidify the tissues and body fluids.
• Use Cobo-12™ cobalt/vitamin B-12 creme.
• Avoid sugar, soft drinks and artificial sweetners.
• Make and drink Kombucha Tea.
• Do the *Young Again Tissue & Liver Protocol™* .
• Use VZ™ SOC™ and L_sP_cC™ **every** day.

"Hanging" s-t-r-e-t-c-h-e-s the spine and joints. Hanging by the ankles and feet is done using an "inversion" table and is extremely helpful for osteoporotic women! Also hang from a trapeze bar, rafter or tree limb. Women must use caution here, as the shoulders are fragile in women after 40 years of age. Hang twice daily. Start slowly. [Those with arthritis, osteoporosis or back pain should also take SOC™, VZ™ and L_sP_cC™ to dissolve scar tissue, open blood and lymph flow, and speed cartilage regeneration. The L/CSF™ machine circulates amyloid, lymph and cerebral-spinal fluids without the time requirement or risk of "abusive" exercise or extreme sports activity.]

Osteoporosis & Calcium

Women are told to take calcium supplements to put minerals into the bones. Unfortunately, this does **NOT** solve the problem because **"lack of"** calcium is **NOT** the cause. A highly **ACID** "terrain" is "why" woman—and men—develop the condition—along with hormonal imbalances and the **inability** to lay-down enough collagen to "offset" collagen loss. [This is a self-cannibalization issue!]

Osteoporosis in women is "typically" diagnosed **after** age 40—when estrogen levels are diminishing and the body has gone "acid!" But the condition **BEGAN** 20+ years earlier when estrogen levels were **"high!"** [The experts just don't get it!]

Osteoporosis is defined as diminished bone "density." Acid bodies "mine" minerals like calcium from the bones to "buffer" acids in the tissues and fluids. Osteoporosis occurs by **"default!"** Medical "experts" and clinical nutritionists don't have a clue about osteoporosis. Osteoporotic people usually have normal to **HIGH** calcium levels in their blood (**hyper**calcemia). [Calcium's primary job—both in the body and in the soil—is that of a "buffer" against **excess** "acids!"]

If your *present* height is LESS than it was at your peak, you need to take ACTION today! [See page 100.]

Rouleau & Dowager's Hump *Connection*

Deterioration of the bones and connective tissues, in general, is **serious** business—and it plagues millions of people. The dowager's hump is a **SIGN!** The "Rouleau effect" in the blood is **symptomatic!** [See page 136.] Pronounced "roo -low," the condition is a forerunner of all dis-ease and is seen under the microscope as "sticky" waste filled blood with "clumped" red blood corpuscles. Blood with Rouleau means that **less** oxygen and nutrients reach the cells—and **less** carbon dioxide and **acidic** amyloid wastes exit the tissues and the body. The end-result is **"acidification"** and **"calcification"** of the connective tissues, scalp, eyes, ears and nerves. [Racemized™ liquid sea minerals eliminate the "Rouleau" effect—and the *Young Again Protocol*™ deacidfies the "terrain!"]

Rouleau appears 5-20 years BEFORE the doctor can render a diagnosis of a life-threatening condition.

SUMMARY: Aging reversal is a one-step-at-a-time project—in REVERSE! Apply what you have learned thus far and you will be on your way to becoming—and perpetually staying—*Young Again!*

PREVIEW: *Our next chapter looks at the world of "shadows" and commonly held beliefs. Jesus and the Great Pyramid of Cheops have much in common—as you will see.*

| Magnesium |

The "experts" **push** calcium and **"IGNORE"** magnesium! Calcium taken without a "viable" form of magnesium in "balanced" ratio **"seeds"** dis-ease. Magnesium affects diabetes [insulin resistance, insulin dependence and glucose intolerance], heart problems, high blood pressure, blood clots, stroke, cortisol and adrenalin production, "stress," thyroid response, osteoporosis, fat "metabolism" and mitochondrial activity and ATP production in the cells. [Racemized sea minerals supply a full spectrum of all mineral electrolytes to offset the Rouleau effect. Taoist TCM™ provides a balanced ratio of magnesium to calcium in a body friendly and usable molecular form.]

| Loss of Vision |

Deterioration of vision does **NOT** "occur" because of poor genes or bad luck! Eye problems have **nothing** to do with "genetics!" Macular degeneration and glaucoma are **"avoidable"** and **"reversable!"** Cataract formation is a "waste" issue! An **"acid"** terrain and poor blood and lymphatic flow in the capillary beds servicing the back of the eyes is a "waste" issue! Behind each eye is 80 miles of **capillaries!** Sluggish blood and lymphatic "flow" and amyloid plaque formation in the tissues servicing the eyes eventually conjures a "diagnosis" from the doctor. Problem is, the doctor's solution is **no** solution at all! [Follow the *Young Again! Protocol*™ and you won't develop eye "conditions!" Eye problems are confirmation of a highly **ACID** "terrain!" Prevention is the best solution! Action is a requirement!]

| Popcorn • Oil • Brewers Yeast |

Popcorn is a good food—as long as it's **not** cooked in soy or canola oil and covered with common table salt and margarine. And for a real treat, liberally sprinkle brewers yeast on "buttered" popcorn for some zest! You will love it!

| Healthy Baby Formula |

3 1/2 C. "healthy" water™, 1 each: racemized™ liver & algae tabs, 1 Disorb Aid™, 1 tbsp. coconut/olive oil, 1 tsp. each of TRP™, cod liver oil, & "blackstrap" molasses, plus "contents" of 1 SOC™ cap, 1 R/C™ cap and a few drops of L_sP_cC.™ Crush/soak/liquify; thin with water as desired; perforate bottle nipple as needed, keep refrigerated, warm slightly, use within 48 hours. Raw "goat milk" is next best to mother's milk. [Local "feed" stores can tell you **"who"** in your area raises goats.]

Fats & Hormones

The body needs dietary "fats" to heal and stay healthy. Fats and oils are the **basis** of hormone production—as is "cholesterol." Eat butter, raw virgin coconut oil and olive oil. Use R/EFA™ to provide racemized™ essential fatty acids. **Avoid** fat-free diets and foods. Fat-free diets are killing women! Eat fats!

Soluble & Structural Waste

"Soluble" acid waste production is part of body metabolism—and the body has **no choice** but to deal with it. The liver filters waste from the blood and stores it as **bile** in the gallbladder. Bile is critical to "digestion!" It also "activates" the bowels. If the liver is **unable** to remove waste from the blood, it is forced—by default—to store those highly acid wastes in the fat-layer beneath the skin—safely out of the loop! Storage of "soluble" acid waste is a **"DEFENSIVE"** tactic! The body stores it to keep us alive **IF** it is unable to send it down the toilet in the bile! Structural" waste is called **amyloid plaque!** It can **ONLY** exit the body with the help of VZ™, Yucca Blend™ and L_sP_cC™. **Why** amyloid plaque forms and **what** to do about it is a "core" issue—and the subject of *SilkWorm Blues*, Chapter 36.

Alkalinity vs. Acidity

The "pH" of body tissues and fluids is a huge issue for anyone wishing to enjoy a long and healthy life. The "pH" of **"circulating"** body fluids tells us *"where we are at"* while the "pH" of **"non-circulating"** fluids tells us *"where we are going!"* The sicker a person is, the more acid is their body "terrain"—and visa versa. After age 25, everyone's body turns more and more acid until we reach the "change" years of menopause and andropause and life becomes difficult. Aging "symptoms" in women come **sooner** than for men—beginning around age "30." Men age more slowly. Officially, dis-ease *"knocks"* when we **"CROSS"** the acid waste "threshold" and the body breaks-down. "Terrain" management is about being **"less acid"—NOT** more alkaline! They are **not** the same concept. [See pages 109, 117, 126,171, 219, 258, 306 and 354.]

Racemized™ Asparagus

Racemized™ asparagus (Aspar-Max™) is good for heart arrythmias, lung, bronchial and sinus issues. Use with MX™ to break-up "mucous!" Aspar-Max™ is also good for bowel and bladder problems and hyper-active children, too! Behind all of these "conditions" is **insufficient** bile-flow and an "acid" terrain. [The *Young Again (Tissue & Liver) Protocol*™ deals with "terrain" problems that underscore mucous and congestion issues. VZ™ "digests" amyloid waste and **denies** microbes the mucous "breeding" ground that accompanies illness.

10

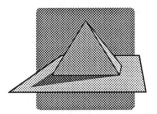

Shadow Land

"Most people would rather swallow lies than truth, especially if the liar has authority and the dis-information is soothing, like a fine liqueur."
Charles Walters

As Pontius Pilate passed by the side of Jesus at His trial, it was reported that he asked the great teacher *"What is Truth?"* The Roman propounded a timely question that went unanswered—at least from the lips of Jesus. Pilate posed his question to Jesus—not as an interrogatory—but as a statement **about** "The Christ."

Socrates maintained that "TRUTH" could **neither** be proved nor disproved. Rather, it formed the **basis** of our beliefs by the **reality of its existence!** The Great Pyramid of Cheops is such a **TRUTH.** It cannot be denied because it is **"THERE!"**

Earlier your author posed the questions *"Why do people like experts and expert opinions?"* *"How could anyone trust their most prized asset—their "health"—to the throw of the dice by medical "experts" who can't even help themselves and suffer and die just like their patients?"*

The answer to **both** questions is that the individual is relieved of personal responsibility when the decision process is given over to "experts." Forfeiture of responsibility provides an **excuse** and someone to **blame** when things go "sour." Unfortunately, blaming others will **NOT** keep you young—*or alive!*

The "Expert" Syndrome

Medical science generally tells us to do exactly the **opposite** of what we should do. Today, its theories are gospel; tomorrow, it casts them aside for newer versions. In the process, it issues the proclamation "magic bullet!"

An unsuspecting public buys into **THEORIES** that were **never** true in the first place—like fluoridation of water and toothpaste; the Cholesterol and Germ Theories of Disease; the idea that estrogen "deficiency" causes osteoporosis; the need for calcium to "prevent" osteoporosis; the "benefits" of soy consumption; the "need" for vaccinations and immunizations—and so much other "hogwash!" We are trained to **ACCEPT** and **NOT TO THINK** and to **IGNORE** our "instincts" and instead rely on "experts" in medicine, government, law, religion and industry—experts who are "expert" at **manipulating** us. The government school system "trains" us **NOT** to think!

Mass Delusions

In 1850, Charles MacKay wrote *Extraordinary Mass Delusions and the Madness of Crowds.* In it, he showed how unbelievably gullible we are—and that the more desperate the circumstances, the greater is our propensity to make unsound decisions "in mass"—usually with the help of the *experts.*

People go crazy in mass, but they return to their senses one at a time. This is why committee mentality manifests itself whenever three or more people get together! "Idiots of 3, they be!"

People seek health care *experts* because they are ignorant of how to solve their own health issues. They don't know where to turn; they're in trouble and they want a fix—*now!*

If people would learn to **"read"** their body's **SIGNS** and **listen** to their **symptoms,** they could prevent health problems and save a lot of pain, suffering—and money!

An **ENDLESS** supply of money—**in the form of medical insurance**—allows the "experts" to keep their hooks in us. Few people escape medical science's tentacles except under three conditions: When we are healthy; when we have no money; or, when we are dead! Medical "decisions" should **NEVER** be based on "who" is paying the bill. The better your insurance, the worse it is for you. "Experts" get the money and you get a "bone" in exchange—if they don't destroy you first!

By definition, an expert is someone from more than 50 miles away. Our fascination with **EXPERTS** convinces me that this is the **SAME** phenomenon causing the Law of Bureaucracy to work flawlessly—and **without** exception. It says *"Regardless of the intended result, exactly the opposite will result."*

We **CANNOT** rely on experts. The experts teach us to **doubt** our intuitions and ignore good sense. Experts practice tunnel vision; that is why they are called "experts!"

We live in a world of shadows—where what we see and hear only "appear" to be the truth; where the more something is believed to be true and the more people who believe it, the greater are the odds that it's NOT true.

Allopathic medicine is in trouble—and so are people who rely on it. Medicine's "model" is based on the Germ Theory of Disease and the Scientific Method. Neither is valid!

Consider the difference between conventional medicine's

approach and vibrational medicine's approach to solving the hearing problem for the deaf. At the age of 15, Dr. Patrick Flanagan invented the **neurophone**—a device to help the deaf hear. Flanagan "sensed" that the brain is a *hologram* with areas capable of performing **multiple** or **duplicate** functions. Consequently, Flanagan used the skin as **both** a pathway to the brain and as an organ with which to "hear!"

Flanagan solved the hearing problem through visualization rather than surgical intervention. The brain is **not** hard wired as taught in the medical schools. The body **can** *regenerate* new brain cells. We **do** have the ability to grow new limbs, bones, cartilage, nerve fibers, skin and connective tissues. Flanagan had **vision.** He understood the Creator's handiwork—as all great men and women do.

The problem for people of science and medicine is they forget they are not GOD! So, their "egos" take over!

Cause & Effect

Earlier, your author mentioned something called "single factor analysis" which translates: "for every effect there is **single** cause; for every disease there is a **single** pathogen that is responsible." This kind of academic tunnel vision has gotten us into a lot of trouble. It is **unrealistic** and it is **NOT** true. Whenever the facts are **FORCED** to fit a pet theory, **TRUTH becomes** the victim; *legitimate* science suffers; and lots of troubles magically appear. So it is with the "scientific method."

Charles Walters summed-up the problems inherent in the scientific method when he stated "Most of what is generally called the scientific system is not science at all, but merely a procedural aspect that calls for setting up experiments that eliminate other possibilities, or it deals with making instruments that enable the investigator to find what he/she is looking for. [Can the reader see the connection here with "statistics?"]

*[But].....there is a **second scientific method** that, although unwritten, has far greater impact on scientists and their findings. This is the reality of project funding, "peer" review and the publishing of scientific papers."* Walters went on to say, *"The backbone of the scientific system has to do with asking the **right** questions, and a scientist can **only** ask the right questions **after** his or her life has **absorbed** the experiences that lead to a **vision** of the Creator's handiwork—hence the right question.* [And].... *"discovery is accomplished by the mind and soul of the whole person and cannot be reduced to a mechanical scientific (by-the-numbers) procedure. It stands to reason that you can't get the answers if you don't know the questions [to ask].*

The Double Helix & The Germ Theory

It was this "second" method that caused James D.

Watson—one of the discoverers of the DNA molecule—to rock the scientific world when he disclosed the behind-the-scenes power plays, jealousy and fights for "funding" in his book *The Double Helix.* Watson also offered an antidote—the observation that *"[True] scientific" discovery involves human* **thought** *and* **vision** *more than test tubes, procedures and microscopes.*

The Germ Theory of Disease (GTD) is very much part of the aging process because it influences the way we **perceive** dis-ease. The GTD so **completely** colors our thought processes that we are blind to the subtleties and cumulative effects of bad living habits and poor diet. The "men of science" do **NOT** understand that the battle for life and health vs. death and disease is won or lost on a playing field that has absolutely **NOTHING** to do with the GTD. **Blind men, they be!**....with fat egos—stumbling in the dark—fearful of the light of **TRUTH!**

We cannot rely on medical science to solve our problems because "they **don't know** what the problem is!" They do not understand life at the subtle energy level—nor the genesis and manifestation of dis-ease." And here is proof!

Experts suffer from the SAME problems as the rest of the population. They grow old. They succumb to the same dis-eases. Their "magic bullets" do NOT save them!

The GTD is a "theory"—yet medical science treats it as holy writ. It is the cornerstone of the archaic medical model under which medicine labors. It is a stone around science's neck! The GTD is so "accepted" that 99.99999% of the medical community own "stock" in it and "live" by it. Perhaps the reader does, too! Conventional medical modalities—from diagnosis to treatment—are based on a **false, theoretical** dis-ease "model."

The model says *"We are nothing but a bundle of chemicals, proteins, fats, water, nucleic acids, flesh and blood— and dis-ease is the product of microbial "invasion!"* The model says that "Dis-ease erupts out of *nowhere!"* These things are not true. Loyalty to the model stands in the way of change.

Regardless of medical science's bullheadedness, we are moving into an era where the **"reality"** of the Third Dimension **physical** body and the Fourth Dimension **energy** body will be be recognized and brought together—so healing can be achieved on a multi-level "total" basis.

The healthy, bio-electric body is a synthesis of energy fields vibrating in concert with Mother Earth and the environment—the internal and external "terrains!"

Things Are Changing

Recognized medical journals now carry alternative articles—a "calculated" move! The press is signalling the **BIG** "players" to position themselves for **control** over of the transition from allopathic to alternative medicine. The driving force behind these moves are the pharmaceutical companies. They are the "forces" behind the GATT, NAFTA and CAFTA "agreements"—as well as CODEX—which limit people's access and freedom of choice. Hobbling the health industry via "mandatory" prescription of health supplements—with the help of bureaucrats to implement and enforce Big Pharma's wonderful little scheme—is the game!

[There are ways to fight back—but they require "thinking" outside the box; methods NOT printed in this book, but there just the same. Never try to go through a wall when you can simply "go around it!"]

Alternative medicine is growing at an exponential rate. It's **NO** accident that present medical and economic systems are being systematically stifled. Consider that in 1994, 40% of the people in the uSA used some form of *alternative* medicine. By 2004, the number was 75%. People are "instinctively" moving away from the "medical model."

Natural healing is "the" thing to be into these days. "Conventional" doctors are authoring books and mailing newsletters "trumpeting" their **CHARADE!** Few physicians can think outside the box. "Few" alternative practitioners escape "schooling" in the medical "model." Licenses and bloated egos are stumbling blocks to real progress. Sadly, it's the way it is.

Translation! You are on your own! The experts can ignore **TRUTH**—but they can't deny it for **TRUTH** is there like the Great Pyramid—etched in stone and timeless. Recognition of TRUTH over theory is how you become *Young Again!*

PREVIEW: *Our next chapter looks at HOW water functions in the bio-electric body. It is a foundation chapter. Please study the chapter carefully—and enjoy!*

Food Poisoning

If poisoned, immediately take "charcoal" tablets and fresh lemon juice followed by a colonic or series of coffee enemas. Most drugstores sell charcoal. Never travel without it!

Prostate Inflammation & Pain

Every man **will** deal with prostate problems—sooner or later! To avoid prostate "misery," use R/Prostate™ I & II. Pain, inflammation, urination issues, impotence and sexual dysfunction should **NOT** be ignored! So-called medical "options" are a cruel joke for men! Better to **avoid** the knife and the laser! Alternative approaches like saw palmetto, zinc and selenium are "good" band-aids—but they do **NOT** explain "why" men's prostate "act-up," and they definitely do **NOT** restore function and integrity to a prostate that is in "serious" trouble. Avoidance is the issue! [See pages 113, 159, 177-8, 185 and 292.]

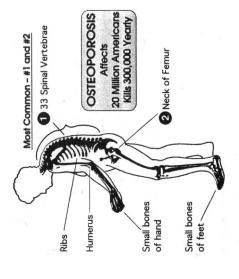

OSTEOPOROSIS
Affects
20 Million Americans
Kills 300,000 Yearly

Most Common – #1 and #2

❶ 33 Spinal Vertebrae

❷ Neck of Femur

Ribs

Humerus

Small bones of hand

Small bones of feet

**LOCATIONS IN THE BODY
WHERE PAIN AND MISERY HIT HARDEST**

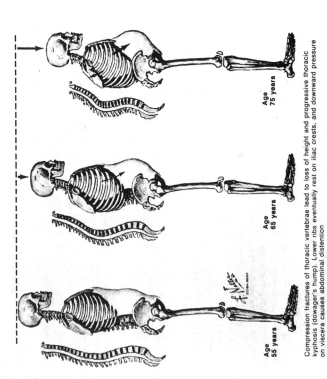

Age 55 years

Age 65 years

Age 75 years

Compression fractures of thoracic vertebrae lead to loss of height and progressive thoracic kyphosis (dowager's hump). Lower ribs eventually rest on iliac crests, and downward pressure on viscera causes abdominal distention

Progressive Spinal Deformation In Osteoporosis

11

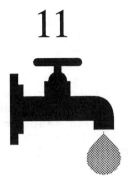

Elixir Of The Ageless

"In health and in sickness, pure water is one of the choicest blessings. It is the beverage given by God to quench the thirst of man and animal, and to cleanse the poisons from our system." Byrne

At birth, the human body is over 90% water. By age 3, *average* body hydration level **should be** 75% water. Adult hydration levels often dip to 65% in men and 52% in women. At death, hydration level can be 5-10%. Fat holds 55% water; muscle 75%; and brain tissue up to 85%. Water **definitely** affects the rate and severity of the way people age.

The **bio-electric** body requires water to function. When we are water-deficient, it's called **neglect!** When we drink contaminated water, it's called **abuse!** Most people's bodies suffer from both abuse and neglect. The *bio-electric* body can bounce back from abuse and neglect—but it can't do it without the help of **biologically friendly** water!

Water has many faces: some wet, some dry, some heavy, some structured. Water has different names. There is distilled water, reverse osmosis water, deionized water, carbon block and ceramic filtered water, hard water, soft water, tap water, ionized water, Grander water, Ludwig water, Ange water, Pi water, Living water, Miracle water, Willard water, Medical Grade Ionized Water,™ saline water, electrostatic water and BFRV™ water. Some waters are pure, but not healthful, while others are the harbinger of dis-ease and death.

Water is a controlling dietary factor in the aging process. Water underwrites health and vitality.

Water Questions

Some water is so dry, you can hardly get wet, while other water is very *wet.* Many factors affect water's qualities: ORP (oxidation reduction potential), pH, mineral load, chemical load, bond angle, vibrational memory, smell, feel, hardness, softness, molecular size, hydroxal load, etc.

Why does some water taste good and some not? Why does some water quench your thirst while another water satisfies so poorly that we avoid it? Why do some religions erect shrines around *certain* waters? Why are certain water holes around the world called *health* spas? Why is water used in the rite of baptism? Why do plants grow better when it rains than when irrigated? Is all rain water the same? Why is water used as the transport medium for pesticides and herbicides? Why are "poisons"—like fluoride and chlorine—added to drinking water? Why do people camp near lakes and rivers? Lastly, what does water have to do with **reversing** the aging process?

Water & Body Fluids

There are **THREE** body fluids: **blood, lymph and amyloid.** Blood and lymph are "classified" as liquid "**tissues**"—and **water** is their "foundation!" Both tissues are "soluble!" They are the body's primary **"protein"** communication system as opposed to the endocrine and nervous systems which are electrical and hormone-based systems

The **"third"** body fluid is called **"amyloid"** fluid. About 85-90% of this fluid "circulates!" The remaining 10-15% is of **IMMENSE** importance to the aging process. [Please refer to Chapter 36, *SilkWorm Blues* for a full discussion.]

All four waste corridors—**SKIN, LUNGS, KIDNEYS** and **BOWELS**—rely on water! We need water to sweat, bleed, blow our nose, breathe, menstruate, spit, cough, and defecate. Without water, the mucous membranes lining the air passages and gastrointestinal tract cannot function.

Water is the ONLY dietary substance over which we can exercise complete and total control.

BFRV™ Water

➡ **Please Note:** The BFRV™ trademark replaces the *"abandoned"* BEV acronym *DUE TO ongoing infringement and "bootlegging"* by individual(s) offering water processing equipment under the "pretense" their equipment fulfills the "terrain" management **CONCEPTS** of the *Young Again Protocol.*™

Water & Conception

Water interfaces with every system in the body at the most fundamental level of human existence. "Choice" in drinking water is of immense importance.

Your author's choice of **drinking** water is called BFRV™ water. It has a "conception point"™ ORP (oxidation/reduction potential)—which is where the egg and sperm were when they "joined!" This gives new meaning to the word **"water!"** [See page 306 for a diagram of core issues surrounding "water!"

Your authors choice of **"therapeutic"** water is Medical

Grade Ionized Water™ ("MGIW™")—which is made from BFRV™ water and racemized™ sea minerals. MGIW™ water has an extremely high ORP! [Your author does **not** care about alkalinity—only the "ORP." [Please see and study page 306.]

"Pure" vs. Body-Friendly Water

Experts like to talk about "pure" water, but they can't agree on exactly what *pure* water is. Chemists claim distilled water is "pure"—and it is "purer" than raw tap water—but it's not particularly healthy as a *drinking* water.

"Pure" water is void of **ALL** substances except one oxygen and two hydrogen atoms and their respective electrons. Pure water should be **"FREE"** of sick vibrational memories imposed on it by the contaminants that were part of the water prior to processing.

BFRV™ water is pure and does not carry pollutant "memory!" It is also "restructured"—and has a right-spin energy "footprint" that acts as a liquid magnet for the release of tissue waste—and as a "transport" for shuttling tissue waste out of the system.

Cohesion & Adhesion

Please refer to the water molecule diagram on page 79. Notice the **hydrogen bonds** *connecting* the H_2O water molecule *inside* the box "linking" to molecules *outside* the box. *Hydrogen bonds* cause water molecules to **stick** together. The effect is called **"cohesion."** The stronger the hydrogen and molecular bonds, the more *cohesive* is water. The more *cohesive* water is, the more **ENERGY** it contains, the more waste it can transport out of the body, and the better people feel when they drink it. BFRV™ water is **VERY** "cohesive!"

High-energy water **"coats"** things. The phenomenon is called **"adhesion."** The stronger the hydrogen and molecular bonds, the greater water's *adhesion* qualities and its affects on health and longevity. BFRV™ water is **VERY** "adhesive."

BFRV™ water is further enhanced by manipulation of the *hydrogen* and *molecular* bond angles within and between water molecules. The drawing on page 79 shows a hydrogen atom connected to an oxygen atom at a **"angle."** So-called **"normal"** bonding angle is 104.5^0 at room temperature and 109^0 when frozen. The BFRV™ protocol™ enhances the "life-force" and energy "footprint" and "signature" of water molecules so inter molecular and intra molecular bonding **angles** *within* and *between* molecules can "float" and the water can do its job when taken into the body.

Water containing inorganic minerals, toxic chemicals, viruses, bacteria, radioactivity, etc. has **POOR** cohesion and adhesion qualities—as well as WEAK hydrogen and molecular bonds. These are a few reasons "why" raw tap water is unhealthy to drink. "Leaky-gut" is another serious side effect of raw city water. [See pages 69, 85, 94, 135, 180, 237 and 243.]

Pollutants "hitching" a ride on the H_2O (water) molecule **weaken** water's magnetic *footprint* and electrical *signature*, leaving water with **little** energy to donate to the body and even **less** energy for transporting wastes out of the system. [See bent/polar water molecule diagram on page 79.]

*[BFRV™ water should **NOT** be left exposed to air or stored in metal or common plastics because it "attracts" contaminants. BFRV™ water is either stored in its own system, in glass bottles, or in special BFRV™ containers.]*

[It is not unusual for people who drink BFRV™ water to experience easing of sinus and lung congestion. Most people feel better and have more energy when they drink more water and add racemized™ mineral electrolytes. Bowel habits also change. Non-water drinkers become water lovers!]

People say "This water feels different in my mouth and body. I feel good when I drink it!"

Rules Of Water • Alkalinity/Acidity

Your author has three **"STRICT"** rules regarding water. **Rule #1:** Get people "off" city water! **Rule #2:** Get people to drink more water. **Rule #3:** Get people to use racemized™ sea minerals in whatever water they choose to drink. Follow these rules—and the rest is easy!

Distilled and common reverse osmosis waters are **NOT** particularly good for the body—although they are far better than "raw" city tap water. Still, purity is questionable and their ORP is **NOT** good. These waters **must** be "restructured" before the body can "effectively" use them. Instead of energy donors, these waters "rob" your body of vital "chi" energy!

High "ORP" MGIW™ water carries **ENERGY** in the form of "free" electrons. **Oxidized** city water is "dead" water. **Reduced** MGIW™ water is "live" water. [Mitochondria within the cells use MGIW™ water's extra "electrons" to produce ATP—the body's energy molecule.]

The "pH" of drinking water is **NOT** the issue—but the ORP is! Alkaline water does **not** make the body "alkaline" any more than vinegar, Kombucha tea, saurkraut and lemon make the body "acid." High ORP "reduced" water causes the body to **"deacidify"**—which is **NOT** the same as being more "alkaline!" [See pages 94, 109, 117, 126,171, 219, 258, 306 and 354.]

We want the body to be less acid, NOT more alkaline. They are NOT the same concept.

Skin • Sweat • Lungs

The skin is a mechanical barrier to infection from

outside elements and pathogenic organisms. Insufficient water **intake** and **bathing** in polluted, highly oxidized city water stresses the skin and ages the vital organs.

Failure to drink enough water **denies** the body the opportunity to **"shed"** waste by sweating. Sweat carries toxic waste energy out of our body. The ability to **freely** sweat is a good **SIGN**. Otherwise, waste builds up in the subcutaneous tissues, closing waste exit portals and forcing the waste "load" onto the kidneys, lungs, bowels and liver!

Soluble waste that is not **"exported"** from the tissues is **"stored"** in fatty tissue beneath the skin. Failure to drink enough water "stifles" waste fluid circulation. Low hydration levels result in low blood and lymph fluid volumes and decreased oxygen levels—**raising** blood pressure and pulse rate.

Water & The Lungs

The lungs rid the body of waste "energy." The lungs are **VERY** dependent on mucous secretions to protect delicate tissues from airborne contaminants. Mucous production is dependent on water intake. Low hydration levels in the tissues cause the mucous membranes lining the mouth, throat, respiratory system, vagina and GI tract to come under severe "stress!" Mucous lubricates the nasal passages, bronchials and lungs, transporting wastes **OUT** of the body. Mucous coats and protects the lining of the vagina, stomach and intestines. Conditions like colitis, diverticulitis, leaky-gut and irritable-bowel have their **roots** in "stressed" mucosa lining. Many disease symptoms **vanish** when water intake increases.

"Cries" For Water

The term **hypo**volemia comes to mind. It refers to a condition of low fluid [blood and lymph] volume in the body. Sexually "impotent" men and women [yes, women!] often suffer because of insufficient "water" in the blood and lymphatic systems. If hydration levels are low, the pulse rate is usually elevated. *Underhydration* is a problem of **EPIDEMIC** proportions for much of the population—particularly among the elderly and sick. Both are *notorious* for **NOT** drinking enough water—and their health problems are a direct reflection of it. Low fluid **"electrolyte"** levels goes with this problem. [These are a few more good reasons "why" everyone should drink plenty of water and use racemized™ sea mineral electrolytes.]

The body responds to fluids containing **"water"** such as milk, juice, soft drinks and beer as **"food."** This is *"why"* they should be "chewed" and mixed with saliva. All food—even good food—imposes stress on the system. [Eating "healthy" and "chewing" food are fundamental concepts.]

Avoid raw city water for drinking, bathing —and

especially for enemas and High Enema Therapy.™

Illness & High Enema Therapy™

"Bile" production and flow are dependent upon water intake—and without enough water, liver and gall stones form and indigestion and kidney problems develop. Other water "related" conditions are arthritis, fibromyalgia, gout, lupus, leaky-gut, sinus issues and asthma—just to mention a few!

One of the **VERY** best "water" remedies for any health problem—and especially bowel and digestion issues—is High Enema Therapy.™ Some people have "hang-ups" about this simple procedure. They think it's *weird*—even *"unnatural!"* But it's not a big deal—just a new experience done privately in your own bathroom. Besides, growing old and suffering and losing control of your life is **NOT** natural, either! So *"get used to the idea!"* It's a simple and inexpensive water-based health procedure that is both "preventative" and "therapeutic!"

[Common cleanse programs do **NOT** cause the body to release **soluble** waste "stored" in the fat beneath the skin—where it is under "lock and key!" That is the purpose of High Enema Therapy™ and the Young Again Protocol(s).™]

People often say *"Oh! I don't need High Enema Therapy!™ I go every day!"* Regularity is **NOT** the issue here. Moreover, properly done High Enema Therapy™ is **NOT** about "cleaning" of the colon. The primary purpose is to **"stimulate"** the nerve plexus feeding from the bowel wall to the vital organs. The second purpose is to increase the flow of **"bile."** [This procedure is the **MOST** "crucial" health maintenance technique your author teaches people. Nothing is more "fundamental!]

Consumption of 14-day old Kombucha tea increases bile-flow and helps to deacidify the "terrain."

When the most popular cowboy in movie history died, over 70 pounds of **mucoid matter** was removed from his colon upon autopsy. The odor was *beyond* description! The great actor's transverse colon—the part that hangs over men's belt line—was almost **12"** in diameter—but the lumen [opening] through which waste flowed was only one **"inch"** in diameter! Elvis suffered similarly. The lumen of a "healthy" colon should be fully "open" and the colon should not "sag." [To tighten-up the waistline, do High Enema Therapy,™ get plenty of exercise, and do lots of load-bearing activity! A "pot belly" on a man is also "linked" to a sluggish thyroid. Use HST™ for this!]

When a man's belly hangs-over his beltline, or fills a women's pelvic area, you are seeing a VERY engorged and prolapsed (sagging) colon—full of waste!

Deep Breathing • Aerobic Exercise

Deep breathing provides wonderful benefits—as does

aerobic exercise in "moderation!" Both procedures are dependent upon proper hydration and blood electrolyte levels. These are simple and effective ways to increase oxygen levels in the blood and tissues, stimulate immune acitvity, and circulate lymphatic fluid movement. Deep breathing also builds mental focus and a sense of well being. Both Yoga and Pilates utilize breathing techniques.

"*Use it or lose it!*" sums up the problem of insufficient physical activity. Low fluid volume, low oxygen levels and sluggish lymph circulation go with an "acidic" terrain. The L/CSF™ machine solves waste, oxygen and circulation issues with very little effort—especially for the sick, elderly and obese. [See pages 132-3, 160, 195, 261, 382 and drawing on 385!]

Soft Drinks

People "think" soft drinks and alcohol are substitutes for "water"—but they are not! Soft drink consumption is epidemic, and the problems that spring from it are as **SERIOUS** as heavy alcohol usage—and far more *insidious, too!* Soft drinks upset the body's calcium:phosphorous ratio and are highly "acidic"—playing havoc with body chemistry and pH. Sugar in soft drinks "**steals**" mineral electrolytes and speeds aging. The **negative** effects of "artificial sweetners" on the "terrain" is *beyond description!* [The name "*soda pop*" derives from the high sodium levels they contain.]

It takes 40 glasses of high ORP Medical Grade Ionized Water™ [with a pH of 10+] to offset the pH plunging effects of one can of soda. [See pages 220 and 306.]

Soft drinks are socially acceptable and are believed to be safe to drink. They are "different" than cigarettes, coffee, drugs and alcohol because their "long-term" effects **DO NOT** manifest in "real time"—avoiding any "aging" connection!

Soft drinks accelerate aging by "chelating" minerals out of the body—especially in women!

Energy Production & Water

Water supplies oxygen that is used in respiration at the "cellular" level—in addition to the air we breathe. Cellular mitochondria use oxygen to burn [oxidize] glucose sugars during the Krebs Cycle and glycolysis. The Krebs Cycle is a "flameless" catalytic process that "frees" hydrogen ions from the water molecule in the electron transport chain within the mitochondria where "**cellular**" respiration occurs and where our energy molecule "ATP" is produced. [Sore muscles from overactivity are the product of lactic-acid formation due to oxygen shortfall during strenuous activity.]

BFRV™ water—and *especially* high ORP Medical Grade Ionized Water™—supply free electrons used in the Krebs

Cycle—fueling cellular metabolism. When people drink these waters, they say **"WOW!"** Purity, ORP, memory and molecular size are the issues here. Water affects the "terrain!"

Ionized "Therapeutic" Water

Therapeutic water is used in special Japanese clinics to restore the health of people suffering from deadly dis-eases. In a "clinical setting," clinical equipment is used to produce high "ORP" water with "therapeutic" qualities. In the home setting, small-scale laboratory equipment is used to create Medical Grade Ionized Water.™

To make MGIW™ water, BFRV™ water is ionized with racemized™ sea minerals to raise electrolyte levels high enough to provide an electron "substrate." Next, electrical current "frees" mineral electrons and concentrates them, creating MGIW™ water. Processing time is 10 minutes. When done, you have one-half gallon of water; one quart each of oxidized and reduced waters. One is drunk; the other is used for the skin and hair—and for "misting" leaves of ornamental and food plants.

Electrons "stripped" from the racemized™ acid elements like sulfur and phosphorous are super bonded to alkaline elements like calcium, magnesium and potassium. The process is simple and has **nothing** to do with "alkalinity." It is the high "ORP" that we are after—**NOT** alkalinity. "ORP" potential is a measure of the free electrons water is carrying. "ORP" restores the "terrain"—not alkalinity!

Medical Grade Ionized Water™ *defies all the laws of physics, chemistry and valence. It is "strange" stuff!*

[Medical Grade Ionized Water™ **CANNOT** *be made from raw city water because the electron substrate is insufficient to produce the desired "ORP!" Besides, water-borne contaminants are concentrated and made worse using "raw" city water. These are the "problems" that are encountered when making so-called "alkaline" water from raw or filtered waters.]*

pH & ORP

pH is a measure of acidity and alkalinity. ORP is a measure of free electrons in solution. Raise the ORP potential of BFRV™ water, and you drive-up the pH as well. "ORP" provides the benefit associated with so-called "alkaline" water.

Medical grade "reduced" water has a pH of 10-11 and ORP potential around <-> 900. Without a highly elevated "ORP," pH is **meaningless!** Water choice based on "pH" is a "moot" issue! We do **NOT** want the "terrain" to be "alkaline;" we want it be "less acid"—and these are **NOT** the same concepts. Drinking alkaline water to become "alkaline" is ludicrous! "Bile-flow" and "release" of tissue-bound acid waste is the path.

"Oxidized" acid water is for external use, with a pH

between 1.5-2.4 and ORP of (+)1200. Despite the very low pH, the water does **NOT** burn delicate tissues like the eyes! What it does do is destroy **ALL** pathogenic organisms like bacteria, viruses, yeast and fungi by stealing their "electrons!"

[High ORP oxidized (acid) water creates beautiful skin, heals wounds and infections, and promotes a youthful appearance. A video showing a Japanese man growing a new "foot" with **"water"** *is available, along with documentation of the water's effect on pathogenic organisms. See Source Page 400.]*

High ORP alkaline water is the exact **opposite** of high ORP acid water. Acid water is highly *oxidized* [stripped of its electrons] while high ORP alkaline water is highly *reduced* [loaded with extra electrons]. "Reduction" is an organic biochemistry concept and term indicating that a substance **gained** electrons and its positive valence is increased. Electrons are the "key!" With the marriage of BFRV™ and Medical Grade Ionized Water(s),™ many benefits are available in the home!

[MGIW™ water does **NOT** *cure dis-ease! It restores the* "terrain!" *Controlling the terrain is central to the development of the BFRV™ Protocol™ as documented in the BFRV™* **manuscript.** *[See pages 104, 117, 126 and 306.]*

Fatigue & Water

"**Under**hydration" goes hand-in-hand with fatigue. So does **excess** acid waste accumulation. Fatigue and muscle **soreness** generally follow strenuous activity, due to depletion of ATP reserves and slowing of mitochondrial activity. When we "overdo," we experience muscle *soreness* because "acid" wastes have overloaded the tissues. **Lactate** formation occurs when there is a **shortfall** of available oxygen at the cellular level, leading to **incomplete** oxidation of glucose sugars. Lactate is the salt of lactic acid which is the waste byproduct of **fermentation** in the presence of **insufficient** oxygen within the cells. During the sleep cycle, the body breaks down lactate and other wastes and soreness eases. The healthier you are, the more efficiently your body will burn glucose and the more efficient the vital organs function—and the less "acid" you will be!

Drinking Medical Grade Ionized Water™ helps reverse the aging process.

Urine

Urine is the metabolic waste byproduct of the kidneys. An examination of urine produces clues as to "what" is happening in the body. Blood pH is "critical" and is maintained with extremely narrow ranges. Urine and saliva pH are less critical— but they are excellent "indicators" of "**circulating**" acid waste that is easy to measure at home without medical oversight. "**Structural**" tissue waste is a totally **DIFFERENT** issue and is

outside the pH of circulating body "fluids" The pH story as it relates to "structural" acid waste is discussed in Chapter 36. Most people's urine pH is **below** 6.0. According to a nurse friend of mine, 90% of the people she checks have a pH between 5.0 - 5.5. She says this is **"normal."** Looks to me like she is prophesying a nation of sick and dying people. [Your author's urine pH raised from 5.1 over a period of **eight years** and finally stabilized at pH 6.8. This is ideal!]

Low urine pH is a **RED FLAG** for cancer and hundreds of other age-related dis-eases. Cancer usually manifests when urine pH drops to 4.5. Saliva pH is usually one point higher.

Low body fluid(s) pH is **NOT** desirable unless the body is "cleansing." It's common for urine and saliva pH to "go acid" for **5-10 YEARS** when following the *Young Again Protocol.*™ It takes **YEARS** for tissue "acids" to release and exit the body. Eventually "terrain" and fluid pH normalize.

Water pH • Sodium

Most city tap water is has a pH of 7-9 and is in a highly *oxidized* state with no life-force and very toxic! "Drinkability" is not the issue here! Please "study" page 306.]

For each **whole** number up or down the pH scale, acidity or alkalinity is ten times greater or lesser. At pH of 8, tap water is 10 times more alkaline than at pH 7. But at pH 9, it is 100 times more alkaline. The pH scale is "logarithmic" by a factor of "10!" To raise the pH of water from 7 to 8 requires large amounts of "buffers!" Lime (calcium carbonate), sodium, magnesium, aluminum and potassium all raise pH. Cities use sodium hydroxide (lye) to manipulate pH. Sodium hydroxide (NaOH) is **extremely** alkaline (pH 12) and sodium is toxic to the cells. People with cancer should **NEVER** drink "raw" city water—nor should anyone else who wants to stay healthy and live a long life. "Choice" of water has consequences!

Casts & Albumin In Urine

Casts are sometimes found in urine. They are aptly named. Casts are deposits of mineral salts (like the ones in city drinking water), hyaline and plasma proteins (albumin) that have taken on the shape of the kidney's "tubules." The tubules filter urine wastes and form "casts." Casts are a **RED FLAG!** They're indicative of pH imbalance, high cholesterol, underhydration, **excess** waste and mineral salt overload.

Albumin is a blood and lymph *plasma* "protein." Excess albumin in urine says *"kidney trouble!* [See A/G ratio on page 113.] Carbamide is **"lost"** in urine—and some folks drink their urine to recover lost carbamide. This **ancient** practice **"SHOCKS"** the system and gets **GOOD** results—but few people are willing to use the procedure unless they are "dying!"

Urine tells a story. If you drink plenty of water, it should be straw colored between meals and bright yellow after meals. The doctor usually wants a urine sample from the first urination of the day. The first urination is usually dark with strong odor and cloudy. Failure to drink enough water will give a similar effect. Too much table salt and a bio-junk diet and poor digestion compounds the problem. If you sweat heavily and don't offset fluid and electrolyte loss, strong, dark colored urine appears—and urination may even be painful!

[Go on a "strict" three-day, fresh lemon juice, honey/ maple syrup and cayenne pepper fast! The first urination on the second day will be **extremely** *dark. Collect it in a small "clear" bottle and set on a shelf and it will form dark brown diamond shaped CRYSTALS of plasma protein waste byproducts—such as uric acid. Read The Miracle of Fasting and Your Own Perfect Medicine. See Source Page 400.]*

Kidneys & "Heart" Connection
The blood is filtered by the kidney's nephrons at the rate of 250 gallons a day or 1000 quarts every 24 hours. A weak liver is unable to do its job and filter-out blood-borne wastes— greatly burdening the heart and causing kidney "overload!"

Build-up of amyloid tissue waste and a sluggish lymph system is the perfect old age recipe!

When you hear of someone with congestive heart failure, **"KNOW"** that their heart muscle is growing **"weak"** and "tissue-bound" amyloid waste is "holding" water. A sluggish lymphatic system and poor kidney overload go with the territory as the lungs **"fill"** with **excess** fluid—and eventually the sick person slowly "suffocates!" [Congestive heart failure **IS** a very **nice** way to die. In the old days the condition was called *"dying of old age!"*] Congestive heart failure is **NOT** a dis-ease. It can be reversed if the body terrain is restored "quickly!" Total cooperation of the individual is needed—along with a very strong will to live. *"A horse cannot be made to drink!"*

God is more inclined to answer prayers when people take charge of their lives and do their part.

The Bowel
When we are young and healthy, we experience good bowel movements because bile flow is strong, muscle tone is good, and we get lots of exercise. But, as we grow older the story changes—and so does our health! Visit a doctor who thinks "basic" and one of the first questions he will ask is ""*How often do you move your bowels?"* Your answer tells a story.

The word *bowel* comes from the French and Latin. It means *sausage* [intestines resemble sausage]. Next time the question is asked, your response should be *"I move my sau-*

sage, ..." Better yet, **stay away** from doctors!

Freud said we are obsessed by **defecation** in our early years of development. He called it the "Anal Stage." Gandhi was once described as a man who had been "over potty trained." Perhaps great people are "anal retentive?"

Even Lawrence Welk had a thing with constipation. He pushed a laxative on his show. The laxative company had a smart marketing team. They knew that people over age 40 were the **"target"** audience! Today, the target audience is anyone over five years. Bowel and digestion problems are liver problems! [See pages 46, 69, 150, 178-180, 195, 240, 318, and 234.]

High Enema Therapy™ • Fever • Illness

Water has many uses besides drinking and bathing. It can be used to break fevers, relieve constipation, cleanse the colon, and stimulate flow-bile from the liver. The first thing mom did when we children were sick was to give us an enema and "empty" the lower bowel. It worked well!

[In 1983 your author pushed himself too hard and became very ill with the flu. My temperature reached 106⁰ F. I was in serious trouble! At two in the morning all I could think of was to crawl into the bathtub and turn on the cold water. It didn't help! In desperation, I gave myself a warm water "enema" and emptied my lower bowel. Within 15 minutes the fever dropped to 100⁰ F and I recovered quickly!]

Hemorrhoids • Constipation • Prostate • Acid Reflux

Hemorrhoids and appendicitis are first cousins—as are colitis and diverticulitis and acid-reflux! Each sets up house for the other. Constipation [less than 3 bowel movements per day] underwrites these miserable conditions. Poor bile-flow and a messed-up liver are **"THE"** central issues!

Adequate water intake insures a soft, moist stool—and without it the stool is hard and dry. Dietary fiber holds water—making defecation easier—and acts as an intestinal broom.

A hemorrhoid is an engorged, swollen rectal vein—and people have all kinds of crazy ideas about them. Bottom line, hemorrhoids result from insufficient hydration, poor bile-flow, constipation and **"failure"** to get into the native "squat" position when defecating on the toilet!

To solve the hydration issue, drink 2 **BIG** glasses of water with racemized™ sea minerals immediately upon rising! Then, at each urination, drink water and minerals. Frequent urination "robs" you of bowel activity. A full bladder puts **pressure** on the colon, stimulates peristalsis, and produces the gas and cramps associated with a bowel movement. Also, eat plenty of raw vegetables, apples and dried prunes, get adequate exercise, drink lots of Kombucha tea, and use Colon

Prep Formula™ and Yucca Blend™ to increase bile-flow!
50% of men between 35 and 50 years of age have **sub-clinical** prostate issues. Eventually every man deals with this "male" issue. Obesity, underhydration and poor diet are factors as are dysfunctional liver, hormonal imbalance, constipation, and lack of essential fatty acids. [A backed-up bowel pushes against the prostate allowing bacteria **to migrate** into the prostate and create inflammation and swelling called *prostatitis.*]
An enlarged, hardened prostate is the male "equivalent" of thyroid problems in woman. Men who **fail** to expell semen regularly have far more problems. Older men are known for "dribbling" when urinating. They can't "make water!"
When a man is young, all he thinks about is making love. In his middle years, all he thinks about is making money. When he becomes OLD, all he thinks about is making water!
Become *Young Again* and you can have it all!

PREVIEW: *In our next chapter you will learn how to take better care of your teeth and gums, and save thousands of dollars in dental bills. You will also learn how to feel good!*

Fix The Problem!

Men who want to "fix" their prostate will cooperate and do High Enema Therapy™ and take R/Prostate 1 & ll. They will also learn how to "milk" their prostate—at home in a hot bath—the same way that you "milk" the gallbladder! These days, young men as early as age 32 are "suffering" and it gets worse the older you get—unless you do something to change the "script!" Surgery—by knife or laser—is a crummy option—and very high risk, too! So what's it going to be, fellas? Prostate is a "terrain" issue! [See pages 77, 99, 105, 159, 185 and 292.]

Stones & Nails

"Stones" in the gallbladder and "nails" in the liver are "calcified" waste material removed from the blood by the liver—waste that "stagnates" instead of leaving the body every day so the body will not turn overly "acid!" [See pages 245 and 343.]

CRP & A/G Ratio

"C" Reactive Protein (CRP) measures "infection" without "fever"—as in "infected" teeth and prostate. Ideal score: "0." A/G Ratio measures where you are "at" between birth and death. [Scale: 1.0—2.32; the higher the better!] Most folks are 1.25—1.6. Your author is at 2.32—and it took 8 years to get there! [See pages 179 and 296.]

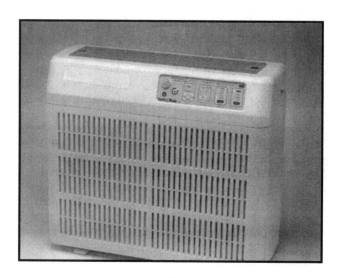

BFRV™ "Home & Office" Air Processor

There are **TWO** things that **"dominate"** daily life. One is the quality of the air we breathe—and the other is our choice of drinking water. Your author considers **both** air and water to be major "terrain" management "factors" for a healthy life.

The BFRV™ Air Processor fulfills the terrain management concepts of the *Young Again! Protocol*™ as outlined in this book. **Look what a BFRV™ air processor does.**

• Stage 1: Filters particulates out of air.
• Stage 2: Absorbs toxic chemical off-gases.
• Stage 3: Hospital-grade HEPA filter removes allergens.
• Stage 4: Oxidizes and absorbs "acidic" ambient air waste.
• Stage 5: Germicidal & ultraviolet destruction of microbes.
• Stage 6: Photo-Catalytic Oxidation for "absolute" air quality.

The BFRV™ Air Processor is absolutely "effective" on circulating in-house air pollutants—and it is very economical to own. Considering how much time people spend "indoors," "healthy" air has profound "health" implications.

Your author has **never before** offered an air "processor" with the quality BFRV™ trademark. This extremely high-tech, economical unit is a 21st Century solution to a very old problem affecting people's lives and "terrains!" Terrain management includes the water we drink **AND** the air we breathe!

Specifications: Dimensions: 22" x 18" x 8." Weight: 23 lbs. Air Flow: 400 cfm free; 265 cfm loaded. 110v. Warranty: 2 years.

[See Source Page 400 for your Source Packet!]

12

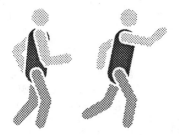

I Feel Good

"Stress is like a chicken. It always comes home to roost!"
John Thomas

We describe the way we feel in terms of black and white. *"I feel good!" "I'm sick!"* People don't like shades of *gray* when it comes to the way they feel.

If we substitute the word *aerobic* for good and *anaerobic* for sick, our descriptions shift from black and white to *gray*. Our words no longer *appear* to carry the same meaning, but they do help us better understand **WHY** we feel *good* or *sick*.

Breathing • Respiration

When we are **aerobic,** we are "with air." When we are **anaerobic,** we are "without air." Both of these states of being are influenced by the way we breathe.

Shallow breathing encourages the accumulation of wastes in the tissues and accelerates aging, while deep breathing causes the body to shed its wastes and rejuvenate itself.

Shallow breathing creates an oxygen-starved body, windedness, low energy and poor focus. Deep breathing produces an oxygen surplus, endurance, high energy and a steely focus. Breathing is central to the yoga experience.

Exercise and strenuous activity promote deep breathing and endurance. Endurance **implies** that a person is in an "aerobic" state—mentally and physically.

"Respiration" takes place on two levels: external and internal. **External** respiration is somewhat of a mechanical process that occurs in the lungs—while **internal** respiration is more esoteric; it takes place in the cells.

The exchange of carbon dioxide (CO_2) and oxygen (O_2) in the lungs is called external respiration. The exchange of CO_2 and O_2 at the cellular level is called internal respiration. Both processes are of great importance.

Glucose [Blood sugar!] is burned [Oxidized!] at the

cellular level within the electron transport chain of the mitochondria. The production of the energy molecule "ATP" is **WHY** we eat food and drink water. Food should produce energy! 40% of our energy *should* derive from fats and oils; 40% from proteins, and the balance from carbohydrates. How efficiently these energy "sources" are processed depends on the "terrain!'

Clinical vs. Subclinical

Aging occurs at the cellular level **BEFORE** it appears in the mirror. We "see" aging on the physical —Third Dimension level—but we need to understand "aging" as an energy "concept" rooted in other "dimensions." Aging **transcends** the Third Dimension where we live out our lives.

Doctors use "observable" **SIGNS** to diagnose dis-ease because they are *clinical* proof. Symptoms are **not** observable—but they are **sub**clinical **evidence** that things are amiss.

When you are *clinically* ill, you are usually under a doctor's care, in the bed or perhaps in a hospital. **Clinical illness is OFFICIAL!** "Clinical" means you are in trouble! The doctor uses **SIGNS** to conjure a "diagnosis," moving the patient from "**sub**clinical" to **clinical** status. [People **"THINK"** they go to the doctor to find out what is wrong with them—when they really want to know "what" to do to regain control of their lives. There is a **"disconnect"** in the doctor/patient relationship!]

Subclinical illness is the "occult" or hidden stage of dis-ease—and takes place at the *subtle-energy level* of our existence. It is a *gray* state of being—often described as *"Feeling a little off!"* People tend to ignore these "off" feelings—hoping they will go away. In time, however, symptoms give way to **SIGNS**—and an official diagnosis from the doctor.

*[Most people live out their lives at the **sub**clinical level— in the twilight zone **between** true health and official dis-ease. At the **sub**clinical level, abnormal is normal and black and white become blurred among shades of gray!]*

Aerobic/Anaerobic Microbes

Aerobic and *anaerobic* "states of being" influence health and dis-ease. The *aerobic* state is a *right-spin* condition, while the **anaerobic** state is a *left-spin* condition. These energy "states" dictate the **type** of microbe (bacteria, virus, yeast or fungus) that **develops, inhabits** and **prospers** in the "terrain!"

Pathogenic microbes LOVE an anaerobic environment. They are blamed for causing dis-ease, but they are blamed unfairly . The microbes are only actors fulfilling their assigned roles—roles dictated by our chosen lifestyles and the "state" of our terrains.

If we dissect the word pathogenic, we get: *path*-suffering, disease; *gen*-producing, giving rise to; *ic*-pertaining to.

When a condition is described as "pathogenic"—it displays certain **"agreed-upon" SIGNS** that elevate the situation to "clinical" status. Pathogenic conditions are "morbid" conditions—hence the term *morbidity*—as used in life insurance company morbidity tables to predict death rates among a population. A *pathologist* is a specialist in *pathology*, which is the study of the nature of dis-ease; its causes, processes, effects and alterations of tissue structure and function.

Microbes And The Terrain
Microbes "change" form according to the environment of the host's terrain. Hence, they are referred to as "poly" or "pleo" morphic because they "adapt" to their environment and only "appear" to be different species of organisms—medical opinion to the contrary not withstanding!

The bio-electric body depends upon non-pathogenic "aerobes" to maintain peak health. **Aerobes** are non-pathogenic bacteria that **LIKE** an oxygen **RICH** environment. Stressed acid-waste filled terrain environments cause aerobes to "mutate"—and become **an**aerobic organisms that prefer oxygen-**less** environments, [The prefix **an** means "without!"] or "facultative" **an**aerobes that can **tolerate** oxygen—but don't require it. A sluggish or constipated bowel is "freindly" to **an**aerobes—and pathogenic microbes take full advantage of it!

When "aerobes" morph into "**an**aerobes," they turn against and **ATTACK** the host—you and me! Included here are bacteria, viruses, yeast and fungi—all of which live in the blood, which is **NOT** a sterile medium as believed by "experts!" These organisms are forever **PRESENT** in the terrain—"waiting" only for a signal to trigger proliferation and take over of the terrain!

From the moment of conception, our blood carries the SEEDS of our own destruction!

Microbes common to the human body include *staphylococcus* —an **aerobe** often involved in skin infections; *andclostridium* —a facultative **an**aerobe that produces **en**terotoxins [*Entero*: related to toxins of intestinal origin; clostridium is responsible for deadly botulism]; *E. coli* is a very "good" colon facultative **an**aerobe—but one that kills when in "pathogenic" form! The job of pathogenic life forms is to **"attack"** and **"remove"** weak organisms from the Earth. Circulation of blood and lymphatic fluids is central to waste management. The heart "pumps" blood—but lymphatic fluids only circulate through movement, stretching and exercise. [The L/CSF™ machine circulates body "fluids!" See pages 107, 132-3, 160, 195, 261 and 382.]

Cavities • Dental Plaque
Cavities and periodontal "oral" conditions like gingivi-

tis, pyorrhea and bleeding gums indicate pathogenic activity—and a very **acid** body terrain! Streptococcus "mutens" bacteria secrete a protective substance to shield themselves from air [oxygen] while they dissolve tooth enamel. These facultative bacteria **create** and **control** their own environment so they can do their dirty work—and they **NEED** an **acid** saliva environment to do it! Teeth "become" a **MAJOR** issue—sooner or later! [Use a Bio-Magnetic™ dental irrigator and Oral Advantage to avoid and treat pathogenic "oral" conditions! [See pages 51 (photo), 79, 149, 187, 204, 233 & 329-30 and 351.]

[The Young Again Protocol™ deacidfies an acid terrain by dissolving and moving soluble acid wastes out of the body fat beneath the skin and down the toilet. Reduce acid waste levels in the terrain and you eliminate dental problems.]

[When the hygienist removes "plaque" from the teeth, she is "altering" the bacteria's anaerobic environment. But cleaning does NOT stop new plaque from building-up again. In time, you must return and repeat the process.]

[Some hygienists and dentists coat the teeth with plastic to discourage bacteria from "etching" tooth enamel and creating cavities. If utilized as soon a child gets their adult teeth, 98% of decay issues can be avoided for an entire lifetime! Coating the teeth only works if used early-on!]

Equip your home with a bio-magnetic irrigator and you will save a fortune in dental bills. The irrigator also works on your dog's teeth—that is with the animal's own cleaning tip! Veterinarians charge $150 + to clean an animal's teeth. [Your author went over 8 years without need of teeth or root "cleanings!" Here's how the dental irrigator works—and why every family should be own one.

Magneto-Hydro-Dynamics

Dental plaque is the "coating" secreted by bacteria to insulate themselves. Plaque has a negative (-) electrical charge on its surface—as do decay—creating bacteria!

When hydrogen ions are "freed" from the H_2O water molecule, they have a positive (+) "charge" that is the exact **"opposite"** electrical "charge" of dental plaque and associated bacteria. [Please review the diagram on page 79.]

The Bio-magnetic™ Irrigator uses magneto-hydro-dynamics™ (MHD)™ to keep teeth and gums healthy. MHD produces "free" hydrogen ions (H+) that "react" with negatively charged (-) plaque and bacteria as the "(+)" charged hydrogen protons wash against the culprits—**oxidizing** the bacteria's and plaque's negatively charged protective surfaces. It does this by **"STEALING"** electrons—a process referred to as **"oxidation!"** When plaque loses its "protective shield" the bacteria disappear! "Pic-type" dental devices are nothing but fancy squirt guns—whereas a Bio-Magnetic™ dental irrigator uses therapeutically "charged" water for a superior dental care!

[The process just described is an electrical event not unlike the rusting of iron or disappearance of aluminum window screens in a salty, ocean air environment. Transference of electrons is the name of the game. Medical Grade Ionized Water™ also involves the transfer of electrons.]

Magneto-Hydro-Dynamics™ is a blend of vibrational medicine and technology! Do **NOT** expect your friendly dentist's office to tell you about this device. The industry will lose revenue if people realize they can care for their teeth and gums without them!

The smell of decay between the teeth disappears when you use the dental irrigator daily.

Birds Of A Feather "FLOCK" Together

Dis-ease is the **"expression"** of negative energy dominance! Contrary to conventional thought, "like" energy attracts "like" energy. The sick body becomes **SICKER** unless action is taken to change the "terrain" and break the cycle!

Low "vitality" indicates a negative energy "state" of being—and a "negative" energy body terrain **"ACTIVATES"** pathogenic microbes that "feed" on acidic, tissue-boundwaste energy. An acid body **CANNOT** restore itself until wastes are "purged" from the system. The **LIVER** is the **"door"** out of the body for 90% of waste flow. Bile is the "transport" vehicle!

Deacidification of the terrain is AS fundamental to restoration of health as good food and water. Believe it!

The *terrain* of the *bio-electric* body dictates the **EFFECT** that food and water produce. The "terrain"—**NOT** the microbes—determines **when, where** and **how** dis-ease manifests itself. "Tuning-in" to your *bio-electric* **terrain** is a "proxy" for resetting your bio-electric **clock!**

Stress & Attitude

Put a person under mental or physical stress and dis-ease will **"take form"**—not because of the presence of microbes and "bugs"—but because stress is an *energy condition* that caters to pathogenic life forms that need an **"acid"** environment to do their job. Stress **IS** negative acid energy! Stress **always** seeks an outlet—and it chooses the **course of least resistance** to express itself. The healthier the "terrain," the less affect stress has on the body and the more resistance pathogenic organisms face. **The terrain controls!**

Stress "attacks" old injury sites and settles into areas where there is weakness! Conditions like hepatitis, chronic fatigue, leaky-gut, asthma, arthritis, lupis, MS, fibromyalgia are **antagonized** by stress. Dis-ease only "seems" to appear out of nowhere. Dis-ease is a "terrain" issue!

Stress of "any" kind impacts the adrenal glands—causing them to produce **EXCESS** cortisol. Cortisol puts the body into "overdrive" and devastates women's hormonal balance! Life today in 2006 is so stressful that people live in quasi-permanent **"OVERDRIVE!"** They are **NOT** able to "unwind" at the end of each day—or during the sleep cycle. So they "wake up" in **overdrive**—tired and stressed-out from yesterday—as they prepare for more stress today! Stress is the ultimate "wild card"—and its affects on woman's hormones is devastating. **STRESS** is the absolute worst factor in modern day life! Burn-out and physical collapse are the product of **EXCESS** stress!

Stress affects conditions like diabetes, lupis, fibromyalgia, Alzheimers and MS because all have hormonal "links" to deterioration of the "neurilemma" (myelin "sheath" protecting the nerve fibers). Deterioration of Schwann's cell activity at the "synapses" along nerve axons is **BOTH** a terrain and a hormonal issue. Behind the deterioration is an **"ACID"** terrain! [See synapse drawing on page 248.]

Schwann's cells are responsible for keeping the receptor sites open for nerve signal Transmission. Maintenance of these specialized cells is crucial to good health— especially in women over age 35.

People "handle" stress when they are "under fire"—but when the heat is "off," illness erupts and settles the score. Weight gain is very much a stress issue. Thoughts and attitude affect health—but attitude "alone" **cannot** overcome physical issues rooted in an **"acidic"** terrain. **Excess** cortisol levels go with suffering and adrenal **"burn-out!"** [PU™ **de-**stresses the system and gets the body **"OUT"** of overdrive! CWD™ is used to control blood sugar "swings!" "Low enema" therapy done morning and evening keeps the lower bowel empty and gets the "bile" out of the body. Dump the bile and you **automatically** "de-stress" the system.]

*[As an aside, when on the verge of a **complete** nervous breakdown and collapse, retire to a **completely dark room void of all light** for 48 hours. Sleep, do enemas, take PU,™ fast and allow the body to "reset" itself **before** emerging!]*

Dark Territory: Fever!

There are two kinds of "clinical" conditions: localized and systemic. A localized condition is specific to one area, while a systemic condition has the **WHOLE** body under siege. Systemic symptoms are things like vomiting, loose-bowels, rubber-legs, chills, fever, horrid gas and severe cramping.

Fever is the body's reaction to a major **terrain** "assault!" Contrary to popular belief, fever serves a useful purpose by killing pathogenic organisms **breeding** and **feeding** on mucous congestion and tissue acid waste in the body. Fever is a hyper (elevated) *thermogenic* (*thermo:* heat-producing; *gen:* origin of; *ic:* pertaining to) condition. Fever is the **EFFECT!** Antibiotics are useful against bacterial infections—but worthless against viruses. Even when antibiotic use is justified, there is a short-term/long-term trade-off! Better to use High Enema Therapy™ and deal with illness **BEFORE** a high fever occurs or antibiotics are required. "Post" antibiotic use calls for use of R/C™ and MZ™ to repair damage to the gut wall.

[MX™ is the Young Again™ answer to mucous congestion for ear ache, sinus and lungs. MX™ is modified DNA that causes mucous to "flow" and deny microbes a "breeding ground." MX™ is not a drug. Mucous is one way the body expels waste. Mucous congestion occurs when acid waste levels **overload** *the terrain. Clear Head™ is used to kill and destory microbial overgrowth in the sinus cavities for instant releif.]*

If fever is not allowed to go above 106⁰ degrees, it will **de**nature and destroy bacterial and viral "proteins." [The sick person must be kept fully hydrated and fluid electrolyte levels must be maintained with racemized™ sea minerals.]

[Drop the contents of a raw egg into boiling water and the egg "protein" will change form—becoming firm and solid. This is what a febrile (fever-producing) condition does to proteins of **pathogenic** *organisms. Fever alters* **protein** *enzymes and structure—causing pathogenic organisms to die.]*

[Historically, society has held strange views about the nature of fever over the years. For example, at the time of the American Revolution, people associated body lice with health. When fever got too high, the lice would leave and the person usually died. People came to associate the presence of lice with health. Lice = life. No lice = death. This is a good example of faulty thinking based on a faulty "model" which perpetuates an endless cycle of misery and dis-ease!]

High Enema Therapy™ is direct, physical intervention for restoring balance to the terrain.

Muscle Tone
When mineral **electrolyte** levels "collapse"—as in heat stroke or heat exhaustion—the effect is **similar** to the effects produced by microbial infection. Fever depletes mineral electrolytes responsible for maintaining **muscle tone.**

"Tone" allows us to maintain position and form. Without tone, we would be like a jellyfish. "Tone" of the connective tissues also affects vital organ function—and the vital organs are "vital!" These organs [heart, brain, lungs, liver, kidneys, pancreas, etc.) receive their orders from the ***involuntary*** parasympathetic nervous system and the **voluntary** central nervous nervous system. Acupuncture, reflexology, chiropractic and High Enema Therapy™ *stimulate* vital organ activity by stimulating nerve-evergy **"flow."** "Tone" is very much a terrain issue affecting health and longevity. Exercise and hard physical work help maintain tone—as does terrain **de**acidification.

Medications

Drug usage is **"chemotherapy"** without the **nuclear** word attached! Drugs "alter" vital organ function and accelerate aging. Drugs are **NOT** safe! All drugs have **"known"** side effects as detailed in the "fine print" and verbal warnings on TV. Drugs are prescribed and justified on the same basis as chlorination and fluoridation of public water supplies and the spraying of food crops with "known" poisons.

If the "hoped-for" benefit outweighs the "supposed" known risks—drugs will be prescribed based on what the medical folks call "the standard of care."

What is **NEVER** talked about is the long-term "toxic" effects of drugs on the vital organs. **Contra**indications associated with pharmaceutical drugs as listed in drug *reference* manuals and on product literature is enough to cause any thinking person to **"opt out"** of the conventional medical approach and go "alternative!" Medical care should be sought when life and death is the issue. Otherwise, why put yourself in harm's way with drugs that carry **"WARNINGS"**?

"New" drugs are pushed by the pharmaceutical companies to replace drugs whose patents have expired. New drugs are **MORE** expensive and generally come with ever increasing **RISK!** People "differentiate" between *prescription* drugs and illegal drugs—but there is little difference between them! Drugs devastate liver function by compromising the **hepatocytes.** They do violence to the kidney **nephrons** (filters). These "functional" cells and tissues perform thousands of biochemical reactions necessary for maintaining a healthy **"terrain!"**

The Young Again Protocol™ avoids drug use by eliminating the need to resort to them.

Staying Healthy Until You Die!

Good health and longevity dictate that we live our lives in harmony with nature so we will have **NO** need of "drugs!"

Do you know anyone who has suffered from the side effects of drug therapy, or maybe someone who walked into the hospital or clinic for testing and was carried out—feet first? Apply the lessons in this book and you won't need the medical system—and you will **NOT** become a medical statistic, either!

A dis-eased body is under "siege!" A healthy liver is **fundamental** to health, and **any** treatment modality—conventional or alternative—that fails to restore **LIVER** function, increase **bile flow** and **de**acidification of the terrain is **DOOMED** from the start. [Remember, 90% of the waste exiting the body is contained in the "bile"—and if bile-flow is not increased, the body is forced to "store" the waste in the fatty tissues.]

High Enema/Colon Irrigation Therapy

An enema is a "quick"—but incomplete—version of a colonic. A colonic is a DEEP enema. This book will only refer to High Enema Therapy™ **(HET)** since the bureaucrats seem to think they "own" the word "colon."

Properly executed High Enema Therapy™ avoids the aging problems associated with sluggish bowels—which is just about every **clinical** and **sub**clinical condition known!

One very interesting bowel issue is when the ileocecal valve becomes **"LOCKED"** in the "open" position. [The *Young Again (Tissue and Liver) Protocol*™ causes the ileocecal valve to restore itself.]

People with cancer usually have their ileocecal valve "locked" in the OPEN position.

The ileocecal valve **CONTROLS** fecal movement between the small and large intestine—as well as orchestrating digestion and absorption of food energy. The valve is located inside the cecum which is the fist-sized pouch from which the appendix "dangles," six feet up from the anus.[See page 46.]

Properly executed HET causes the body to release the **"chocolate pudding."** The pudding is the "stuff" of old age and dis-ease; its the stuff that feeds cancer! All bowel waste enters the colon by way of the *ileocecal valve.* The small intestine ["gut!"] **ends** and the large intestine ["colon!"] **begins** at the cecum—extending six feet to the anus. [See page 46.]

HET stimulates peristaltic activity and increases bile-flow from the liver and gallbladder while stimulating the nerve complex flowing from the intestinal wall to the vital organs. An enema is **NOT** a substitute for High Enema Therapy™—but enemas are very useful when traveling or where bathroom space is cramped or when a **"quickie"** is needed and there is not enough time or energy to do HET. [The *Young Again*™ Enema Kit is the perfect answer. See pages 70, and 399.]

HET equipment is **NOT** expensive and it is the **ultimate** health management tool. Your author has used the same equipment for 30 years! The *Young Again! Protocol* ™ calls for HET 2 times a week for **life!** [Some people consider HET to be "unnatural"—but it's better and less expensive than losing control of your life!

Begin today and you will **SHOUT** "I feel good!"—as you become *Young Again!*

PREVIEW: Our next chapter deals with the HIV virus and the connection between "weeds" and viruses.

Cancer

Cancer is no different than other dis-ease "conditions" in that if you **re**create the conditions in your body that caused it to appear the first time, it will **come back** to haunt you. Cancer is a "terrain" issue. It is **NOT** something you "catch!" Like malaria, hepatitis and other "liver" conditions, cancer just has a different name. The price that each of us must be willing to pay to avoid major dis-ease is **"ETERNAL VIGILANCE!"** Give your body the opportunity to show you what it can do!

Body Fluid Circulation

Circulation of body fluids is dependent upon physical move-ment, exercise, activity and work. Lymph and cerebral spinal fluids **must** circulate or the body grows "old!" One of the best ways to circulate these fluids without "exercise" is to use the L/CSF™ machine. [See pages 107, 132, 160, 195, 261 and 382.]

The Golden Years!

"The 'golden years' have come at last! I cannot see; I cannot pee; I cannot chew; I cannot do; my memory shrinks; my hearing stinks; no sense of smell; I look like hell; my body's drooping; got trouble pooping. The 'golden years' have come at last!" The "golden years" come **earlier** than they used to—and *"They are NOT golden!"* Aging is the *nice way* of describing the ultimate dilemma. Having **"control"** of one's health **IS** as golden as it gets! Apply the lessons in this book and you will realize your wishes and enjoy a golden, healthy future, too!

People & Pets

Dogs and cats are people with "four legs." They suffer from the same problems that humans do—and their bodies respond and rejuvenate similarly, too! Because pets live shorter lives, they age and respond faster than do humans to simple lifestyle and dietary changes. Hormone issues are part of animal aging and longevity as they are in humans. Acid "excess" destroys animal health—and the animal liver fails just like the human liver. Animals get fat and go down to diabetes, arthritis, heart attack, stroke and cancer—just like humans do! Treat your pets like you would treat yourself with the following items: Pac's, R/C,™ racemized™ algae, liver, Yucca Blend™—and racemized™ sea minerals in their water. It's easier to keep pets—and people—"healthy" than it is to restore their "terrain" late in the game. **Tip:** watch for **SIGNS** and symptoms. Pets depend on us!

➥ *If your author can practice what's in this book, so can you! All it takes is some effort!*

Statistics & Palliation

It's difficult to discuss "health" with people who have been schooled in the scientific method. It's not that they are anti-health—they are not! Rather, their world is built upon medical statistics and studies. Theirs is a world of numbers— numbers that prove something is or isn't so. The *passwords* into their world are "statistics show" and "scientific proof."

Medical science sees dis-ease in terms of single issues demanding single answers—based on "findings." Medical science demands that "health-minded" people play their statistical **game** or suffer ridicule for *"No scientific proof!"*

Anyone with a lick of sense knows that you must take care of yourself or good health falters and dis-ease results. Health minded people know that nourishing food, drinking plenty of water, getting exercise and rest, entertaining positive thoughts, keeping the bowels open and the "bile" flowing—and doing the things discussed in this book can greatly improve one's quality of life. **"Our" PROOF is *healthy* human beings that don't need a doctor or the 'sick care' system!**

Medical science sees "health" as a numbers game. Their game is designed to keep the public confused by dazzling them with skewed studies and statistical gymnastics. **"Their" PROOF is millions of subclinically sick people who *bear witness* to medicine's "findings."**

Palliation lends itself to the numbers game called "statistics." *Palliation* [See page 23.] is a powerful tool of *manipulation* in the hands of medical science. *Palliation* allows science to state its case in the short run with **little risk** that the public will ever discover that they have been "duped!"

Medical science **KNOWS** the risks that accompany drug usage. However, drugs provide credibility and "scientific proof." Without tools of manipulation—like statistics and studies—medical science cannot maintain its **"strangle hold"** on the people, and the endless flow of money will **CEASE!**

Health-minded people do not live in fear of medical science's statistics and studies. Rather, we **ignore** them—for their **game** is an exercise in futility. We enjoy health and vitality by living according to nature's way. Nature rewards our efforts with **PEAK** health *instead* of statistics and illness.

Health-minded people measure results in years YOUNG. "My" goal is 250 years YOUNG! How about "you?"

Reality!

Food additives and colorings have the same effect as rogue, zeno estrogens found in the environment. Turn these harmful molecules "loose" in the body, crank up the heat and pressure of daily life along with a poor diet, and you have the perfect recipe for dis-ease! Failure to understand the rules of the game means loss of health and the realization that money is **NOT** enough to recover your health in the "sick care" system!

BFRV™ Water

➡ **Please Note:** The BFRV™ trademark replaces the *"abandoned"* BEV acronym, **DUE TO ongoing infringement and *"bootlegging"*** by individual(s) offering water processing equipment under the "pretense" their equipment fulfills the "terrain" management **CONCEPTS** of the *Young Again Protocol™*.

Consider these points about BFRV™ water:
•BFRV™ water promotes cellular metabolism. Its molecules cause the body to "dump" cellular waste and fuels mitochondrial production of the high energy molecule "ATP" within the electron transport chain of the mitochondria.

•BFRV™ water is a naturally potent biological solvent of body wastes and toxins.

•BFRV™ water stops the flow of waste minerals, trihalomethanes, bacteria, viruses, chlorine, chloramines, fluorides and toxic chemical wastes into the body.

•BFRV™water is very aggressive and acts as a liquid magnetic transport medium to the tissues and cells.

•BFRV™ water effectively hydrates the tissues due to its bonding angles, conception point "ORP" and low resistivity. It's ORP is very close to where the egg and sperm were when life was conceived [Please study diagram on page 306.]

•BFRV™ water uses the homeopathic principles of *resonance* and *transference* to bring "life" into the body.

•BFRV™ water-processing units do not require electricity and there are no elements to clean.

•BFRV™ water helps maintain control of body "terrain"—and its enjoyable to drink, too! Non-water drinkers become water drinkers with their very first glass!

•BFRV™ water is the ultimate biologically friendly drinking water and is the basis of Medical Grade Ionized Water.™ [See Chapter 11 and pages 71, 220, 306 and 400.]

Alzheimers!

Alzheimers is "old-age autism!" Alzheimers dis-ease should be **THE** household topic! Sadly, the medical folks don't have a clue about **HOW** to **"prevent"** it. As of 2005, 4 million people in the USA suffer from progressive mental deterioration and memory loss—and three out of four are women! [There **IS** a hormone "connection" in the Alzheimers story.] By 2010, 100 million will succumb. **Prevention** is the issue! Don't allow yourself to slip away. [See pages 173, 177, 374 and Chapters 36 and 37.]

Warning!

After age 40, men suffer from depression, loss of muscle mass, impotence, low sex drive, pot belly, loss and thinning of hair and low energy. It's called "male menopause," guys—and what you do about it is a very BIG DEAL! [More as we go along.]

13

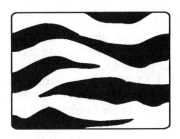

Viruses & Weeds

"There is no difference between plant and animal."
Dr. Guenther Enderlein, 1898

Medical science knows little about viruses. The average person knows almost nothing about them. Most folks think a virus is like a bacterium—a "bug" that you somehow "catch!"

Antibiotics hold **NO** power against viruses. If you are sick with a viral infection, "they" tell you to stay warm and drink lots of fluids. So much for the experts!

There is a better way to deal with viral infections! The **informed** person will perform High Enema Therapy™ and take MX™ to breaks up mucous and cause it to "flow!" The **informed** person uses Yucca Blend™ to increase bile flow; L_sP_cC™ and L_sP_cB™ to achieve "therapeutic" levels of vitamins B and C in the **blood stream** "without" need of an intravenous needle; and consumes fresh beet, carrot and celery juices [plus other vegetable juices as desired] daily, and eats low stress foods sparingly until recovery begins.

The informed person does NOT wait to be told to clean the bowel, restore bile flow, and flush the lungs, ears and sinuses of mucous waste—waste that provides the PERFECT breeding ground for viral and bacterial infections—and the misery that goes with it!

Colleges and medical schools do not see viruses for what they are. Viruses are poorly understood by the student and by instructors alike. **NOTHING** is taught about **where** viruses come from or **how** and **why** they proliferate. [Students are taught to *"sing!"* the party line—and that's about it!]

Viruses Today

We hear a lot about AIDS, influenza, herpes, hepatitis (A, B,C, D, & E), shingles and mononucleosis. These are **here and now** viral conditions afflicting millions of people.

Prevention is **always** the best approach to dis-ease—

viral or otherwise. The controlling "factor" before or after infection is the *"terrain!"* An acid, mucous-filled *terrain* is perfect for "opportunistic" viral outbreaks. The link between fringe life forms—like viruses—and aging is spelled **"terrain."**
The virus is an anomaly, a paradox and a slave master. It is the point man of nature's garbage crew. Science does NOT classify viruses as *life forms*—but they are NOT dead either. They are **OPPORTUNISTIC** organisms—as are bacteria. Create a suitable environment, lose control of the terrain—and viruses will **appear**, and **seize control** of cellular machinery as well as life at the *subtle energy* level.

Viruses are energy fields—and they have an energy *footprint*. A virus is a strand of either DNA (deoxyribonucleic acid) or RNA (ribonucleic acid) that is protected by a protein "capsule" or shield. Viruses exist in the **gray area** between living and non-living things—and can **neither** reproduce nor perform normal life functions on their own. Viruses are **entirely** dependent on energy generated **INSIDE** the cells of the host's body. Viruses are classified based on their composition (DNA or RNA), origin, mode of transportation, reproduction methods, and **where** they first break out in the host's body.

[Viruses are so small that "science" needs an electron microscope to view them—but only in a "dead" state. Seeing viruses "live" and "active" was overcome with a Nassens condensor microscope—but mainstream science ignores it!]

Because viruses are ubiquitous, there is **NO** avoiding them. But in a healthy body, viruses do **NOT** threaten the host because the "terrain" is unfriendly and they *cannot* gain access to cellular machinery. [Acid, mucous-filled terrains forfeit control and allow viruses to take over and proliferate.]

Mental and physical "stress" disrupts our energy fields, and the body's protective systems are **"sabotaged!"** The immune system is such a system and a waste laden terrain imposes "stress!" The immune system can overcome viral invasion if the "terrain" is restored. Getting rid of mucous and acid waste is KEY! [Plants respond to stress similarly. Healthy, nutritious, bug and dis-ease free crops are the product of a balanced "terrain" environment.]

Viruses—like their cousins bacteria and fungi—have a job to do. Their job is to rid the Earth of weak life forms, be they plant, animal or human!

HIV & AIDS

HIV (human immunodeficiency virus) is the virus associated with the manifestation of AIDS (Auto Immune Deficiency Syndrome). The HIV virus uses an enzyme called *reverse transcriptase* that allows it to infect the host *in reverse*. This is why HIV is called a **"retrovirus"** (*retro* means after the fact; in reverse). As the HIV virus mutates, it is given other names like HTLV 1, ll, or lll, etc. HTLV stands for human T-cell **lymphotrophic** virus. [Disected: **lymph**-plasma protein fluid scavenged from the tissue spaces by the lymphatic system; **troph**-a change or a turning; **ic**-pertaining to.] So a "lymphotrophic" virus causes a *change* **within** the **lymphatic** fluids and in the lymphatic system. *Cancer uses the lymphatic system to travel and to "metastasize" to other parts of the body.*

[The lymphatic system is central to aging and dis-ease Not all tissue fluids return to the blood via the lymphatic system. Fluid left behind is called "amyloid" fluid. In time, amyloid fluid "morphs" into amyloid "plaque" that is "structural" in nature—before morphing into SCAR tissue. The product VZ™ "eats" and "digests" amyloid tissue and returns it to a soluble fluid "state" so it can "exit" the body. Amyloid plaque is what "invades" the brain of Alzheimers patients. Amyloid is behind loss of hearing and vision, joint deterioration, aging skin and arthritic bodies. L_sP_cC™ works exactly the "opposite" of VZ™ by causing the body to lay-down massive amounts of new collagen—the structural foundation of the body's connective tissues [bones, ligaments, muscles, tendons, cartilage, skin and gums]. Without new collagen formation on a daily basis, the body grows old and "osteoporosis" and arthritis take over.]

The T-Cells

The HIV virus has an affinity for "T helper cells." These are lympho**cytes** that originate in the heart of the immune system—the thymus gland. *Cyte* means cell. So a "T" lymphocyte is a cell circulating in lymph fluid. Viruses wage war in the plasma proteins of the lymphatic system long **BEFORE** viruses appear in the blood—which explains why blood samples often test negative for the presence of HIV virus. As tissue plasma proteins "stagnate," the body's "defense system" shifts from right to left spin—causing the body to **"drop"** its defenses. [Once the body is in trouble, a bad diet, lack of sleep, insufficient water intake and poor bile-flow impose massive stress upon an already out-of-control "terrain!" The sick person who wants to recover **MUST** have a strong desire to "live!"]

AIDS Not A Virus

AIDS is not a virus. It is a *"syndrome"* of secondary "conditions" brought on by a **weakened** immune system. HIV is an **adeno**virus (*aden*—a cavity in the body). This class of viruses is **"OPPORTUNISTIC"** and takes advantage of a weakened "terrain." We do not die from AIDS, but from secondary complications like pneumonia. [Actually, we die when the mitochondria within the cells **fail** to produce sufficient ATP to keep us alive.] As HIV infects the system, a "syndrome" of problems called AIDS develops. Contrary to popular belief, AIDS is **not** a dis-ease of homosexual origin—though it is prevalent among gays. [The bureaucrats *lie* and disseminate *disinformation* to purposely keep the public confused.]

[People who suffer with viral infections—and other conditions like herpes, strep, STD's, hepatitis, athletes foot, pink eye, ring worm, fever blisters, insect bites, yeast infections, human papilloma virus (HPV), etc. find "relief" with Herpo-Max™, Yucca Blend,™ High Enema Therapy™ and Medical Grade Ionized Water.™ All of these are "terrrain" issues, and a sick liver and poor bile-flow are behind all of them!]

Sabotage

Retroviruses like "HIV" sabotage the cell's DNA and RNA genetic information base in order to redirect and siphon away the ATP "energy" molecule produced by the mitochondria. Once in control of the body's "energy" generating capabilities, viruses "morph" into virulent, pathogenic forms.

The virus' job is to kill the host and rid the Earth of weak organisms. Viruses are **NOT** the enemy! They and their cousins—the bacteria, fungi, and yeasts—are "present" the moment the egg and sperm join. They are polymorphic "mutant" life forms that **ONLY** morph into into their *"pathogenic form"* when the host loses control of the "terrain!"

Viral infection is *confirmation* things are not right and should **cause** the **THINKING** person to recognize that their terrain is *"au fait"* (favorable) for viral take-over. Viruses **only** attack people who are acid and toxic; who fail to eat live food; who do not digest well; and who have stressed livers and poor bile-flow and an acid, **an**aerobic "terrain!"

The *Young Again Protocol*™ **is designed to restore the terrain and give back control of your life!**

Blood NOT Sterile

Contrary to medical myth, blood is **NOT** a sterile medium. Medical science has perpetuated this mistruth in the face of *irrefutable* evidence to the contrary, as proved by Dr. Guenther Enderlein and Gaston Nassens over 100 years ago!

"All life contains the seeds of its own destruction WITHIN its own fluids."

That is what Dr. Enderlein meant when he said, *"There is NO difference between plants and animals."* He discovered that when the energy balance of the terrain is lost, the microbes **automatically** emerge **from** their "healthy" 3-stage **CLOSED** "loop" into a "21 stage" path leading directly to the grave yard.

The pharmaceutical companies and the medical system stand to lose trillions of dollars if the above information was taught in medical schools—something that will never happen! *Recognition that the blood is NOT sterile is tantamount to open refutation of the Germ Theory of Disease— and allopathic medicine knows it!* Pride and greed prevent medical science from "rescinding" its false theories. Millions of people have suffered and died needlessly because medicine labors under the shadow of lies and withheld information. As Christ said in Luke *"Woe be unto you lawyers, scribes, hypocrites, Pharisees; you hold the keys of knowledge; you yourself will not enter and you prevent those who would enter from entering."* Life was meant to be a celebration—not a requiem! Hosea said *"My people are destroyed for lack of KNOWLEDGE."*

Cellular Energy

Strong, positively charged cells and tissues are **NOT** affected by viruses. "Acidic" tissues are waste-stressed tissues in a **an**aerobic, compromised "state." Under these conditions, viruses take over the cell's "energy" machinery and replicate themselves for further advances throughout the body.

Rogue viruses *steal* the body's production of ATP and use the energy molecule to grow and form "cancer(s)." Cancer tumors and masses are **HUGE** fields of *negative* energy controlling all *metabolism* within their sphere of influence. [Please refer to page 307 for graphic understanding of this concept.] *Cancer viruses proliferate in a body where tissues are anaerobic, acid and loaded with sodium.*

An *anaerobic* body is an old body. Old bodies are unable to rejuvenate for lack of sufficient ATP production and **extreme** acid-waste overload. Dis-eases are "energy wars" and the bullets used are negative energy bullets. Conventional medicine's "magic bullets" are "futile!" The **PROOF** is all the dead and dying people! [Implementation of the *Young Again Protocol*™ **restores** the "terrain!"

Useful Forms of Oxygen

Hydrogen peroxide (H_2O_2) and "medical grade" ozone [triatomic oxygen or O_3] are useful products. Their effectiveness is related to the amount of available oxygen present and their molecular instability. Instability allows them to give up oxygen atoms freely. Oxygen is a highly magnetic element which accounts for the bent shape of the water molecules on page 79.

Oxygen therapy is useful in the treatment of cancer **masses** and **tumors.** Skilled healers sometimes inject H_2O_2 or O_3 directly into cancer masses with good results. Given intravenously or by water infusion in the rectum or vagina, ozone therapy can be effective—but requires *supervision!*

In the home, a "medical grade" ozone generator purifies

air and eases respiratory problems. Emphysema patients respond well to whole-house **ozone therapy**—partly due to ozone's ability to **OXIDIZE** toxic "off gassing" of airborne chemical molecules—and partly due to the elimination of microbial "breeding grounds"—like carpets and drapes!

Medical grade ozone destroys pathogenic molds, fungi, yeasts, dust mites and viruses and oxidizes [burns-up!] food supplies these organisms feed on. Cigarette odor disappears from clothes, house and car. These devices are GOOD protection against winter illness, too! Every home should have one!

Use "medical grade" ozone equipment only. Ozone in the **WRONG** molecular form irritates the mucous membranes of the sinus cavities and lungs. [See pages 188 and 196. For filtering of air particulates and microbial "spores" in the home, see the BFRV™ Air Processor shown on page 114.]

*[As noted earlier, the product MX™—a modified DNA formula—offers wonderful results on mucous congestion in the lungs, ears and sinuses of adults, children and pets. Best of all, it is **not** a drug! It causes mucous to break-up and "flow." High Enema Therapy™ is another effective congestion "tool."]*

Exercise & Viruses

Aerobic exercise is crucial to long-term good health. Exercise increases lymph and blood fluid circulation and raises plasma and cellular **oxygen** levels. Exercise revitalizes the body's organs by speeding deacidification of the tissues. **People who exercise regularly experience less sickness, too!**

Much has been written on the benefits of aerobic exercise. Recently, however, the press is parroting the idea that we don't need aerobic exercise. Equally bad are those who promote **hyper** aerobic [Think, "abusive!"] exercise. Ignore them all by seeking **moderation** and **balance** in your life. Good circulation is a prerequisite to good health. Blood and lymph movement reduces waste build-up in the system and creates an environment that is **HOSTILE** to pathogens. A "lymph roller" or L/CSF™ machine greatly improves fluid and tissue waste circulation. **Extreme "anything" translates: abuse!**

Rebounder

A rebounder [See page 382.] is a simple piece of health equipment available from most discount stores. The "correct" way to use a rebounder is to stand flat footed on the mat, gently swing both arms to the front and then the rear **"together"** as you add a little "flex" to your knees developing a slight "pulse" sensation in the head as you motion "up-and-down." Your feet should **NEVER** leave the mat. The "pulsing" sensation is produced by the movement of lymphatic fluids. The body depends on **MOVEMENT** to circulate lymph fluid—where the blood is "pumped" by the heart. [An L/CSF™ machine is FAR superior in every respect to a "rebounder" and can be used by elderly and bed-ridden patients, too! Simply lie down and relax. [See pages 107, 132-3, 160, 195, 261, 310, 382 and 385.]

Increased lymphatic circulation is pivotal in restoring hair, hearing and eyesight, and improving skin tone. "Movement" **prevents** stagnation of plasma protein wastes—particularly in the legs. Edema (water retention) is a **SIGN** of fluid "stagnation." Do **NOT** ignore it! Edema is influenced by bowel activity, bile flow, exercise, hormones, diet, a weak heart and acid waste overload. [Puffiness in women prior to a menstrual period is common and is not necessarily a health issue.]

The head receives 40% of waste laden arterial blood leaving the heart each time the heart "pumps!" Over time, the VERY fine capillaries of the scalp, eyes, and ears become clogged with amyloid plaque which brings on balding, gray hair, wrinkles, poor hearing and loss of vision.

*[After "rebounding" or an L/CSF™ workout, use the Biogenic™ body roller to stimulate subcutaneous nerves, break-up **cellulite** and circulate waste so the liver can remove it from the body. A hot bath with a cup of epsom salts is also very good. Kombucha Tea helps deacidify the body and is inexpensive to make at home. Many professional football and hocke players take a gallon of it to their games for increased energy and stamina. Your author drinks 2 gallons a week. It is good stuff if made correctly.]*

Viruses • Molds On Food

Have you noticed the vegetables and fruits from the store are growing strange molds and fungi? Molds tell a story. They are the lowest level of parasitic growth and their color indicates the toxicity level. White is the least toxic; red the most toxic; green, gray and black are in between. Fuzzy, smooth, and shiny tell a similar story. [Failure to rot says "irradiation!"]

The *experts* have been in charge of our food supply for a very long time. They have convinced the farmer to use hard chemical fertilizers, pesticides and herbicides—the latter two contain VERY potent "zeno" estrogen analogs that foul the planet and create "hormonal" complications for adults and children alike! [Read *Our Stolen Future;* see Source Page 400.]

The *experts* have upset nature's balance and—in so doing—have brought marginal health and dis-ease upon us all. People are aging faster and becoming **sub**clinically sick because they eat what the experts "call" food! These are the same *experts* whom Rachel Carson vilified in her 1959 blockbuster book, *Silent Spring.* The book is must reading if you want to better understand the nature of the dilemma we face. *Silent Spring* is more pertinent today than when it first appeared.

Fruit in grocery stores has little flavor because it contains few minerals and vitamins. Is it any wonder people are sick! The *experts* tell farmers to use chemicals to ward off bugs and weeds. The more they use, the worse the food quality! Nature will **NOT** be mocked—and mankind is paying the price!

Weeds & Aging

Look at the weeds! They proliferate in the face of voluminous amounts of herbicides. Each year, the weeds grow bigger. They are **mutating!** They have a job to do. They are getting ready.

Leonard Ridzon was a very savvy farmer. He was close to the Earth. He was a Wizard and one of the most original thinkers I have known. He authored *The Carbon Cycle* which is must reading. [See Source Page 400.]

Ridzon recorded ragweed over forty feet tall! Weeds are to the soil what pathogenic life forms are to the body. They proliferate and take over when the conditions are "ripe!" Weeds **appear** to be the problem, but they are only reacting to changes in the "terrain"—the soil and air in this case! Their job is to protect Mother Earth and to reclaim abused soil and air with the help of the microbes. The weed's job is to **absorb** toxic energy in the atmosphere and soil and make it "available" so the microbes can break-it-down and return the soil and air to a healthy "state."

Weeds are not plants out of place. The proliferation of noxious weeds is no more an accident than the molds and fungi on our food or the viruses in our body. They are **"SIGNS"**—and SIGNS give rise to diagnosis of dis-ease. Dis-ease at the **sub**clinical level means a population of sick people and escalating violence in society—and that is now taking place!

Answers & Overview

Asking a question implies there is an answer. Incorrect questions generate incorrect answers. There are plenty of **CORRECT** answers to the questions we have raised thus far—but you will not find them in the press, scientific literature or college texts. You will only find pieces—and incomplete answers. Science asks piecemeal questions—usually the wrong questions—and *pontificates* piecemeal answers.

When we use poisons against the Earth, we wage war! When we poison plants that God put on this earth and foul our air, we wage war! We are at war with every living thing on this planet—including ourselves—and we are paying the price!

Rachel Carson, author of *Silent Spring*, died shortly after her book was released, saving her from immense hatred by "interests" she opposed. She came from **within** science's camp and science proclaimed her a **witch**. They burned her at the stake for the TRUTH she heralded. They are still trying to burn her memory from our consciousness—but TRUTH does not go away. Like the Great Pyramid, it is there!

Anyone with a lick of sense knows that things are not right. The hole in the ozone layer is no accident. The hurricanes are not accidents. The floods, crop circles and crop disasters are not accidents. These things are the direct result of science and money turned to **EVIL** purposes—and all of the inhabitants of the Earth are paying the price.

Mother Earth Is Vomiting

Mother Earth is deathly sick! She is vomiting her guts out. She is fighting back the only way she knows how—with viruses and bacteria, abnormal weather patterns, floods and weeds. She will overcome the arrogance of our attacks.

The abnormal pressure created by negative energy forces cause the Ozone Layer to periodically open and close. In this way, deadly energy is released into space before every living thing on the planet Earth dies! Industrialization as we know it is incompatible with Earth. Man's toxic energy fields alter life at the *subtle*-energy level of our existence. These abnormal energies produce mutations in our children.

And Mother Earth and Her inhabitants CRY OUT— *"Dear God we are sick!"*

*[A Word from the Author. The aging process is so well camouflaged that when we come to understand how and why we age, it **appears** as oversimplification—but it is not! TRUTH is simple, and straight is the path and narrow is the gate that leads to* **TRUTH.** *Few people find the path—especially the "experts"—for they have knowledge without understanding.]*

If "you" follow the straight and narrow path to TRUTH, you are likely to get your wish and become *Young Again!*

PREVIEW: *The next chapter deals with the transfer of energy: Laying on of hands, cell phones, microwave ovens, Carpal Tunnel Syndrome, radiation and irradiation of food.*

Leaky-Gut

Leaky gut affects **99.9%** of the population—*from birth to death!* **All** auto immune dis-eases and "conditions" involve a leaky "gut" wall that allows overly large food molecules to "leak" directly into the blood, causing the immune system to "attack" the host. Leaky gut is **behind** sinus problems, so-called allergies and asthma! [R/C™ and M/Z™ help close a leaky gut wall. Yucca Blend™ increases bile-flow. Enema therapy speeds the process. [See pages 69, 85, 94, 135, 180, 237, and 243.]

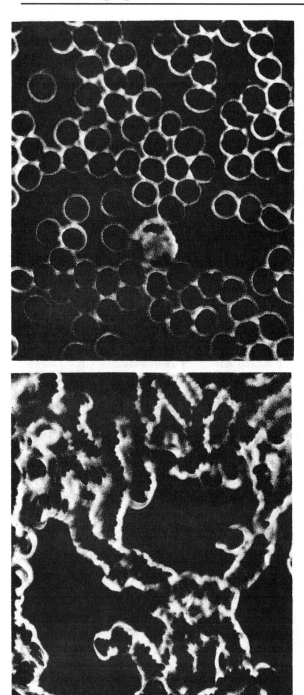

Before

After

Elimination of ***Rouleau*** from *live* blood one hour after drinking water with racemized™ ionic sea minerals. "Sticky" blood looks like rolls of pennies stacked together. The effect is due to negative energy "acid" wastes in the blood. Healthy blood does not stick together and is free to access the fine capillaries of the body delivering oxygen and nutrients and removing toxic wastes. Photos are of "live" red blood corpuscles (red blood cells without a nucleus). Medical grade magnets produce a similar effect on body tissues and fluids accounting for their therapeutic effect. Taken on a Nikon Opithat microscope with a 100 watt lamp and a Naessens condenser at 15,000 magnification.

Water Comparison

➽ **Please Note:** The BFRV™ trademark replaces the *"abandoned"* BEV acronym, **DUE TO ongoing infringement and "bootlegging"** by individual(s) offering water processing equipment under the "pretense" their equipment fulfills the "terrain" management **CONCEPTS** of the *Young Again Protocol*™.

Medical Grade Ionized Water™: BFRV™ water acts as the foundation water for this product; ORP potential **beyond** conception point; *oxidized* output used for topical skin infections and assists with venereal infections (syphilis, herpes, warts, etc.); *reduced* output assists with arthritis, diabetes and heart issues; fuels the production of mitochondrial ATP; costly to set up; inexpensive to operate; long-term health implications quite exciting; book and video available; a good investment for forward-thinking people. [See page 306.]

BFRV™ **Water:** Biologically friendly to body; extremely pure water (up to 99.5% contaminant removal, including parasites, viruses, bacteria, heavy metals, radioactivity, toxic organic chemicals); flushes contaminants as it works; superb flavor; feels "silky" in mouth; conception point ORP; energizes body; uses principle of *resonance* to boost health aspects and principle of *transference* to boost body metabolism; hydrogen and molecular bond angle restructuring; cost per gallon about 20¢. No electricity required; works anywhere worldwide.

Distilled Water: Biologically dead water; partial purification; water unfriendly to body; concentrates volatile gases (PCBs, THMs, TCEs, chlorine, chloramines); microbe growth problems; consumes lots of electricity; very slow; requires continuous maintenance; flat taste; negative ORP potential; water structure destroyed; diminishes body vibratory rate; zero carbon exposure time; cost per gallon approximately 50-80 cents; high parts replacement cost.

Reverse Osmosis: Partial purification (75-90%); quality and flavor better than distilled water; incomplete removal of bacteria, viruses, and parasites; does not provide BFRV™ restructuring; okay taste; *resonance* and *transference* zero to poor; limited carbon exposure time; cost per gallon 30 cents; no conception point ORP; wide variation in quality of water produced; superior to city "tap" water.

Carbon Block/Ceramic Cartridge: Purification fair; not self-cleaning; microbe & toxic waste build up; cost per gallon about 15-40 cents. **Ceramic Cartridge:** Marginal purification; fair taste; not self cleaning; cartridge subject to fracture and leakage; expensive; poor ORP. **Bottled Water:** Questionable purity; expensive to use.

"Water is MORE than wet! Water is FOOD!"

Hormone "Analogs"

Radiomimetic substances are everywhere around us. Pesticides, herbicides, plastics, food additives and dyes are good examples. These "zeno" molecules *act like* the real hormones—but they are **NOT** the real thing. And once they attach to the "receptor" sites, you become a prisoner unto yourself—unable to monitor and regulate your hormonal system. Radiomimetic chemicals "mimic" nuclear radiation. DDT is a good example. Chemical analogs have serious hormonal overtones. Remove them for your "receptor sites" with FG™ Creme (females) and MG™ Creme (males). [See pages 46, 72-6, 152, 164, 178, 194, 212, 268,362, 374 and 378.]

Soluble vs. Non-Soluble

Soluble and *non-soluble* tissue wastes are **NOT** the same thing. They affect the "terrain" in two different ways. *Soluble* waste is stored in the body fat beneath the skin—safely out of the loop to keep the body "alive." *Non-soluble* waste is residual; it is a stagnant, tissue fluid called "amyloid" fluid. When amyloid fluid "morphs" into "structural" acid waste, it is called amyloid "plaque." What you do about **BOTH** of these types of acidic body wastes is central to aging and longevity. Please read "MoonShine" Chapter 37.

180⁰ Off Course

We are told to stay out of the sun because it causes cancer; that soy and canola are good for us; to take aspirin to thin the blood; that "liquid" foods substitute for water, that science's version of a *balanced* diet is good for us; that routine work is as good as aerobic exercise; to not eat butter and avoid eggs; that there is no difference between "synthesized" vitamins and those in real, "live" food; that tobacco and second hand smoke are behind the proliferation of lung cancer; to take calcium supplements to avoid osteoporosis; that red meat is bad for us; that commercial chicken is good for us; to eat fish in lieu of both; that healthy "processed" foods are just as good as real, fresh food; that dis-ease is the product of microbial invasion; that vaccinations are good and genetics controls all. **None** of these things are true. Follow the experts advice and you will grow old fast and **die** early. All of the above is *disinformation* and *misinformation* emanating from the halls of science, medicine and the media. **If you want proof** that what your author is saying is **true** and what "they" are saying is **false** take a good look at the "experts." They become sickly, grow old and die from the very "conditions" that they purport to "cure!" **Ignore the experts and help your body heal itself!**

14

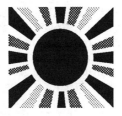

One Day At A Time

"The highest [energy] form of hostile organisms are fungi that are always present in the tissues of a corpse, and often in the tissues of sick patients."

Dr. Guenther Enderlein 1916

We live in a physical world, and we perceive dis-ease to be a **"physical"** process because we can *see* and *feel* and *measure* dis-ease's **EFFECT** on the "physical" body. We know that the *bio-electric* body is a *composite* body—part physical, part energy. We know that dis-ease is the ***manifestation*** of conflicting energy fields where left-spin energy has dominance.

The **"real"** conflict between energy fields occurs in the invisible world—a world that we do **NOT** see even though it is there! The process we call **aging** occurs in the invisible realm—and it occurs **one day at a time!**

Laying On Of Hands

An example of *positive* energy flow between the visible and invisible is the practice of ***Laying On Of Hands.*** Most religions have some version of their own.

Laying On Of Hands (LOH) couples the power of prayer with the physical body. It involves the *transfer* of positive energy from *healthy* people to the body of the sick person. It is a practice that demands tremendous focus.

Laying On Of Hands can spontaneously heal a sick person and although LOH is not a science, it is a **religious** healing "modality" involving the transfer of **energy!**

LOH often fails to produce positive change in the sick person, eliciting skepticism and mockery when the effort should be recognized for what it is—people with good intentions trying to help an ailing fellow traveler. Few participants understand the electrical phenomena taking place, but they devoutly care about their friend or loved one.

The phenomenon called "LOH" is a **"manipulation"** of

electrical **"ENERGY!"** The principle involved is a version of what occurs when dowsing for water or differentiating between left vs. right-spin foods or measuring energy fields with an aurameter—except that LOH takes place in a religious setting where positive "energy" and "love" are the controlling factors. Positive results of LOH are called *miracles!*

In the religious arena, people accept healing on its "face"—without explanation—and give God "credit!" Seeking and accepting the benefits that derive from other forms of "alternative" energy manipulation is a worthwhile goal.

If we could heal with a **black box** that had bells and flashing lights, no one would question it. We need the same openness when considering energy phenomena and paranormal healing where the manipulation of energy, good intent and focus are involved—be it in a church, a hospital or in the presence of a godly, gifted "healer!"

*["Black Magic" is the **exact opposite** of what we are discussing. That craft uses negative energy for **EVIL** purposes. Sticking pins in dolls should not be dismissed! It represents the **"dark side"** of energy manipulation.]*

Therapeutic Touch
"Therapeutic touch" is taught in nursing school curriculums—and is very similar to LOH.

"Touch" is our most highly developed sense. A baby's response to touch is indisputable. Combine touch with loving care and a nurse can "open" congested energy centers in the body and redirect the flow of energy to promote healing. Both parties must "focus" their mental and spiritual energies for healing to occur. Disbelief, negativity or disdain can **BLOCK** energy flow. [Wise nurses practice this technique "below radar" to avoid criticism by ignorant cohorts and egotistical doctors.]

First, the nurse assesses the person's energy state using *gut* instinct and by "reading" energy auras. The nurse then opens the body's energy **meridians** so **"chi"** [pronounced *chee]* can flow. Chi is what the Chinese call **"life force!"**

We are talking about energy "manipulation" for the purpose of health and healing. Science pronounces these techniques "quackery"—but vibrational healers and recovered patients think otherwise. Therapeutic touch, dowsing, LOH, pendulum or vibration chain techniques, magnetic therapy and Gua Sha are all energy phenomenoa.

Manipulation of energy for good purposes is a good thing. Learning when, where and how to use these skills is another. "Gut" instinct is the healer's compass.

Energy Abuse
The proliferation of *negative* electrical energy pollution

is a serious problem. Electrical pollution is **subtle**—and it can have disastrous effects on people's health.
Consider the "modern" microwave oven. Froth and excitement accompanied its introduction to a "gullible" public. It was touted as "the" answer for homemakers and for conserving energy—along with its **"health"** benefits! Where I lived, utility companies assigned an "expert" to help people transition to the "modern" way of cooking. Microwave cooking recipes appeared in the bulletin accompaning the utility bill.
These days—year 2006—it's "cell" and "cordless" phones. And like microwave ovens, there will be a price to pay for using them **"unprotected!"** The threat is **VERY REAL** and involves alteration of brain tissue and function along with serious dental consequences—and like microwave ovens, it will be "years" before the public wakes up! By then the damage will have been done. [A practical and inexpensive solution to "microwave" cordless phones is found on page 59.]

Few People Questioned
In those days 30 years ago, few people questioned the idea of the microwave energy cooking—except a few "cranks," and everyone knew "they" were nuts. "Demurs" were ignored!
Microwave ovens initially made their way into schools and government operations in the name of *efficiency*. Soon, they appeared in restaurants across the country. Owners and cooks alike loved them because they were so *people-friendly!* Food and plates were piping hot when served—and preparation became faster and easier!
Today, you belong to the stone age if you do not own and use a microwave oven. These **"safe"** appliances are now considered a necessity. People love them because they equate nourishment with a hot meal. But microwave cooked food is **NEITHER** alive nor life supporting. Microwaves **destroy** "lifeforce" in healthy food and **imposes** negative effects on the *bio-electric* body—accelerating the aging process. **Avoiding** "microwaved" food is something over which we have **TOTAL** control—if we choose to exercise it! Avoiding it will improve your chances for good health and longevity.

Effects Of The Microwave
Microwave ovens produce left-spin energy frequencies and are dangerous to adults and children who are in the same room. The energy **"ZAPS"** people's immune system and **destroys** food enzymes by altering their molecular "structure." Microwave energy is *anti-life* and incompatible with living things. When healthy people are exposed to **"freak"** energy, they become **sub**clinically ill—with symptoms the medical folks call "syndromes"—due to the **"subtle"** effects imposed on

natural body rhythms and enzymes. Enzymes make life possible! Enzymes in "healthy" food are right-spin energy—and the body uses them to digest very same food to fuel the process called "anabolism." When microwaves **"ZAP"** "living" molecules, life-force is scrambled and lost and biochemical reactions **FAIL** to occur! The effect is called "catabolism!" [See pages 21, 22 and 198.]

Two Seconds

Food cooked in a microwave oven for as little as two seconds takes on a **"skewed"** energy footprint. "Freak" microwave generated energy **"FORCES"** the *bio-electric* body into a catabolic "state!"

All microwave ovens **leak** unhealthy, "invisible" energy that "alters" body frequency and function in the "invisible" realm. When you eat microwaved food and water, the homeopathic "principles" of *resonance* and *transference* come into play—diminishing *life force* to such a negative energy "state" that so-called "food" becomes a huge burden on the body.

Microwaved Blood

Microwave ENERGY destroys water's molecular structure—turning what **should be** a life-giving substance into something antagonistic to life. Microwaved "water" *denatures* enzymes in the blood and lymph fluid which should be 90% water by volume. Drinking "microwaved" water imposes stress on the "terrain!" Biologically friendly water is **crucial** to good health—so why drink water that is long-term *lethal?*

[In Oklahoma, a nurse used a microwave oven to warm blood. When the blood was given to the patient—he died! As little as two seconds in a microwave is all it takes to "destroy" the life-force in blood. I doubt any "expert" would personally use microwaved blood to prove this statement wrong!]

Police • Carpal Tunnel Syndrome

Policemen using RADAR guns for traffic control are **"at risk"** for cancer, cataracts and connective tissue degeneration. These disorders are the "predictable" outcome of microwave exposure. Microwave-created degenerative dis-ease has **MANY** faces—and all of them take form in the "invisible" realm quietly and slowly—making work-related lawsuits "moot!"

[Do not expect the courts to protect people from microwave devices. Doing so means biting the hand of powerful interests. Faceless "experts" with CREDENTIALS will testify that there is "No scientific evidence!"]

Carpal Tunnel Syndrome (CTS) is a big problem for tens of thousands of people. Repetitive activity is often blamed as the controlling factor. Yet where microwave exposure is part of the person's health history, the problems are worse—and 100% predictable for those incurring daily exposure. That is why "CTS" is especially prevalent among supermarket checkers and computer operators—people who are exposed to small but continuous amounts of microwave energy. Microwaves "antagonize" nerve fibers and connective tissues (bones, ligaments, tendons, muscles and cartilage). Some people are affected more than others and develop "syndromes." We are concerned with the **"LONG-TERM"** effects of microwave exposure—regardless if it emanates from cooking ovens, cell phones or cordless phones. Short-term effects can't be measured—providing the *experts* with a "cover!"

Computer Terminals

Little is said about computer-induced health problems—except for eye strain. But have you noticed how you feel after several hours in front of one? **Tired? Drained?** Computer operators suffer from Carpal Tunnel Syndrome and immune system problems because of their **exposure** to errant energies emanating from electrical devices surrounding them.

[A Biogenic™ Super Magnet™ worn over the thymus gland is a very practical way to protect the immune system and vital organs. Super Magnets™ neutralize the effects of 110v, 60 cycle alternating current from fluorescent lighting and computers terminals. They are 12,000 gauss "permanent" open-field magnets.]

Not everyone experiences the same problems from exposure to alternating current energy fields—at least not in the beginning. For most people, the effects are *subtle* and *slow* to manifest. When the *bio-electric* body can't take any more, **"SIGNS"** of dis-ease magically appear out of nowhere and the doctor provides a diagnosis.

Symptoms of electromagnetic pollution are generally **"sub**clinical." Pay attention to stiff body and joints, low energy, sleep disorders, mental lethargy, menstrual irregularities, menopausal complaints and weakened immune function.

[Your author wears a Super Magnet™ pendant suspended over his thymus gland. He also sleeps on a medical-grade magnetic sleep pad. Some women tape Super Magnets™ directly over their ovaries monthly. Cancer patients find them useful. Alzheimers patients "settle" and sleep better. Sinus congestion, earaches and headaches also respond.]

FOOD: Radiation & Irradiation

The word "radiation" hints at the idea of energy flowing outward from a central point—like light from a light bulb. The word "radiation" also hints at energy as a **"substance."**

Fission energy is **"RADIATION"** deriving from a

"nuclear" source—like recycled radioactive waste used in the medical arena or in "spent" uranium military ammunition. Fission energy does "violence" to healthy tissue through "ionization!" Ionizing **"radiation"** destroys healthy tissue—creating "cancer" where none previously existed. A synonym for ionization is "scramble!" *Scrambling* one's DNA is a good way to ensure your life will end in "misery!"

Irradiation is a term that describes the **"act"** of directing nuclear *ionizing radiation* at living things. By inference, the word "irradiation" implies that radiation has **"substance"**—a footprint of sorts—and therefore is **MORE** than just an act of directing "invisible energy" at living tissue. In other words, radiation has **"physical consequences."** It kills healthy tissue and plants the seeds of cancer in its wake!

"Irradiation" of food is done with ionizing, nuclear radiation that scrambles and destroys the "life-force" of food molecules—making irradiated food **unfit** for human or animal consumption. Cooking food in a microwave oven does the exact same thing without the word "nuclear!" Eat irradiated food and you will grow old and die early.

The word **"irradiation"** is a *bastard* term that confuses people who are not wise in the ways of crafty wordsmiths. Irradiation is a *quasi-scientific* term used to **"disguise"** and **"distort"** the facts. Irradiation focuses on the *act* involved, rather than on the *effect* the act produces. In the public eye, *irradiation* does **NOT** mean the same thing as *radiation*. The word irradiation is a *grey* word—a mixture of black and white.

People think "nuclear" when they her the word radiation. When they hear the word irradiation, they don't know what to think.

Avoid microwave radiation; refuse to consume "freak" food and water—and avoid subjecting your body to the effects of 110 volt, 60 cycle, alternating current energy radiating from computer terminals and fluorescent lighting. In the book *Vibrations*, [See pages 57, 144, 188 & 283-4.] the author offers practical ways to "neutralize" a home at the power panel. Everyone should take a **defensive** posture on this subject and wear a Super Magnet.™ See pages 49, 81,144 and 233.]

Genetically "Engineered" Food

The terms "genetically engineered" and "irradiation" are **not** threatening to the public because they "sound" scientific and do **NOT** hint of the word "radiation." In future chapters on hair loss, balding and blindness, the reader will discover that there is "no difference" between radiated and irradiated food because both are poisons!

The **"experts"** talk of the wonders of food preservation through *irradiation.* They talk of bacterial contamination of food and water from microbes like E. coli O158.H7 and Cryptosporidium and scare us with "bogie-man" stories. What they *intentionally* don't mention are the *real* reasons behind the drive to irradiate America's food. They *know* chemically grown food grown on sick soil has poor shelf life and must be *treated* to keep it from spoiling. So they give us the "industry's" version of a **forever** shelf life. Eat "processed" food and you will experience the **graveyard** version of forever!

Neglecting to inform people of the consequences of eating microwaved food is a "sin" of omission!

Irradiated food has a "forever" shelf life. Whatever *living* enzyme molecules the food may have had are destroyed by *irradiation.* And the **"proof"** is that bugs and microbes will **NOT** eat food energy molecules that have been **"scrambled!"** They can "read" the energy signals given off by left-spin foodstuffs and they follow their "instincts." People do not!

Don't buy or eat irradiated food, microwaved food or processed food. Think, cook and eat simple.

Measuring Energy Fields

It is easy to verify the presence of stray energy fields emanating from electrical appliances and equipment. The following method measures *SOME* negative energy frequencies—but there are many. For example, connect a radio to a long extension cord and locate a spot on the dial *between* two stations that is *silent.* Next, turn-up the volume to maximum, and with the radio held in front of you, approach your computer, monitor, TV or microwave oven. When the radio begins to buzz, you have entered that device's *field of electrical influence.* Remember, you are only measuring **SOME** of the errant frequencies. The concern here is the *length of time* people spend in "negative" energy force fields—as well as the **"strength"** of the field itself!

When using a computer—stay *beyond* its "field" and wear a Super Magnet.™ The effects of negative energy forcefields is subtle—like eating irradiated and microwaved food or using cell and cordless phones. Short-term effects go unnoticed—but **LONG-TERM** effects eventually take "form"—**FIRST** as **sub**clinical illness and **LATER** as "clinical" dis-ease!

A two-inch thick slab of LEAD blocks nuclear radiation, YET it **cannot** block 110v alternating current force-fields. **Never** use an electric blanket! If you are cold, take an epsom salt bath or soak your feet and hands in a basin of hot water or drink a cup of hot herbal tea to warm your tissue "fluids."

Medicine & Radiation

Radiation "therapy" and *radioactive* "chemotherapy" used in the treatment of cancer are **devastating** to the body.

People believe allopathic medicine's magic-bullet "fairy tales" and line up at the medical clinic for their "opportunity." People are confused and **fail to differentiate** between diagnostic X-rays and the overkill effect of "radiation" therapy. Radiation is **NOT** a "therapy" because it is anti-life! Rather, it is *palliative,* treating **SIGNS** and symptoms without cure of the underlying causes. Patients are **"TRAINED"** to focus on **"hope"** of cure—instead of being "told" of the violence *ionizing radiation* inflicts upon their bodies. [It's nothing but a game!]

The government school system is designed to prevent people from thinking outside the box!

Ask The Experts

If the things we are discussing are true—and they are—then we must learn to *live defensively and think independently!* "Experts" in science and government are not allowed to study or divulge anything that might quash monopolistic control over energy, medicine, the money system—or the courts and schools.

Ignorance is a "lame" excuse that will **NOT** keep you healthy or young. Aging is the "total" of all *negative* forces in your life—so live and think OUTSIDE the box!

You become young the **opposite** way that you grow old. You become Young Again—*one day at a time!*

PREVIEW: *Our next chapter looks at wrinkled skin—WHY it occurs and WHAT you can do about it. It also discusses body odor as it relates to aging.*

"B" Vitamin Absorption

"B" vitamins are important! Ideally, they should come from healthy food and fresh vegetable juices. Unfortunately, digestion and absorption "issues" **STOP** them from achieving **"therapeutic"** levels in the blood—where it counts! The *Young Again*™ solution to this problem is called L_sP_cB.™ The "surprise" is the transport "vehicle" used to shuttle these life-sustaining molecules directly to the liver and blood. In Chapter 37 you will learn the details of this incredible story and what it means for you. [See pages 59, 127, 162, 177 and 205.]

Acne & The Terrain!

Puberty imposes "stress" on the liver that often manifests as acne! Acne is a "liver" and "leaky-gut" issue. The *Young Again Protocol*™ remedies liver and terrain problems like "acne!"

The word death is mostly "eat."

"Eat your vaccine, dear!"

Government, the medical and pharmaceutical complex and multinational food giants have implemented a **devilish** plan that will have **disastrous** effects on the health of people worldwide—and especially in the USA.

The scheme involves using **genetically altered** fruits and vegetables to shuttle the likes of hepatitis B, polio, measles, mumps, tetanus, swine flu and rubella into **YOUR** body—via the food you eat—supposedly to "immunize" against dis-ease! *Gene splicing of the food supply will produce millions of sick people. It will render "forced" immunization moot while it keeps the hospital rooms full!*

If you want to live a healthy, happy life, you **MUST** plant a garden or grow food in containers on your patio or share a community plot or hire someone to grow "safe" vaccine-free and chemical-free food for you and your family.

Home-grown food—even in small quantities—produces astounding effects on health! The best way to get into gardening is to start today! All it takes is some "dirt," a bag of chicken manure compost from garden suppliers plus some gypsum, sand and vermiculite. Your author also recommends a product called Bio-Grow™ [See pages 80, 147, 231, 305 and 370.]—along with liquid kelp and fish fertilizer for a foliar mix and spray. This recipe converts dirt into live soil overnight using the foliar-to-root pathway. Create a positive **energy** environment where microbes and plants prosper and you get "healthy" food. This is a Fourth Dimension **ENERGY** "concept!"

Sexual Dysfunction & The Terrain

Loss of sex drive is a **symptom** that indicates deterioration and atrophy of vital organ function. The problem, therefore, is "systemic" and goes *beyond* just sexual malaise.

Conditions like obesity, skin disorders, thinning hair and balding, thinning and dryness in vagina, yeast infections, bowel disorders, poor digestion, pot belly, acid reflux, sagging facial tissue, low of muscle mass and wrinkles are "first cousins" to loss of sex drive. Impotence in men is a dead give-away of **prostate** trouble and **diabetes** in the making. Central to these "conditions" is a poorly functioning liver, poor bile flow and a **sub**clinical thyroid condition.

To restore health and sex drive, the reader should follow the *Young Again Protocol(s).*™ Liver function absolutely **must** be restored. Thyroid function in women **must** be addressed. Finally, the puberty "window" **must** be reopened. **Deacidification** of the terrain and restoration of the female hormone cycle are a **must.** Old age will fade away—if you are willing to do what must be done! [See pages 72, 164, 212 and 292.]

Understanding Diabetes

Diabetes plagues millions of people in industrial societies. Yet in third-world countries—where people eat traditional diets—the incidence of diabetes is very low. Medical science blames genetics for the rise in diabetes. They are wrong! The problem is fivefold and **genetics is NOT one of them!**

Diabetes results from toxic **excesses** within the system, loss of the gallbladder, hormonal imbalance, **IMMUNIZATIONS,** a good dose of "leaky-gut"—and low magnesium!

Diabetes is **proof** of severe vital organ **stress** and hormonal issues in adults over age "35"—and especially in women as hormone production slows. When **excess** acid waste reaches crisis levels in the system, the threshold is crossed and dis-ease announces itself!

Type II diabetes is the most common type and is often referred to as *old age* or *sugar diabetes.* It typically occurs between ages 35 and 50—**the years when women and men "slide into" old age** and the "window" that **opened** at puberty officially **CLOSES!** The following **SIGNS** and **symptoms** shed light on the "auto-immune" nature of Type ll diabetes. Hair, energy, sex drive, fat, thyroid problems, nerves issues, wrinkled skin and flabby muscles—are some of the complaints!

Type I "juvenile diabetes" is a **severe** condition where the child's immune system "attacks" the pancreas cells responsible for insulin production. Diabetes Type l is **DEFINITELY** an **"auto-immune"** condition brought on by vaccination-induced **SUPER antigens** in"foreign" serum proteins—with a dose of "mercury" that drives the immune system absolutely wild!

DAPT (diphtheria and pertussis + tetanus) and polio vaccines contain **SUPER antigens** and mercury that turn the body "upside down!" [Racemized™ sea minerals provide **magnesium** and trece mineral electrolytes in balanced form. It is **VERY** useful for dealing with all forms of "diabetes!"]

"Attenuated" strains of the polio virus **can and do** mutate once inside the body! So do hepatitis B and flu vaccines! Flu shots are a total scam because viruses mutate by the minute—rendering vaccinations a "moot" issue! Vaccinations do **NOT** provide immunity—so why expose yourself?

Loss of the gallbladder is a 99% guarantee of diabetes within 20 years—**unless** protective measures are taken. Ten women to every man suffers gallbladder surgery. These ladies often have the **"same"** complaints **"after"** the surgery! Sadly, 8 out of 10 women did **NOT** need the surgery in the first place. Gallbladder surgery is BIG business. The *Young Again Protocol*™ avoids the need to subject oneself to surgical abuse. Understanding health in terms of the **"terrain"** is the issue!

"Always drink upstream from the herd!"

Skin & Body Toner™

Look in the mirror. Do you see sagging skin hanging from your arms and sagging cheeks? Are you sporting "Howdie Doodie" lines from the corners of your mouth to the sides of your chin? Are those tell-tale lines forming on your upper lip? And do you see crows feet around your eyes? And what about your torso and legs? Do they bear excess fat or cellulite? Has muscle mass turned to flab? Do you have a pot belly or saddle bags on your hips? Drooping, deflated breasts? Do you remember when your body was "younger?" When you were developing in your mother's womb, you were fed a steady supply of "**ante**genic" protein and hormones. **Ante**genic protein is very special stuff. The body uses **ante**genic protein to grow "new" tissue and vital organs. Provide your body with racemized™ **ante**genic protein and the "transformaton" into a more youthful body accelerates!

*[The combined effects of Skin & Body Toner™ & Bio-genic™ hGH are "**cumulative**" when taken consistently, each night before bed—along with R/J Factors I & II™ and L$_S$P$_C$C.™ VZ II™ "digests" amyloid and scar tissues and lays-down new, collagen for "younger" tissue. (See pages 127, 149, 152, 162, 177, 247, 261, 292 and Chapter 37 for more details and further discussion of these interrelated subjects.)]*

Prostatitis • Thyroid • Sex

Prostate issues in men are similar to thyroid issues in women—and behind both are "liver" and thyroid issues. Sexual disfunction, skin and hair, brain fog, depression, loss of muscle mass and coldness are all connected. Don't let these problems steal your life away. Deal with them! [See pages 99, 113, 147, 152, 160, 178, 185 and 292.]

Smoke-Out™

Do **NOT** put up with the "**effects**" of second-hand smoke—at home or the office. Ditto for automotive pollutants when unavoidably stuck in traffic. Remove the "**residues**" of airborne pollutants and carcinogens from your "tissues" with Smoke-Out.™ For children and adults, alike! Enhance the process with Yucca Blend™ for increased "bile flow."

Teeth & Gums

Teeth and gums are BIG issues—especially after age 25! Periodontal problems, decay, plaque, root-cleanings—are addressed with the Bio-Magnetic™ Dental Irrigator and Oral Advantage! The irrigator transforms "water" into an effective dental remedy—and when combined with nightly use of **Oral Advantage,**™ the results are dramatic! Oral Advantage™ "pulls-out" infection, tames inflammated gums and tightens loose teeth—fast! Dental issues are "aging" issues. Don't ignore them! [See pages 79, 149, 187, 204, 233 and 351.]

Stool Analysis

Gusher—the "ideal" bowel movement! Quick call; no effort; very loose; "unformed;" similar to diarrhea *without* characteristic "burn" associated with it. A very "rewarding" experience that "ideally" should occur 3-5 times per day!

Bear Poop—stool should resemble a pile of mush and should pass in 2-3 seconds. Sit down, stand up, its over.

Normal Stool (so called)—formed stool; medium brown color; easy passage; little taper; ends with gas pocket.

Floaters—stools that float in the toilet. Indicative of poor fat metabolism; poor bile flow; poor digestion.

Stringers—stringy stools that are both narrow and fat. Indicative of a spastic and kinked colon, poor muscle tone in colon wall; high-stress personality; negative thinking; poor bile flow.

Pelleted Stool—Indicates slow transit time; poor bile flow; under-hydration; poor diet; inadequate fiber; lack of rhythm in daily life; stress issues.

Pale-Colored Stools—Indicative of liver malfunction, poor bile flow, viral activity (white stools are seen with hepatitis). Stools should be medium brown.

Bloody Stools—Indicative of hemorrhoids, diverticulitis, colitis, irritable bowel and Leaky Gut Syndrome(s); under hydration; stressful life or personality.

Dark Colored Stools—Sluggish gut and bowel; old blood from ulcers and colitis; under-hydration; dietary influence of prunes, beet juice, and greens.

Fat-Headed Stools w/Tapered End—"Pooling" at rectum; under-hydration; ignoring nature's call; lack of fiber and exercise; incomplete evacuation; poor bile flow.

Complete Stool Evacuation—characteristics of "bear poop" stool with nothing *held back*. Bowel movement often ends with distinctive pocket of gas.

NOTE: To improve your "poop" characteristics, speed **de**acidification of the terrain and **increase bile-flow:** Drink 2 glasses of water with racemized™ sea minerals upon rising and one glass at each urination; take one tablespoon of Yucca Blend™ with each meal; drink fresh vegetable juices daily, preferably with breakfast; eat dried prunes; do High Enema Therapy™ 1-2 times weekly and low enemas daily; eat healthy food and avoid junk and snacks; eat meals on schedule; get "non-abusive" exercise daily; sleep 8+ hours nightly.

15

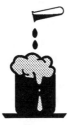

Grandma's Lye Soap

"Oh, little Herman and brother Therman,
Had an aversion to washing their ears.
Grandma scrubbed them with lye soap,
And they haven't heard a word in years."
            Dr. Roger Lent

The **"integument"** ("skin") is the largest organ of the body in surface area. **Hair** and **nails** are extensions of skin—skin being one of **FOUR** exit portals for the elimination of toxins and acid wastes. The skin is the **FIRST** organ to form after "conception"—all of other organs and tissues "derive" from skin by a process called *differentiation.* To say that skin is important is an "understatement!"

The skin's has three **siblings** that also work the "waste" venue: the **bowel, kidneys** and **lungs.** This group of four manages acid-waste "storage" and "disposal" within the body's "terrain!" **SOLUBLE** waste that fails to exit the body each day is "removed" from circulation and stored in fatty tissue beneath the skin. In some people, stored "soluble" waste manifests as acne, psoriasis, liver spots, discoloration, dryness, wrinkles and boils—just to name a few! Skin is the body's **"first line"** of defense against dis-ease and infection.

Skin functions much like the lungs. It **breathes, absorbs** and **releases** waste through **perspiration** and secretion of **oils** and **fats** and through the growth of **hair** and **nails.** Blood and lymphatic fluids provide moisture given off as sweat. Sebaceous glands secrete "waste-laden" oils and fats. **"Soluble"** waste that does not exit the body through the skin becomes **"trapped"** in the tissues **"beneath"** the skin. [The *Young Again! Tissue and Liver Protocol*™ **releases** stored soluble waste and provides safety **"buffers"** while waste is in circulation. Waste exits the body in the "bile" by way of the bowel.

"Soluble" waste that collects in the joints and tissues is called **"amyloid"** fluid. Amyloid fluid is highly "acid" cellular waste that eventually **"MORPHS"** into **"structural"** waste.

Structural waste is called **amyloid** "**PLAQUE.**" It is the tissue "equivalent" of **brick and mortar!** Amyloid plaque also "**MOR-PHS**—by forming "scar" tissue.

Tissue "**calcification**" is a related concept better known by the name "arthritis!" Stiffness and loss of elasticity are **SIGNS** of "old age" —as are wrinkled skin, sagging face and breasts and sore feet. "Feet" problems in the elderly are confirmation of a **VERY** acid "terrain"—plus the effects of gravity, collapsing arches, acid-waste "crystallization" and nerve deterioration. [The connective tissues of the feet repair slowly due to the distance from the heart and waste levels.]

Connective Tissue

Connective tissue comprises 90% of total body tissues, and collagen comprises about 30% of connective tissue. Collagen is the "**SUBSTRATE**" and "**MATRIX**" for mineral deposition and bone creation. Collagen is "**FOUNDATION**" tissue.

"**Ongoing**" collagen formation is crucial to healing broken and aged bodies. Hormones play a part here—as does **de**acidification of the "terrain." Therapeutic "blood" levels of Vitamin-C provides a "spark plug" effect to collagen formation—something that **UNTIL NOW** could only be achieved intravenously with a "needle!" $L_sP_cC^{TM}$ is the *Young Again*™ solution to **avoiding** Vitamin-C administration by needle. Oral pills and powder forms of Vitamin-C are a "moot" approach. [These concepts are covered in greater detail in Chapter 38.]

Dissolving "structural" waste tissue and building healthy new tissue is done with SOC,™ *L_sP_cC*™ *and VZ II*™.

Osteoarthritis is *calcification* of the joints. Tuberculosis is *calcification* of the lungs. Calcification follows "alteration" of healthy tissue. Calcification of "tumors" is the body's way of "containing" highly concentrated waste energy. **Calcification is PROGRESSIVE!** [Osteopenia refers to failure to lay down collagen and new bone as fast as old tissue is breaking-down!]

Waste & Hormones

Hormones, sleep, diet and exercise affect the connective tissues because they affect the "terrain!" The **inability** to dissolve amyloid plaque and move acid wastes **OUT** of the body "speeds" connective tissue breakdown and "calcification. So does hormonal "stallout!" Hormonal activity keeps the puberty window "open!" Synthesized hormones "skew" the system and stress the liver. A better approach is to use racemized™ hormonal precursors and make your "own" hormones!

There is "**little**" difference in the effects of so called "**natural**" synthesized hormone and pharmaceutical versions. There are thousands of chemicals —from pesticides and plastics to food additives and sweeteners—that "**mimic**" real hormones. Crafty chemists move the reactive "-R" group on molecules so they can "patent" them. "Real" molecules cannot be patented!

Avoiding analogous substances that "lock-up" body receptor sites and regulatory centers in the brain is a good idea, considering that **"analogs"** have a "forever" life and do **NOT** break down or release from receptors on their own. ["Polishing" receptor sites and flushing chemical analogs from the system is part of the *Young Again! Protocol.*]

Once analogous hormones attach to your receptor sites, you become a "prisoner" in your own body.
Thyroid activity affects the "rate" of connective tissue formation. "Sluggish" thyroid activity affects 99% of younger women—partly due to menstrual/hormone issues—and **MOSTLY** due to the mercury in women's teeth. [HST™ Creme is used to "perk up" metabolism in both sexes over age "40."

After age "40," thyroid activity in women progressively "slows." Conventional blood lab tests look for "clinical" thyroid dis-ease while ignoring associated **"symptoms"** like cold hands and feet, low body temperature, weight-gain, falling and thinning hair, brain-fog and memory complaints, low energy, sagging and wrinkled skin, loss of muscle mass and tone, sore joints and dry skin. [Both BT™ and HST™ Creme are the *Young Again*™ answer to these complaints.]

Tissues & Remedies

There are two classes of tissue. Healthy, **"functional"** tissue and non healthy **"scar"** tissue. Scar tissue is the body's response to **trauma** and **acid-waste** accumulation—and the **INABILITY** to lay down healthy "new" tissue. Scar tissue can be an internal or external issue. Scars and skin "blemishes" are versions of scar tissue. Scarring of "vital" organ tissue is an internal issue that is "central" to aging and longevity!

SOC,™ *RJ Factors*™ *l & ll and L$_s$P$_c$C*™ *provide needed "materials" for growing healthy tissue. So does Skin and Body Toner*™ *and racemized*™ *hGH.*

[Vitamin B-12 affects the connective tissues. Exhaustion of vitamin B-12 from the vital organs is a big issue for women beginning in the mid-twenties, due to loss of menstrual blood. Dietary intake of B-12 suffices to about age 30 until "diminished" production of intrinsic factor from the stomach wall and "insufficient" hydrogen chloride production prevents women from absorbing B-12. Vitamin pills, mouth sprays and sublingual tablets are NOT a viable B-12 source, any more than synthetic B-12 shots.The Young Again Protocol™ uses Cobo-12™ *racemized*™ *transdermal creme that absorbs directly into the blood. Symptoms associated with a B-12 shortfall number in the "hundreds" and generally manifest after age 35 and*

worsen after age "40" as menopause gets into full swing.]

Wrinkles bother people who want to look young. The beauty industry uses the "mud-against-the-wall" approach by putting "collagen" in skin and hair products. Applying collagen to skin is similar to taking **glucosamine** and **condroitin** sulfates to build cartilage—which they **do not!**

*[The body "makes" collagen when provided with **BOTH** the stimulus and the raw materials as noted above. [VZ™ is used to "eat" structural waste and get the digested "sludge" down the toilet.]*

Movie Stars • Skin • Hair

As we age, the skin becomes stiff and leathery—indicating cross-linking of the collagen matrix. Sometimes, cracking and bleeding occurs on the chafe points as conditions worsen—especially with the elderly.

Movie stars and the "vain" resort to face-lifts to hide their skin problems. The "stars" understand that a young face "pulls" better at the box office and that the **"younger"** you *look and feel,* the more opportunities you will have and the longer you will be a movie star. Movie star or not—people should **NOT** be resorting to **superficial** body "makeovers" when they are growing old and dying on the **"INSIDE!"** [Your author's vanity secrets are outlined on page 317.]

Face-lifts help appearance, but they are an expensive "cover" for what is "really going on" inside the body—and for what is NOT being addressed!

When SOC™ lotion, R/Skin Creme™ and L_sP_cC™ are used regularly, skin becomes very soft, wrinkles fade and the face takes on a *healthy glow!* These products are **"food"** for the skin—both internal and external. They are **NOT** cosmetics! Your author looks and feels young—as you can tell from the "untouched" photo on the back cover—and his *bio-electric* age is holding at "19!" [Another personal secret for no gray, full color, thick hair is Kombucha tea and GH_3+.]

Society is biased AGAINST the aged. People who look and feel young enjoy a big advantage!

Urine & Your Face • Digestion

The term **"acid"** is a chemical term. An acid—by definition—is a hydrogen donor; a substance that donates "hydrogen" ions to a chemical reaction. Natural vinegar contains natural, organic acids and tastes "sour." Natural acids like those in raw vinegar, Kombucha Tea, lemons and sauerkraut rejuvenate the body by increasing "bile-flow" which **"de**acidifies" the tissues—**despite** these foods having an acid pH. Naturally acidic foods cause the body to become less acid—**NOT** more alkaline! [Please do **NOT** confuse the acid/alkaline

concept of "terrain" management with pH chemistry.]
Natural acids heal. Urine contains "acids" that beautify
the skin. Some Scandinavian women wash their face in their
urine to keep their skin smooth and young looking. Some
people drink their urine daily to rid themselves of cancer and
heal their bodies of dis-ease. [High "stomach" acidity is absolutely **critical** for protein digestion and killing incoming parasites. So-called acid-reflux has "nothing" to do with stomach
acidity. This is a classic liver/bile/bowel problem.]

Reduction in hydrogen chloride and enzyme pro-
duction diminishes rapidly after age 30. Poor digestion
affects 95% of the population—young and old alike!

Protein "digestion" begins in a very "acid" stomach
where the peptide bonds linking amino acid proteins together
are "lysed!" Poor health and "reduced" stomach acidity is
central to protein **mal**nourishment issues. Digestion complaints and "acid reflux" are **BIG RED FLAGS** that things are
very out-of-balance! [Disorb Aid II™ and R/BHC™ help hee!]

Carbohydrate digestion occurs in the **alkaline** environment of the small intestine (the "gut"). Special lymphatic
vessels absorb fats and transports them via the "portal vein" to
the liver for processing. A "leaky-gut" wall allows overly large
food molecules direct access to the blood stream—spawning
autoimmune issues and serious dis-ease!

As people age, digestion "collapses" because the stomach wall **FAILS** to produce enough hydrogen chloride and
intrinsic factor, the pancreas **FAILS** to produce enough pancreatic enzymes, and the liver and gallbladder **FAIL** to produce—and release—enough "bile." The digestion **"dilemma"**
underscores both health and dis-ease—and needs tending if
"restoration" of health is expected.]

A "healthy diet" alone is NOT sufficient to over-
come digestion issues and the poor health it spawns!

As the body grows "older" insufficient intake of quality
proteins **plus** poor protein digestion and assimilation "forces"
the body to **"cannibalize"** itself in an effort to meet its protein
needs. Cancer patients—who are literally starving to death—
are classic examples of auto-cannibalization in progress.

Vegans and vegetarians—with rare exception—
live the slow motion version of "auto-cannibalization"—
and in the end "die" meat-eaters—by default!

Gout • Stones • Toxemia

People with **poor** liver function and **poor** bile flow
CANNOT fully process animal proteins. Poorly digeted proteins
have an **"ACIDIC"** effect on the body's "terrain!" Without hard
physical work and fresh vegetable juices, gout rears its ugly
head! Historically gout was known as a **rich man's dis-ease.**

The rich suffered from inflammation of the feet, toes and hands **partly** because they ate too much animal protein and **mostly** because they **FAILED** to eat fruits and vegetables. [Parasites go with **"ALL"** foods. Sanitation and digestion are the keys here.]

Social pressure makes it difficult for people to maintain a healthy lifestyle—and the wealthier you are, the easier it is to develop bad dietary habits. Alcohol, heavy food and late social engagements sum up the problem. The cliche *"Eating high on the hog!"* is a carryover expression that hints of **"excess!"**

When highly "acidic" tissue fluids combine with waste alkaline earth minerals—like calcium, magnesium and sodium—crystalline precipitates **"settle"** out of solution into the tissues and joints. Poor digestion and leaky-gut issues serve to boost blood protein **metabolites** like "purines." Purines are responsible for the formation of uric acid—and uric acid salt "crystals" are responsible for the painful condition called "gout." Gout medications are "palliative"—and fail to address the causes. Gout medications **destroy** the liver! [Causes of gout are easily remedied by following the *Young Again! Tissue and Liver Protocol.*]

In the past, gout was not a problem for middle class and poor people who did hard, physical, load-bearing work. A sedentary lifestyle belonged to the domain of the wealthy. Today—with the advent of the "service" society and the computer—**sedentary** life styles are epidemic! Wealth and opulence no longer dictate who gets gout and who develops a dowager's hump! The middle class and poor are living longer and are now sharing the misery. The old saying *"Misery loves company!"* sums up the situation. [Gout, gall and kidney stones and spurs are **not** normal. They are **SIGNS** of aging.]

Gout is primarily a "male" condition. The female versions are called "osteoporosis" and "arthritis!"

Gall and kidney stones are "precipitates." Stones can be mineral or cholesterol-based precipitates—or both! The type of stone determines the doctor's remedy short of surgery. With **gall stones**, death occurs with 24 hours if the common duct becomes blocked. Kidney stones damage the kidneys!]

Passing of gall and liver stones is done at home following the Young Again Tissue and Liver Protocol(s).™

Blood poisoning describes a "condition"—not an event. In pregnant women, excess waste accumulation in the blood is called "toxemia" (*tox*-toxic; *emia*-of the blood). The pregnant woman's liver does double duty for mom and baby! Infection causes "sepsis"—which is blood poisoning. The "slow-motion" version of blood poisoning in the average person is called "acidosis"—meaning "acidification" of the terrain. Unchecked accumulation of acid waste in the tissues translates poor health, misery and early death. Movement of waste is **"TO-**

TALLY" dependent upon bile-flow from a healthy, functioning liver. Tissue hydration levels play a part here also.

Bad drinking water loads the body with "useless" mineral salts that "precipitate" and clog the tissues!

[Grandma mixed and heated animal fats with lye (sodium hydroxide) and got "lye soap" through the process of **saponification**. *But, when she used her soap in* **hard mineral tap water**—*she got soap-scum "precipitates" in the tub. The scum was the product of lye soap and the hard water minerals.]*

Dietary oils—like soy and canola—mix with waste mineral salts to form "soap scum" type waste in the body. Clogged and hardened arteries (**athero**sclerosis and **arterio**sclerosis) are filled with "plaques"—like the scum in grandma's tub. **Plaque formation** is a **"symptom"** of trouble. Plaque is spelled ***AMYLOID!*** Amyloid plaque forms in all sectors of the body—and invades the brain in people going down to *Alzheimers!*

Calcium & Osteoporosis

Medical opinion to the contrary, elemental calcium and magnesium supplements taken for arthritis and osteoporosis are **worthless!** They do **NOT** solve the problem and they create new and different issues in the process.

Doctors prescribe "calcium" because they have been **"told"** by the "experts" that females need it to avoid and treat "osteoporosis"—particularly when menopause "manifests!" They try to **FORCE** the body to accept elemental minerals that have not gone through the carbon cycle. In the process, they create imbalances that are "driving" heart attack in women—the #1 killer of women!

Elemental minerals precipitate **OUT** of body fluids and join with other metabolic wastes to form plaques, stones and spurs. When taken with meals, elemental calcium and magnesium interfere with digestion of proteins by neutralizing stomach acids critical to proper digestion.

Diminished bone density is "called" **osteoporosis**. Insufficient bone-building activity is "called" **osteopenia.** Both are primarily **female** issues. Men generally don't become diagnosable until after age "70"—but the process is well on its way after age "40!" In women, onset of osteoporosis occurs in the "pre" menopause years beginning at age "25"—about the same time the "puberty effect" peaks.

[Osteoporosis occurs earlier in women because of a slowdown in the "hormone" cycle, increased tissue acidity, and inability to lay down new collagen as fast as it is breaking down. Fair or not, females turn acidic about **10 TIMES** *faster than men. This is "why" your author has emphasized—**over-and-over** throughout the pages of this book—the **never ending** need for* **DEACDIFICATION** *of the terrain!]*

Deacidification and female health go "together"—as does the "concept" of keeping the middle-years window **"perpetually open"** for as long as a woman wishes to keep her beauty and youthfullness and remain sexually active. Why should a woman allow menopause to "steal away" her life? [Regardless of a woman's age, condition of her parts or menstration issues—the Vorago™ Effect gives women control of their health and longevity. [See Chapter 36, *Vorago SunRise*]

Body Odor

Body odor (BO) is a **symptom** of a *polluted* body! BO is experienced when toxic acid waste **FAILS** to exit the body via the liver, bile and bowels—and instead builds-up in the fatty tissues below the skin—providing food for the bacteria that live on waste. BO is more than socially offensive. It is the **"shadow"** of old age. When you smell BO, you are smelling toxic, aromatic waste evaporating from the tissues!

We first become aware of body odor at puberty. It is usually related to hormonal activity and increased **STRESS** imposed on the **liver** by puberty-related "changes." It's the **same** stress that occurs at menopause and andropause.

In adults, teens and children, BO signals tissue acidification and liver and bowel issues. The stronger the BO, the sicker the person. Strong BO should **not** be ignored!

*[You do **NOT** have to be old to have foul body odor. If you are old in body and young in years, you will "stink!" If you are old in years and old in body, the odor is "suffocating!" A clean body with a efficient liver has little if any BO because the liver is responsible for processing 90% of body waste.]*

Children have a good sense of smell. They can detect toxins escaping from their grandpa's or grandma's body. They can smell old age and sickness—and so can pets! Children smell sweet and fresh because they are **YOUNG** in years—for sure in body. BO is symptomatic of *catabolic* activity. People with potent BO can shower five times a day with **grandma's lye soap,** use the best of deodorants and get **zero** results. BO "oozes" from the body as fast as it is washed off. **The problem of body odor is internal, "NOT" external!**

The quickest way to rid a body of BO is by following the steps outlined in this book. The waste we want to dislodge from the body is **NOT** stored in the liver and colon. It is stored in the **"fat layer"** under the skin. The *Young Again Tissue and Liver Protocol*™ **safely** releases and transports tissue wastes out of the system and down the toilet. As the "terrain" of the body improves, body odor goes *"bye, bye!"*

EVERYTHING in this book relates to control of the "terrain." Restore the TERRAIN and "you" get out of jail. Maintain the terrain and aging reversal is automatic!

Deodorants & The Puberty Window

Anti-perspirant deodorants should **NEVER** be used because they **"BLOCK"** sweat glands and flood the body with heavy metal ions and chemicals. **Anti**perspirants contain toxic ALUMINUM ions that fuel conditions like *Alzheimers!* The areas of the body where sweat is heaviest has "meaning." These areas are very high lymph node concentration—like the groin, arm pits, breasts, neck and head. Inability to freely sweat is **NOT** a good sign—and cancer loves a congested lymphatic system and an "acid" terrain. Remember, cancer "travels" the lymphatic highway. Lymphatic circulation is an extremely **critical** issue.

Everything from constipation and health issues to diet and hormones affects "body odor." Female menstruation and odors associated with it are **similar** to what happens to men during "their" hormone swings. Men have a monthly "hormone cycle"—as their wives and girl friends will confirm! The male equivalent of menopause is **andropause** (*andro*-refers to male hormones; *pause*-cessation of).

Menopause and andropause are a BIG deal! They are the flip side of puberty—one female, the other male. They represent a major **shift** and **slowdown** of body metabolism—particularly in the testicles, ovaries and **liver.** The phrase "the change" does **NOT** fully convey what is really going on. Menopause and andropause should be **INTERPRETED** as **"past tense"** issues because they begin 15-20 years **prior** to manifestation. In other words, humans **PEAK** around age "25!"

The **"puberty window"** opens at puberty and closes at menopause/andropause. **Extending** the "puberty window" should be the name of the game for anyone **under** age "35!" **Reopening** the puberty window IS the name of the game for anyone **over** age "35!"

[The reader will find a complete discussion of the "game" in Chapters 35 entitled Vorago™ SunRise. And as the reader might guess, the Vorago™ Effect is very much a hormonal story. It is a story that only "appears" to pertain to women—but it impacts the life of men, also!]

We are supposed to grow a "new" body every 7 years. The body YOU get depends upon YOUR "choices!"

No Sweat

People sweat! Some people sweat profusely. Other people hardly sweat at all. Sweat is a good indicator of how efficiently the skin is functioning as a waste portal. If you sweat heavily, it's a very good **SIGN**—provided blood and tissues fluid volume levels are kept fully "hydrated" and saturated with racemized™ sea mineral electrolytes so the waste can "flow!" Not until his early "50's" did your author "sweat!" After completing the *Young Again (Tissue and Liver) Protocol*™ —so he could get "out-of-jail" and discovering how to "properly" do High Enema Therapy™ did his body begin to sweat freely! He is now age 61! Exercise is good—but it is **not** sufficient to **free** your body from a "prison" of waste! All acid waste—both soluble and non soluble, liquid and structural—"must" leave the body before it can restore itself to a youthful condition. [Movement of "soluble" tissue-bound acid waste is accelerated with the L/CSF™ Machine. [See pages 133,195,261&382 regarding waste issues—and pages 107,160,310,381&385 for L/CSF.™]

Skin: A Two Way Door

We "absorb" through the skin. Few people realize the amount of chemicals and poisons entering the body through the *swinging door* called *skin.* The skin functions **bi**-directionally—meaning it **BOTH** expels tissue wastes and absorbs toxic substances from perfumes and bathing and drinking water.

[The Young Again Protocol™ utilizes the skin's highly efficient absorption capability to shuttle racemized™ transdermals like SunLight™ Creme [Vorago™ effect]; F/G™ & M/G™ Cremes [female and male]; B.T.™ Creme [thyroid]; HST™ [restoration]; and Cobo-12™ [Vitamin B-12 creme.]

The mucous membranes lining the mouth, throat, lungs and GI tract have a combined surface area **600 times greater** than our skin—and these membranes absorb far more efficiently, too! They the **MOST** efficient "absorption" tissues in the body—and they are the **MOST** "exposed" tissues in the body. "Ask" a beautician or a nail lady how they feel after a few years exposure to hard-core chemicals. **"Look"** at the general population who drink "raw" city water. Fact is, people in general are growing older at an accelerated rate—and the skin and mucous membranes are part of the story.

If chemical exposure is severe, the body will break out in hives or a rash, experience breathing difficulties—and on occasion, "collapse!" The body was **not** meant to deal with the barrage of poisons bombarding it daily—particularly, environmental "zeno" estrogens—and food additives that act like "zenos"—locking up hormonal receptors.

"Exposure" to environmental poisons is **unavoidable!** **"Dislodging"** dangerous chemical molecules that have accumulated in the tissues over many years is a tall order! First, the body must "choose" to **RELEASE** toxins and poisons into circulation. Next, "buffers" are needed to **SAFELY** "shuttle" the waste through the blood and lymph, liver and intestine and finally **"OUT"** of the body and into the toilet!

Environmental, dietary and cellular-generated poisons MUST exit the body "daily" to avoid "aging."

➥ The body has **ONLY** two options when it comes to dealing with incoming poisons and internally generated cellular waste: "pass" them down the toilet via bile flow from the liver—or "store" them in the tissues. If you FAIL to give your body the means of dealing with "waste," and it will be forced to **"STORE!"** *Terrain management is the underlying principle of the Young Again Protocol.*™

Time Bombs
Unless the *Young Again Protocol*™ is **"lived"** on a daily basis, *sick and old* become reality! Your author hopes the reader will opt to follow his lead and enjoy a long and healthy life—instead of facing the "day of reckoning!" **When that day arrives,** you will notice a lump in your breast or bleeding from the vagina or rectum, etc., and the doctor will say: *"YOU HAVE CANCER!".....or "DIABETES!".....or.....?*
And you will say to yourself *"Why me? What did I do to deserve this? I'm not old enough to have?????! I have taken good care of myself! Surely the diagnosis is wrong."*
BUT! You did have a hand in this story, didn't you? Save the excuses—they don't count! Claims of ignorance won't ease the hell you face! Wouldn't it have been better to take responsibility sooner—when you could have restored "your" terrain? *Imprint these thoughts in your memory—and LIVE by them!*
Prevention is better than cure. Neither government nor science can protect you. In matters of health, never blame others. You alone are responsible.
The "sick care" industry is a financially healthy **oxymoron** that perpetuates itself and protects **"its"** health and economic interests. Learn to protect **YOUR** health and economic interests by taking care of yourself—every day!
Be willing to do **whatever is called for!** Good health and longevity are matters of **choice** for those people who want to be *Young Again!*

PREVIEW: *Our next chapter is about "wildcats." It was a favorite of those who reviewed this book prior to publication.*

It is curious how certain lines of thought are off limits to mainstream medicine—so why are we surprised?

Chicken Pox • Herpes • Shingles

Chicken Pox, herpies and shingles are **"terrain"** conditions that "signal" **stressed** liver, **stressed** nerves, an **ACID** terrain environment—and poor "bile flow!" These "conditions" can appear at any age when the acid waste "tipping point" is exceeded! [Solution: Herpo-Max,™ enemas, L_sP_cB,™ and Cobo-12.™ See Pages 59, 127, 152, 177, 185 & Chapter 37.]

| **Hair! What To Do About It!** |

Fourteen-day-old Kombucha tea and GH_3+™ are powerful rejuvenators for clearing **acid** waste from the system, easing aching joints and improving bile-flow. They also help restore natural hair color and regrow hair—especially inconjunction with the use of HST™ Creme.

Loss of hair color, thinning and balding are **SIGNS** that the body's "terrain" is in **trouble!** Hair problems are one of the *first* **"visable"** aging **SIGNS** to appear. Hair is an *extension* of skin, so always think of hair and skin as "one!" [The earliest **"non visable"** aging "symptoms" are dental problems!]

Fast growing hair is a good **SIGN!** Loss of "body" hair tells a story. We "gray"—and lose body hair—from the top down. **Hair goes gray from the "end" back to the root—NOT the other way around as people believe.**

Medical science **ignores** hair—but hair has a "purpose!" Hair removes toxic energy from the tissues **beneath** the skin where the most toxic "soluble" body waste is stored.

Hair issues in women **always** involve female hormones and thyroid issues. Blood tests for **sub**clinical thyroid problems do **NOT** exist. Clinical tests provide a "label" for the ailing person—but labels don't provide a solution or define the cause(s). Kelp and iodine are **NOT** viable "thyroid" remedies. Thyroid activity affects connective tissue **growth-rate** in women—hence thyroid affects hair because hair is an *extension* of skin and skin is a connective tissue. Brain **"fog"** is a **BIG** menopausal-related female complaint involving the thyroid. So is "coldness!" [Men seldom suffer from "clinical" thyroid dis-ease—but all of the **symptoms** associated with male aging after age "45" screams **sub**clinical thyroid!

[Solutions to the above problems are B.T.™ *Creme, HST*™ *Creme, L_sP_cB,*™ *Kombucha Tea, GH_3+,*™ *L_sP_cC*™ *and VZ*™. *SOC*™ *increases blood flow to the scalp. The Young Again (Tissue and Liver) Protocol*™ *deacidifies the "terrain."]*

Kombucha Tea and GH_3+™ are **part of** your author's regimen for natural hair color at calendar age "61!" The tea is **inexpensive** to make at home, so no one can complain they can't afford it! Approximate cost per gallon: "50 cents!" Kombucha reproduces "perpetually" from **certified** "starts."

Deacidification is the **"KEY"** to the "terrain." Later comes hair color. Hair "regrowth" takes longer—but it's worth the effort as your author can **demonstate** and **attest to!**

➡ **Please Note:** According to Hoy Lee of British Columbia, Canada, the name *Kombucha* is of Chinese origin. Kom = gold; bu = precious; cha = tea. Hence, "precious golden tea." *"Thanks for this valuable insight, Hoy!"*   J.T.

High Enema Therapy™ Book

Forty color pictures is **why** this book is included in the *Young Again (High Enema Therapy™) Protocol*™ package. Having performed this therapy for 30 years—and incorrectly for 25 of those years—your author **discovered** the **"secret"** to this simple, inexpensive therapy. If you want to see the the miracle of agelessness manifest in your life—ask for help! [See pages 26, 76, 106, 123, 203, 212, 234, 262-3, 274, 326, 338, 343.]

Ileocecal Valve & Cancer

Six feet *up* from the anus is the "beginning" of the colon (large intestine)—and the end of the small intestine (ileum). **Between** the large and small intestines **"inside"** the cecum is the ileocecal valve that **"controls"** the rate of waste movement and nutrient absorption in the intestinal tract. People with cancer almost **always** have an ileocecal valve "locked" in the **OPEN** position—causing them to **"starve to death!"**

High Enema Therapy™ **"restores"** bowel integrity, **"stimulates"** the colon wall nerve plexus feeding the vital organs—and boosts "bile flow" from the liver/gallbladder.

Babies and children [And dogs and cats, too!] also have bowel and liver issues that need addressing. Mom can help baby with a simple enema—and children learn fast if Mom will "teach" them how to care for themselves. For adults, liver and bile and bowel issues are part of everyone's "aging" story!

So, dear reader, *"Take the leap!"* and ask for guidance with this simple health technique. Consultation is available without charge. There is **no cost** for this one-on-one service— and you will learn plenty, too!

Brain "Fatigue!"

Brain "fatigue" comes with stress, sleep deprivation, emotional issues, hormone "swings" and thyroid problems. Racemized™ Gingko, HST™ and B.T.™ cremes are **MOST** helpful for boosting a "lethargic" mind. [See page 378.]

Enhanced "PAC's"

Enhanced PAC's™ are a complement of biologically acitve **proanthrocyanidins** —all in racemized™ footprint format. PAC's™ "buffer" the body from toxic, acid wastes released into circulation during the **Tissue and Liver Protocol.**™ Without PAC's™ the body will **NOT** release its most toxic **"soluble"**wastes. Taken daily, PAC's™ restore the liver and arteries, lower blood pressure, "moderate" heart and stroke issues, ease eye problems and ease aches and pains. [These complaints are **"symptoms"** of a highly toxic, acid "terrain."] PAC's™ are *fat-and-water soluble* and a **one-of-a-kind** product "without equal," containing **24,660 activity units per bottle** in racemized™ footprint format with a biological activity rating of 10/10! They work for children, pets and adults alike!

Female Issues

1. **"Polycystic"** (*poly:* many; *cyst:*a fluid filled sac.) ovaries are a common diagnosis among women. Unfortunately, the "diagnosis" does **not** tell the patient *why* she suffers and *what* to about the problem. A cyst on the ovary is an **INCOMPLETE** ovulation [The egg never broke through the ovarian wall for deposition into the fallopian tube.]

2. Whenever women experience female discomfort, rest assured that "yeast" is also involved—but yeast is **NOT** the cause! Yeast feeds on acid waste in an out-of-balance "terrain."

3. Adult diabetes Type ll goes with polycystic ovaries, as does a "leaky-gut," sluggish bowels, poor bile flow, congested liver, bad diet—and depletion of vitamin B-12.

4. A vitamin B-12 shortfall affects everything about female metabolism. Women run short of vitamin B-12 due to poor diet, insufficient secretion of "intrinsic factor" from the stomach wall, and blood loss from years of menstruation.

Vitamin pills, sprays and sublinguals do **NOT** solve the B-12 problem. B-12 shots are synthetic band-aids, at best! The *Young Again Protocol*™ calls for the use of Cobo-12™ transdermal B-12 creme for *quick absorption* into the blood. The results can be impressive. When racemized™ algae and liver capsules are taken with Cobo-12,™ their effect on hemoglobin formation, increased oxygen capacity and anemia is "noticeable!"

5. Small amounts of fresh beet juice "daily" accelerates the **de**acidification process—and helps with both menstrual and menopausal issues. The *Young Again (High Enema*™ *& Tissue and Liver*™*) Protocols*™ SPEED **de**acidification of the female "terrain!' [See hormone cycle diagram on page 72.}

6. Thyroid problems are "epidemic" among women. The **sub**clinical **"symptoms"** are cold body, dry skin, joint-pain, wrinkling skin, thinning hair, loss of muscle mass and tone, low energy, brain fog, memory issues and slow metabolism. Excess body fat can also involve a lethargic thyroid gland.

7. Worring about the big "C" word is **NOT** part of the Vorago™ female's "worry" list. The big "C" is **NOT** genetic, but it does have **EVERYTHING** to with lifestyle, hormones—and management of the female "terrain." Follow the *Young Again (Hormone) Protocol*™ and **"IT"** will not become part of your life or **your** vocabulary. Remember, avoiding health issues is easier than trying to solve them after they happen! [See Chapter 35 *Vorago*™ *SunRise* for an expanded discussion.]

About Those "Cravings!"

If you suffer with "cravings" for processed food, cigarettes, alcohol, drugs or chocolate—and you wish to get things under control—all you have to do is **deacidify** your body and eat real food, and your carvings will go *"bye, bye!"*

High Enema Therapy™ is part of the the *Young Again Protocol*™. This simple process may "seem" a bit strange, but it works its "magic!" All you have to do is *"Do it!"*

16

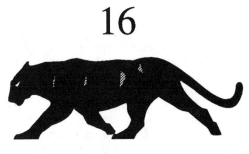

Wildcats

"The skin is to the body what the soil is to the Earth."
John Thomas

The halogens are known as the **"wildcats"** of the earth's elements. They are gases—and "chemically" speaking they are **extremely** reactive! The term *"halogen"* is dissected: *hals*-Greek for salt; *gen*-to produce. The halogens are an important piece of the aging story.

When "acid" halogen gas combines with "alkaline" earth metal ions—like sodium, calcium or magnesium, they form an ***ALKALINE salt*** like sodium chloride (table salt)! When a **halo**gen atom combines with a **hydro**gen atom and a metal ion, an ***ACID salt is formed***—like fluoride—as in tooth paste!

The halogens are part of naturally occurring mineral compounds—as found in sea water or soil and do **NOT** pose a health threat because they are in equilibrium **rather than** in toxic, chemically unstable, reactive "forms."

When man isolates and "frees" the halogens—creating out-of-balance halogen containing waste byproducts—the halogens take on a **"life"** of their own. Rock salt (halite) is sodium chloride otherwise known as "table salt!" Nature isolates this compound and stores it in the earth. Man comes along, mines it, puts it on the dinner table in defiance of nature's dietary laws—giving the halogens a part in the aging process.

Chlor**ine** and fluor**ine** are **"HALOGENS."** They are also gases. When in "solid" form, halogens are "stable." But when these "salts" are **dissolved** in body tissue fluids, the halogens are **released** into "solution" as "dissolved gas ions" that **aggressively** seek to "bond" with enzymes and tissue "proteins" in order to **STABALIZE!** Halogen-altered "protein" structures cause aging of the body's connective tissues to dramatically "accelerate!" [More information coming later in chapter!]

Chlor**ine** gas in water occurs as a chlor**ide**. Fluor**ine** gas in water occurs as fluor**ide**. Chlor**ides** and fluor**ides** in solution have an unbalanced electron valence—and therefore, try to "bond" with other molecules to "stabilize" their unstable molecular structure.

In tissues fluids of **"living"** systems, the chemical bonds binding fluorine in solid salt form are broken by hydrolysis (*hydro*-water; *lysis*-to cleave or break). Fluorine then bonds to proteins in the blood and lymph, forming **unpredictable** compounds that are hostile to delicate life processes. Fluoridated water and tooth paste are **deadly** and the experts know it! [Regardless, "corporate" government forces fluoride upon citizens under the **yellow fringed, national "war" flag** flying above every court house and public place in the union.]

Chlorine
Stabilized chlorine is a bactericidal that **indiscriminately** kills bacteria—and is very effective as a disinfectant. [Think laundry bleach!] Chlorine is used to treat public water supplies. Chlorine is VERY toxic to the liver and does major violence to the delicate mucosal tissues lining the "gut!"

Use of chlorine in public water supplies is justified on the basis of what medical science calls the "benefit-to-risk" ratio—**meaning** if the benefit to the population as a whole outweighs and justifies damage done to the individual, then a chemical or vaccine or whatever is "certified" as safe—usually under authority of "law!" [This type of thinking keeps the hospitals full! It's the reader's job to **avoid** the trap!]

Chlorine's carcinogenic characteristics are well known and are expressed in the body in many **subtle** ways. "Subtle" meaning no one dies **on-the-spot** from drinking chlorinated water. This is called *"Make it to the door science!"* If people can make it to the door, then it must be safe!

For instance, chloroform is a byproduct of chlorinated drinking water. Chloroform is extremely toxic. It is a broad spectrum poison that **indiscriminately** kills friendly "gut" bacteria while "oxidizing" delicate "gut" mucosa. It also destroys the liver! Chloroform replaced ether as a general anesthetic in surgery rooms at the turn of the century. Both have been replaced by safe substances, **"safe"** being a relative term!

There is a strong relationship between chlorine's introduction and use in public water supplies (1908) and the statistical emergence of heart attacks and cardiovascular disease. The relationship is **more** than happenstance.

Prior to 1920, coronary heart disease was not a statistically recognized problem in the United States in spite of heavy meat eating, drinking and smoking.

Atherosclerosis (build-up of plaque and deterioration of the arteries) is **directly** linked to chlorination of public water supplies. Chlorine's initial use must be understood in the wake of the epidemic of water-borne dis-eases that ravaged the United States between 1910 and 1920—infecting and killing tens of thousands of people. There were few alternatives then; but this is "now"—and there are plenty of truely safe alternatives. ***Water contaminated with pathogenic microbes is unacceptable—and so is chemically toxic drinking water. The "personal" answer to both problems is BFRV™ water.*** Due to outbreaks of pathogenic *E. coli* and *cryptosporidium* bacteria in public water supplies, the "Feds" squeeze local "corporate" governments and water districts to use toxic chemicals, chlorine, mercuric acid, etc.

Chlor**amines** are extremely toxic to the liver and are the result of "hard-core" chemical reactions with organic substances in drinking water. [BFRV™ equipment removes chloramines, as well as fluoride, flagellates (amoebas), viruses, bacteria, radioactivity and junk minerals. Once removed, vibrational memory of the contaminants is "erased" and the water "restructured." BFRV™ is **biologically friendly drinking water!**]

[Water for bathing and for High Enema Therapy™ is produced with a 3 stage, oxidation/reduction shower filter. These devices typically last for **5-8 years,** *offer high-volume water flow, and do* **NOT** *use or require cartridge replacement.]*

Sodium Hypochloride
Chlorine is *dissolved* into public water supplies from a stable **salt block** form. The reason chlorine is used in salt form has to do with pH—which we will discuss momentarily.

A salt is a combination of an acid [halogen gas ion] and a base [metal ion]; hence, "sodium fluoride" as found in tooth paste! Municipal water treatment protocol calls for the use of sodium hypo-chlor**ite**—which contains chlor**ine** in salt form. Sodium is a **BASE** alkaline metal and hypochlorite is an **extremely ACID** and unstable chlorine compound. When combined, the new compound is called, sodium hypochlor**ide.**

When the *Jekyll-and-Hyde* sodium hypo-chlorite compound is dissolved in water, it **separates!** Chlorine kills the bacteria and hydroxide raises pH so water will be palatable. The pH of most tap water is between pH 7-9. Biologically friendly drinking water—called BFRV™—is a **combination** of pH, reactivity and ORP potential "factors" that speed restoration of the **"terrain"** and return of health. [See pages 71-8, 102-109, 117, 126, 173, 220, 297, 306 (chart), 378 and Chapter 11.]

Terrain Problems
Toxic chemicals **enter** the body **bonded** to *waste* mineral ions. In the body, **acidic** chlorine and fluorine bond with metabolic wastes and oils [like soy and canola] and form **hybrid** toxins that **ALTER** the terrain and manifesting in the **"electrical"** profile of the blood as "Rouleau." Rouleau appears

as *clumped* red corpuscles. [A corpuscle is a blood cell without a nucleus.] Rouleau is a "marker" condition of a "terrain" that is under **STRESS**—and a red flag of dis-ease in the making! *The word "aging" hints at the problem. The word "degeneration" says it better!*

Sodium is a player in the aging scenario. High sodium levels in the tissues agggrevate "**hyper**tension." As excess sodium **invades** tissue fluids, it *upsets* the sodium : potassium balance in the body—setting the stage for "**cancer!**"

The body requires a **constant** supply of organic potassium to maintain its sodium : potassium balance. [Fresh vegetable juice and home-grown, organic green leafy vegetables are the most "effective" source of organic potassium.] The body "**offsets**" dietary "deficits" of potassium by "stealing" it from inside the cells. The process of "trading sodium for potassium is "**invasive**" and "**cumulative!**" Sodium invasion of the cells slows mitochondrial activity—converting an **aerobic** environment to an **an**aerobic one. The mitochondria **cannot** function in a high sodium **an**aerobic environment. The process sets the stage for **CANCER** at the "cellular level."

Chlorinated tap water is "**weakening**" the entire population. There are better and safer alternatives, but powerful industrial interests—in cahoots with yellow fringed flag "corporate" government—support chlorination. Our situation today is not unlike the outbreaks of Childbirth Fever in Dr. Semmelweis' time. [See pages 43 and 45.] Chlorine and fluoride are good for business. They keep the cattle lines at the clinics and hospitals "filled" with sick and dying people.

Imagine the economic impact that safe, biologically friendly food and drinking water would have on organized medicine, the legal system and the school system!

"Corporate" government is a BOGUS foreign "state" operating under the "yellow fringed flag" with a vested interest in keeping people sick. Sick and dead people are good for litigation, probate, estate taxes and other legal "mewings!" [See pages 196, 229, 292 and 384.]

Public Mentality

Fluoride is an American "institution"—second only to hot dogs and apple pie! Americans have a love affair going with their sweetheart "halogen"—fluorine. [Fluoride is the salt form.] The question is **WHY?** This book provides the answers for those who **CHOOSE** to think *outside the box!*

Industry, medicine, dentistry and the pharmaceutical companies have done a magnificent job of **brainwashing** Americans on the benefits of "fluoride." [Let us not forget the dental industry's "game" of calling "mercury" dental fillings, "silver" amalgams! Mercury is the most toxic element known!]

Fluorine is **THE** wildcat of the halogens. It is numero uno—**number one**—on the list of atomic elements for "reactivity!" God put fluoride under lock and key by isolating it in underground water and mineral deposits. When man discovered fluoride's industrial uses, he opened a Pandora's Box. *Fluorine is toxic to all living things. Fluoride poisoning— "fluorosis" of the tissues—manifests as **HUNDREDS** of "symptoms!" Because fluoride is a "systemic" poison that takes* **YEARS** *to manifest, it escapes blame—along with the **criminals** in government, industry and dentistry that promote it! Medical science's challenge of "No scientific proof!" is an effective cover for poisoning of ignorant, but innocent people. Fluoride is a perpetual money machine for the medical system.*

Fluoridation of water should be "CRIMINALIZED"— as should putting mercury into people's teeth!

HARD (Teeth-Bones-Skin) HEADS

Fluoride hardens the teeth—and the head. The experts fail to mention fluoride's toxic side effects—effects that grossly outweigh any conjured benefit. Theirs is a "sin" of omission! Fluoride has a subduing effect. It "slows" the brain and makes us docile—and easier to manipulate! Fluoride is easily absorbed through the skin and mucous membranes of the mouth, throat and intestines.

Medical insurance creates the "illusion" of security. Reliance on it causes people to forfeit personal responsibility for their health and rely on the system.

*[A certain toothpaste introduced in the late 1950's received the endorsement of the American Dental Association (ADA). It uses fluoride in "stannous" form. Stannous fluoride is a tin-containing compound. Tin is an element and a metal. When you mix acid fluorine gas with the alkaline metal ion of "tin," you get a SALT crystal. Stannous fluoride is a gas in salt form as designated by the -ide on the end of the word "fluoride." The ADA elevated a waste product of the tin industry to the "status" of a medically **endorsed** "therapy!" The profits to be made in a deal like this are beyond the dreams of avarice. Dentists can make a good living without poisoning people!]*

Fluorine is widely used in thousands of industrial processes—and fluoride is the industrial ***spin-off!*** Fluorine-containing compounds are **VERY** powerful left-spin substances that are **VERY** biologically "active"—and **VERY** anti-life!

In living systems, fluoride **dis**associates and becomes **EXTREMELY** unstable and "binds" with **protein enzymes** and connective tissues like bone, muscle, tendon, skin etc.

Fluoride **"attacks"** the **collagen**ous protein matrix that gives connective tissue its *flexibility* and *strength*. Wrinkled skin is a good example of the "fluoride effect." **Acidification** of body tissues only makes things worse. Fluoride is an **acid** gas! *People are rightly concerned about wrinkled skin, brittle bones and falling hair. Yet they use fluoridated water and toothpaste. They need to connect the dots!"*

Place "bone" into muriatic acid and the minerals in it will *go into solution,* leaving behind, a **rubbery-like** substance resembling a piece of spaghetti. This "substance" is the **collagen protein matrix** into which the osteoblasts deposit minerals for the construction of "bone." Fluoride binds to bone collagen proteins and create the perfect aging "crisis!" Fluoride acts similar to the hormones in birth control pills, estrogen replacements and "zeno" hormones in food and water. Fluoride interferes with the osteo**blasts** (bone building cells) and the osteo**clasts** (bone dissolving cells) by slowing repair and reproduction of healthy bone and connective tissue. Fluoride causes them to become **hard and brittle.** Bone is supposed to be **rigid** and **flexible**—like a healthy tree! Fluoridated water and toothpaste causes "brittleness," builds-up in the tissues, and causes serious degeneration. The *experts* **BLAME** osteoporosis, scleroderma, lupus and exposure to the sun. Baloney!

[*Connective Tissue Syndrome* is the latest "buz" syndrome. Broken bones and weak joints are extremely common among adolescents and older people. Something has changed! One of the "somethings" is fluoridated water, toothpaste—and that **not so innocent** little cup of poison from the school nurse and the dental hygienist!]

If you wish to enjoy a healthy life, you must learn to live and think outside the box! The Young Again Protocol™ reverses the aging effects of fluoride and a host of other "conditions!"

Medical science has endorsed the use of fluoride and is too *stubborn* and *proud* to admit its mistake. Please consider what Sir Arthur Edington once said about the scientific mind. *"Verily, it is easier for a camel to pass through the eye of a needle than for a scientific man to walk through an open door."*

The public does **NOT** know that the "famous" fluoride study about natural fluoride in well water and the absence of dental caries (cavities) was bogus! What "experts" **fail** to mention is that man-made *sodium* and *stannous* fluorides are **FAR** more reactive and hostile to living tissues than is naturally occurring fluoride. **"Living" systems are DYNAMIC!** People are not sterile, laboratory test tubes. Fluoride **"reacts"** when heat, pesticides, food additives, soy and canola oils and metabolic wastes are present in the "dynamic" of the body.

Powerful interests in dentistry, medicine and the pharmaceutical houses **influence** public policy on issues like "fluoridation" of public drinking water supplies. The *insidious* *"grant system"* decides **WHO** gets public money and **WHAT** projects "science" will study. Money controls! These same powerful "interests" determine **WHAT** is taught in medical and dental school curriculums—and they see to it that text books are heavily "**biased!**" [Private interests use "corporate" government and the "yellow fringed flag" court system as a "cover"—while foisting their deadly industrial wastes onto a trusting and unsuspecting public.] Bought-and-paid-for "experts" ply their trade—rubber stamping new "cutting edge" drugs for **NEW** dis-eases in an ongoing effort to to keep the public "confused!" **Think about this: "10" years ago,** there was no such thing as "acid reflux;" **"15" years ago,** fibromyalgia and lupus hardly existed. **"25" years ago,** Alzheimers was unknown! The "beat" goes on!

Synthesis, Stress & Acidity
"Synthesis" in chemistry jargon refers to "combining" two or more chemical agents For example, hydrogen + oxygen = water! Synthesis results in a "product" that is **physically** different than—and has different **characteristics** than—the original individual ingredients.

"Synergy" is a closely related term referring to the effects a compound or molecule produces when it interacts with substances in the environment—or in the body environment. In the body, synergism can have positive or negative effects on the terrain!" The word synergism "hints" at the "-R" group location and molecular structure of a compound. The "—R group" defines the **"reactive"** chemical nature and characteristics of a molecule. For instance: DDT vs malathion.

A healthy, youthful body is the result of **anabolic synthesis.** Anabolism is the **building-up** process. Healthy food, fresh vegetable juices, High Enema Therapy™ and bio-friendly water promote "anabolic synthesis."

Fluoride, chlorine, vaccines, pesticides, mercury, toxic air, food dyes and additives, soy and canola oils, chlor*amines* and free radicals "trigger" chain reactions in the body. If the body is under "**STRESS**"—negative synthesis and synergy destroys healthy tissue—causing the body to "go acid" and produce free radical reactions in the "terrain!" When body acid levels "max-out," sickness and dis-ease "manifest!"

Stress is the ultimate ENERGY "wild card" in everyone's life. Stress always seeks an outlet and must be "managed." Energy is NEVER lost, it merely changes form.

Free Radicals • Antioxidants • Organic Food
Toxic substances released in living systems produce "free radicals." Free radicals trigger uncontrolled oxidation of cells and tissues. There are **only** two ways for the body to deal with free-radical molecules: **STOP** their formation or **NEU-**

TRALIZE their effect by "altering" their structure through the addition or subtraction of "electrons!" Free radicals cause **"uncontrolled"** cellular oxidation [catabolism] and the death of healthy cells. [See pages 23, 24 and 198.]

Catabolic, self-cannibalization and aging go hand-in-hand. Catabolism and anabolism are opposites!

A "pesticide" is both an organic poison and a free-radical producing chemical. Pesticides are man-made organic poisons constructed around the "carbon" atom. The public fails to understand the danger of mixing words and concepts like organic, poison and carbon. [**"CARBON"** is atomic element #12. These subjects will be discussed in detail in Capter 21.]

Crafty wordsmiths and bogus science *scramble* terms to create **confusion** and the **impression** in the public's mind that pesticides are **"ORGANIC"**—and therefore are "friendly" to Earth and Her inhabitants. [Your author encourages the reader to ignore the opinions of "experts" in matters of health because they can't even save themselves!]

When the term *organic* is applied to food, the inference is that poisons are not present and the food was grown using natural fertilizers—as opposed to NPK salt fertilizers. Organic food is generally—but not always—better than non-organic food. Home-grown food is the best! [Corporate government—a "pawn" of private interests—took "jurisdiction" over the term "organic" to create the **"PERCEPTION"** of *wholesomeness* and to "license" the the term "organic" for our "protection!" Perception is reality—and the public *swallowed the hook!* Real organic is fine! Government organic is fraud! Believe it!

Everyone should grow some fresh vegetables—be it in pots or a section of the yard. Even small amounts of real "live" food has powerful effects on health.

The Establishment

The entrenched scientific, medical, and pharmaceutical establishment is **"at odds"** with personal health and longevity. They have a vested interest in **keeping** things status quo—so they can bilk the people of their money, limit their freedoms and control their minds.

Professional people often suffer from **professional myopia**—along with a good dose of *professional ego!* They are the product of their training—and few of them venture outside the "box." [In fairness, professionals are **"watched"** by their "state" licensing boards. Those who step-out-of-line or *carelessly* put the patient's best interest "first"—are at odds with fellow practitioners! Doctors and dentists who act upon **TRUTH** must be **very careful** and keep a very low public profile because their "peers" will turn on them like the pack of "devils" they are! Professionals must meet the "standard of care!" Believe it!

It's a good idea to "cultivate" a relationship with an alternative-minded physician in case you are in trouble and want to avoid falling prey to mainstream medicine. Conventional practitioners are **NOT** open to—or free to pursue—alternative healing modalities. They quote chapter and verse from medical literature in their "defense" when they know better! At the same time, they are caught between "ego," insurance companies, government control, an ignorant, lawsuit-happy public—and watchdog medical review boards. No wonder things are such a mess!

Few medical insurance carriers will insure people working in dental offices because of the high incidence of sickness, dis-ease and suicide! The mercury and fluoride they use are to blame—and these professionals pay with their health and lives—even more than their patients!

Mercury • Fluoride • BFRV™

Heavy metal poisoning is a serious and common issue. Toxic metals interfere with brain and nerve function and **must** be purged from the tissues. [The *Young Again Protocol*™ frees and safely passes heavy metals from the *bio-electric* body.]

The USA is experiencing huge increases in neurological **brain disorders** like Alzheimers, Multiple Sclerosis, Muscular Dystrophy and brain tumors. You can "bet" fluoride, toxic heavy metals and "zeno" estrogens are root causes of these horrible maladies! When fluoride combines with mercury residues, the immune system *"takes a hit"* and **Schwann's cell activity** at the nerve "synapses" drops-off! The result is a list of "syndromes" and nerve "disorders." [See page 248.]

Fluoride is a systemic poison that is **"at odds"** with good health and the idea of a healthy, happy life. Avoid it if you wish to become *Young Again!*

PREVIEW: *In our next chapter, you will discover WHY sex hormone production collapses as the bio-electric body ages.*

The God Card

Pull the "God card" whenever medical folks get "pushy!" Tell'em *"I will pray about it and let you know!"* Repeat as necessary!

What is the hardest task in the world to do? Think!
Ralph Waldo Emerson

Source Information Packet
For information, call (800) 659-1882 or (509) 465-4154 or write: John Thomas P.O. Box 1240 Mead Washington 99021-1240 USA fax (509) 466-8103.

Think!

We suffer and die for "failure" to observe the rules of the game—NOT because of what we do!

Did the cancer patient *always* have cancer? **No!** Was the diabetic *always* a diabetic? **No!** Did the lady with arthritis *always* have arthritis? **No!** These people **LOST CONTROL** of their body "terrains" due to:

- **Failure** to observe the "fundamentals."
- **Failure** to deacidify the body's tissues.
- **Failure** to restore the hormonal system.
- **Failure** to drink biologically friendly water.
- **Failure** to eat right-spin, high-energy food.
- **Failure** to live a disciplined, focused life.

Failure to make correct choices is **"THE"** issue. **Failure** is a "self-imposed" choice! If you want God to do you a miracle, you have to do your part. Stop the blame game!

Mind & Body

Never underestimate the power of mind over body. Daily, your author talks with people who **cannot** be helped because they **refuse** to control their thoughts—and labor under **misconceptions** about the **causes** of their problems.

There are many, good books written about the power of the mind. Let's summarize a few points:

1. Negative, unhappy, critical, angry, fearful, depressed and misguided thoughts and "words" manifest in physical form—which affects mood, hormones and immune function—and brings on dis-ease. Thoughts and words have consequences!
2. The aura diminishes in size when we "think" negative thoughts. Dis-ease manifests as "thought" in the flesh.
3. A healthy outlook promotes healing; and a poor emotional/mental attitude blocks healing. Guard your thoughts!
4. Bowel and liver function are affected by emotion and thoughts. Good thoughts are better than laxatives!
5. *Positive-image "visualization"* produces results. What we think, we experience. What we voice, we create.
6. Beliefs about oneself, life and future affects us—and those around us. Refuse to harbor bad thoughts!
7. Exercise is as good for the mind as it is for the body. Exercise daily. Walk, pump iron, do calisthenics and yoga.
8. Good thoughts, kindness to others and self-love "heal!"
9. Forgiveness heals! Do not hold grudges. Forgiveness releases you from the other person's hate! Karma rules!
10. Create the world you want with your thoughts!
11. Protect yourself and loved ones through positive visualization—and by refusing to "focus" on darkness and evil.
12. Love is *light;* hate is *dark!*

Read: *Your Body Believes Every Word You Say!*

17

Diagnosis Or Post Mortems?

*"The organs of the body can be likened to towns on a
map, each being unto itself while each is connected to
the other and ultimately to the composite body."*
Dr. Arnold Lorand

The "golden age" of medicine extended from approximately 1840 to 1930. It was a period that saw an explosion of new knowledge in all fields of science.

"Clinical" observations of the doctors of this period are of particular interest to us—partly because they provide a **fundamental** view of "aging"—and mostly because they *preceded* the advent of modern man's environmental mistakes.

The golden age of medicine was a period of "low-tech," drugless medicine. Doctors relied on astute observation to guide the patient. They also spent more time with patients, often getting to know them better than they knew themselves.

Uncommon good sense was the guiding rule. There was no place to shift the blame if the chosen modality (therapy) failed to cure the patient. The patient was viewed *in camera*— as a unit—**NOT** as "parts," and the word "syndrome" was not yet in fashion. Cause and effect, diagnosis and prognosis, were anchored in **"OBSERVATION"**—rather than endless **"TESTS!"**

Modern Medicine
Present-day medical technology is a *mixed* blessing. It **excels** in diagnosis "after the fact," organ transplants and emergency medicine. Dis-ease "prevention" does **NOT** exist! Modern medicine has become a never-ending "process" of trial and error, hard-core drugs, sharp-scalpels and **"ISOLATED"** **snap-shots** of the "process" called dis-ease. The medical system is "reactive" when it should be "proactive!"

High-tech modern medicine is hopelessly befuddled because doctors and nurses are **NOT** trained to identify and diagnose **sub**clinical illness. Yesteryear's observations are considered "dated"—even primitive—because the new kids on the block learn it all in "college"—using high-tech smoke and mirrors—and the "model" they learn is **DEFECTIVE!**

Allopathic medicine has an **"unholy"** reliance on gadgetry and high-powered drugs—where people are seen as flesh-and-blood machines composed of "replaceable" parts. Medicine does not understand that health and energy are **lost** in the "invisible" realm—before dis-ease **manifests** in the "visible" spectrum. Medicine does **NOT** realize that the body is composed of *energy-dynamic* forces that dictate vital organ function—and that the "terrain" is **"EVERYTHING!"**

Diagnosis Or Post Mortems?

If it were possible to examine the vital organs of the body—particularly the *ductless* glands like the pituitary, thyroid, parathyroid, adrenals, thymus, pancreas, and gonads (testes and ovaries)—the "effects" of our living habits would be plainly evident. But we cannot make such an examination and must, therefore, learn **HOW** to read and interpret **symptoms** and solve our problems before they become **SIGNS!**

Dr. William Albrech, a brilliant professor of soils at the University of Missouri, once commented that we no longer know what healthy animal organs look like because we see only *abnormal* organs. That's the way it is in medicine today.

There was a time when the physician saw **both** healthy and *pathogenic* organs and could compare them. By knowing what "healthy" organs looked like, the doctor could identify disease—and if a good observer—he could identify **sub**clinical symptoms before they became clinical **SIGNS.**

Today, **sub**clinically sick people are the norm—and medical science's efforts are directed at "naming" the dis-ease. The "label," however, is **meaningless** because it does **NOT** explain **"HOW"** and **"WHY"** the dis-ease condition developed—and **most importantly**—what steps must be taken so the body can restore the "terrain!"

"Strange Meanings!"

To compensate for the *universality* of a **sub**clinically sick population, medical schools have rewritten the **STANDARDS** by which they **define** health and dis-ease. This is similar to what is occurring in "government" schools—where today's "A" was yesterday's "C"—and in the financial markets where people rely on "lies" from government statistical bureaus and corporate financial reports based on "pro forma" information. [Think Enron, et al!]

For example, **bogus holistic medicine**—as taught in "traditional" medical schools—defines **"illness"** as an abnormal condition where the *present* level of function has declined compared to a *previous* level. By this definition, *neither* the present level nor the previous level of function meets any defined "**STANDARD.**" No longer is "illness" defined as the **absence** of health or "health" as the **absence** of dis-ease. "Illness" and "health" have lost their meanings.

Today, health and illness are defined in terms of the individual's *personal perception* of their state of being. In other words, how one *feels* about oneself. Trying to make sense of this reminds me of the Chinese journalist who exclaimed, *"Explain please, strange words and meanings!"*

Reversing the aging process requires that we become enlightened as to "**WHY**" we age. We cannot assign responsibility for good health to **experts** and a medical "model" that fails to account for root causes of illness, dis-ease—and aging.

95% of the population suffers with Rouleau in their blood. [See pages 99, 136, 242, 257 and 308.]

Body Communication Systems

The body has six different internal communication systems—and all of them affect the aging process. These systems transmit and coordinate messages to various parts of the body. The names of these systems are the endocrine and exocrine systems, central and peripheral **nervous** systems, and the **blood** and **lymphatic** systems.

[Medical science ignores the lymphatic system which is the body's primary "protein" communication system affecting circulation and stagnation of tissue plasma proteins. Blood plasma proteins "seep" into the tissue spaces between the cells where the exchange of oxygen and carbon dioxide, waste and nourishment takes place. The tissue spaces are where acidic, amyloid waste accumulates and amyloid plaques "form." Old age and dis-ease have their roots in the tissues of the "terrain!"]

The *nervous, exocrine and endocrine* systems are **irrevocably** linked to each other. The nervous system "**transmits**" electrical impulses originating in the neuron's cell body by way of dendritic nerve fibers called "axons." Signals are transmitted in picoseconds—faster than the speed of light—moving along the axon from synapse to synapse with the help of specialized cells called "Schwann's" cells. [See page 248!] Schwann's cells are **critical** to a healthy nerve tissue—and they play an important part in **female** [and male!] physiology and health.

As we age, the neurilemma (the myelin sheath covering the nerve fibers) "deteriorates," paving the way for degenerative nerve conditions like Alzheimers, MS, Cerebral Palsy, peripheral neuropathy and lupus. [F/G™ creme, Cobo-12™ creme, VZ II™, L_sP_cC,™ L_sP_cB™ and SOC™ help **AVOID** and **MANAGE** these ugly conditions by restoring the "terrain!"]

Once a degenerative nerve "condition" displays sufficient **SIGNS** for the doctor to diagnose it—the patient is in deep water. And yet—given the opportunity and the means to recover—the body can **"regenerate"** an entirely new and functional nervous system—but only if "terrain" issues are **"addressed!"** The body can regenerate limbs, grow hair on bald heads, exchange fat for muscle and grow joint cartilage. These miracles require a healthy and functioning endocrine system, **de**acidification of the terrain—and lots of PATIENCE!

Endocrine & Exocrine Systems

The endocrine system makes its wishes known using chemical **and** hormonal messengers! Chemical messengers produce a fast response. Think of an emergency situation where adrenalin is produced to cope with "crisis"—and cortisol for handling the "transition" **after** the crisis is over. Sexual messengers like estrogen and testosterone are different. They require hours-to-days to produce a response—and their effect can last for days and weeks.

Restoration of nerve and hormonal system pathways is fundamental to health and longevity.

Most exocrine glands secrete into **ducts** which in turn flow into body cavities like the stomach or intestines. Exocrine glands like the sudoriferous (sweat) and sebaceous (oil) glands secrete to the skin's surface instead.

The **ductless** glands of the endocrine system secrete their hormones directly into the **tissue spaces** around and between "secreting" cells—instead of into ducts. The tissue spaces **between the cells** are filled with amyloid fluid and blood and lymph "capillary beds."

Some hormones are transported *by the blood* to their destination(s)—which is usually another gland. Hence, the **ductless** glands interact together and in *concert* with the entire body terrain via the "receptors." [Receptor sites *"lock-up"* when zeno analogs "attach!" The **ENTIRE** population suffers from "zeno" estrogen lock-up of critical receptor sites. Lock-up exerts influence over the "terrain" via the vital organs.]

Receptor "lock up" is common in women using—or who have used—birth control pills. HRT (hormone replacement therapy) and steroids—including synthesized DHEA, cortisone and melatonin—cause women to lose control of their "terrains" and become prisoners unto themselves! Synthetic hormones do **NOT** voluntarily release from the "receptors." [That is the purpose of the *Young Again Protocols.*™]

"STRESS" dramatically affects the functions of the ovaries, liver, adrenals and thyroid.

Some endocrine glands are both **duct** and duct**less** glands. Examples are the pancreas, ovaries, testes, kidneys, stomach, small intestine, skin, heart, and placenta.

Hormones maintain health and manage **metabolic rate.** The amount of hormones released into or withdrawn from circulation is based on the body's needs, the secreting gland's ability to produce and/or degrade hormones, and the body's ability to respond to circulating hormones. [The liver "orchestrates" the hormones—and if the liver is in trouble, so is the terrain and the person to whom it belongs.]

Hormonal excess manifests as "deficiencies" when the hormonal system is OUT OF BALANCE!

Some hormones are carried "free form" in the blood; others require blood plasma **carrier proteins** to bind and transport them. For example, insulin. Carrier proteins are made and managed by the liver—and dysfunctional **liver** manifest in unexpected ways, diabetes being one of them!

[Diabetes is an autoimmune condition involving a leaky-gut, a strssed liver and pancreas, and poor "bile flow!"]

Back to the receptors. When receptors on "target" cells respond to a hormone, a message is relayed back to the gland that produced the hormone to **STOP** production. Excess hormones are supposed to be degraded (oxidized) by the targetcells themselves or by the **liver!**

If the LIVER is dysfunctional and cannot do its job—health suffers and dis-ease takes over the terrain.

Old-Age Symptoms In The Young

SIGNS of early senescence (aging) include obesity, hair and skin problems, connective tissue disorders, and gum and teeth problems. ["Aging" begins 20-30 years ahead of manifestation of age-related clinical dis-ease.]

Symptoms that serve as **"markers"** of poor health are amenorrhea (irregular menstruation), low sex drive, impotence, accelerated pulse, cold in the extremities, a tendency to constipation, edema, brain-fog, depression, excess albumin in urine, a low A/G ratio, and elevated "CRP" levels.

Albumin is a blood "serum protein"—and very little of it should get past the kidney's filters. Excess albumin in urine is a serious condition indicating diminished kidney function and deterioration of the kidney's glomeruli.

Casts are composed of salts, hyalin, protein—and chemical and mineral wastes. These wastes "precipitate," taking the shape of the kidney's tubules. Their presence indicates **"catabolic"** activity within the body's "terrain."

Cold in the extremities indicates thyroid **dis**function, stressed ovaries, mercury poisoning and hormonal excess. Central to these conditions is a stressed **LIVER**—the body's "furnace." An accelerated pulse and fever indicates the presence of "infection" **somewhere** in the system! A "non-febrile" infection—an infection **without** a fever—can be detected with a blood test that measures "CRP." Infected "teeth" or an infected prostate often produce a non-febrile, low-grade infection that spill toxins and bacteria into the bloodstream.

Constipation is "systemic" aging **symptom** because it is **central** to **ALL** body functions. Constipation is usually defined as not moving the bowels "regularly"—whatever that means. Moving your bowels is **NOT** the same as a bowel movement that is the result of heavy **"bile flow"** from the liver and gall bladder.

"Frequency" of bowel activity does **NOT** tell the whole story. Yes, it is better to have 2 or 3 bowel movements a day—than only one. But the question is *"As a result of what?"* Water intake? Dietary fiber? Physical activity? Juicing? Nerves? All of these things influence bowel activity—but they do **NOT** "open" the liver's biliary ducts and increase bile "flow."

The MOST critical issue to human health is "bile flow." Bile flow controls deacidification of the "terrain!"

Herbs and laxatives **"make"** the bowels **"move"** without increasing bile flow. Bile carries "acids" and kills parasites, too! **De**acidification is the **primary** issue in maintaining and regaining control of the "terrain." [The *Young Again (Tissue and Liver) Protocol*™ restores and maintains bile flow.]

So-called "acid stomach" is another **aging symptom**. Acid stomach is **NOT** an acid condition. Rather, it is a bile-flow issue that manifests as a digestion problem. Anything involving the bowels or digestion involves bile and the "liver!"

Insufficient production of digestive enzymes in the stomach and intestine is a "given" after age 30—and the older you are, the worse the problem becomes. Hence, the need for racemized™ DiSorb Aid II,™ R/BHCl™ and Yucca Blend.™

Today, everything related to digestion gets the label "Acid Reflux Disorder"—a *ghost-type* condition that everbody seems to have, but none of the "experts" seem to be able to explain **"why?"** Stomach acidity and acid regurgitation into the esophagus are the result, **NOT** the cause, of the condition.

Acid-reflux, leaky-gut, irritable-bowel, diverticulitis, colitis, Crohn's, constipation and hemorrhoids are *birds of a feather*. "Terrain" **de**acidification solves all of them!

Edema (water retention) is an **aging symptom**—and the liver and bile flow are central to it! The accumulation of excess amyloid wastes in the tissue spaces draws and holds **excess** water. Use of diuretics are seldom justified because "water" is **NOT** the problem—**EXCESS** "waste" is! Loss of body hair goes hand-in-hand with an acid terrain. Acid waste settling in the legs of older people is common and goes with edema, swelling, fungus under the nails—and deterioration of the feet. [The L/CSF™ machine circulates lymphatic fluids and moves tissue-bound waste out of the legs.]

Stress • Obesity • Sleep

As early as 1903, it was demonstrated that the **ductless** glands control **ALL** the processes of oxidation—and that diseases of metabolism like diabetes, obesity, gout, arthritis, heart dis-ease, etc. are the direct consequence of *alterations* in the function of these important glands.

"Oxidation" is another word for aging! Oxidation is the opposite of "reduction." Tissue oxidation produces free radicals, slows metabolic rate, and diminishes production of our energy molecule "ATP." Ultimately, the thyroid and liver control metabolic rate—and the **"TERRAIN"** controls both of them!

Hormones play a key role in glandular metabolism—and are also a driving force in the production of ATP. The pancreas, thyroid, testicles, ovaries and liver **"stress out"** whenever the body accumulates **excess CORTISOL** [A non-sexual hormone produced by the adrenal glands that has **profound** influence over female and male sexual hormones!]

The adrenal glands produce adrenaline and cortisol. Adrenaline is a *"fight-or-flight"* hormone offering **instant** response. Cortisol's effect lasts for many hours.

Due to the nature of modern life—with all its stresses [husband, wife, children, financial, work, etc.]—people are **"stressed-out"** 24/7/365! Constant stress causes the body to go into **"overdrive"** and **STAY THERE!** [Stress has **disastrous** effects on the vital organs and greatly interferes with management and maintenance of balance within the "terrain!"]

Elevated cortisol levels absolutely **DEVASTATE** women's and men's sexual hormones. That is why people "lose" their appetite for sexual activity when they are "stressed"—and this is now occurring as early as the mid-twenties!

People think they are doing just fine—until they reach their mid-twenties and thirties and their "adrenals" give-out and their lives come unraveled!

Over-stimulate the body with cortisol and you will go into **"overdrive!"** Stress disrupts normal liver and bowel function—and it totally disrupts the ability to achieve deep, restful sleep! The "stressed" person goes to bed in overdrive—and wakes-up in overdrive—**NOT** fully rested. Each day piles on more and more stress in an endless cycle. [Stress "hammers" the adrenal glands and drives cortisol production—the single biggest stress-related **"wild card"** in the aging process.]

[When your author was a child, mom would talk about poor Mrs. Jones who had a "nervous breakdown." **Translation!** *Mrs. Jones was suffering from adrenal exhaustion with a good "dose" of menopause! The doctor would tell the husband the condition was "mental"—which was a bald-faced lie! These woman needed four things: Sound sleep, liver and adrenal support, zero stress, and help with female hormones!]*

*Sleep is something you CANNOt put into a pill.
Without enough "deep" sleep, the body comes unraveled!*

*[The Young Again Protocol™ destresses the "terrain"
and puts people in control of their lives. Destressing the system
is accomplished with: PU™ and CWD.™ PU™ settles the adrenals
and cuts cortisol production. CWD™ is a multi-function approach. "C" is for cortisol; "W" is for weight; "D" is for depression
and blood-sugar-related "mood swings!" Food-related stress
and cortisol levels affect fat metabolism—and female hormones,
too! When you put people under pressure and turn up the heat—
their terrains "collapse!" Is it any wonder people are having a
difficult time "coping" these days?]*

Scar Tissue • Alcohol • Cirrhosis

Functional cells are called **parenchyma** cells. Dysfunctional cells are called **stroma** cells. As functional cells die,
they are replaced by dysfunctional cells forming **"scar"** tissue.

Stroma cells "encase" the vital organs—but they do not
directly contribute to the organ's functional purpose. For
example, bile production by the liver. The liver's parenchyma
cells are called **hepatocytes** (*hepat*-liver; *cyte*-cell). As the
hepatocytes die, stroma cells **"invade"** along with amyloid
plaque. Alzheimers dis-ease is a classic example!

Alcohol is a poison and causes scar tissue formation in
the liver by "killing" the hepatocytes. The "drunk" is said to be
"in**tox**icated!" **Tox**—as in **tox**in—means **poison!** When you
drink alcohol, you are **poisoning** yourself.

*A healthy, functioning liver is needed to reverse
aging—so avoid alcohol to see your wish fulfilled.*

*[If you know someone who drinks regularly, perform this
liver test on them. First, have the person lie on their back on the
floor and raise their knees to relax their stomach. Then, gently
but deeply, push down on the person's front right side, just
below the rib cage. You will feel a firm to hard "mass"—the
LIVER! Be careful, it may be tender and massaging harshly can
cause the person to become ill—and lose it! The liver should be
soft and hidden up-under the ribs. Or have the person stand and
extend their right arm. Then, gently pull down at the wrist, while
measuring arm "strength" to maintain the horizontal, shoulder-
level position. Next, gently pull down on the arm while your other
hand touches the "liver region." People with stressed, toxic livers
lose strength and their arm cannot resist! Some people become
nauseated and have to lie down because of the surge of
electrical energy into their sick liver—and a "surge" type release
of bile from the gallbaldder.]*

Atrophy Of Sex Glands & Obesity

Atrophy (deterioration) of the sex glands goes hand in

hand with systemic toxicity, obesity, thyroid, and **LIVER** problems. Atrophy of the ovaries and testicles takes **"years"** to fully manifest. Diminished sex drive is a **symptom** of growing older and slowing metabolic rate. A youthful body has a "high" metabolic rate and "recovers" and regenerates quickly. [Return of sexual vigor takes time and is related to "thyroid" issues.] Obesity is a **SIGN** of metabolic slowdown and hormonal imbalance in both sexes—and particularly in women. **Meno**pausal effects are more pronounced in women than are **andro**pausal effects in men! Sadly, doctors think nothing of removing a woman's female organs (uterus and ovaries) with **"LITTLE"** justification! [The female medical "model" is defective. It does **NOT** teach women how things work and what they need to do to care for themselves.]

Removal of woman's ovaries is the equivalent of castration for men. How many men have you seen standing in line to be castrated?

Women must learn **HOW** to stay healthy if they expect to avoid female problems. [See page 72 and the index under "hormones" for a discussion of the "hormone cycle"—which is **NOT** the same as the menstrual cycle.] Maintaining the "cycle" with or without body parts and monthly periods—**regardless of age**—is the focus of the **Vorago**™ effect. Vorago™ women do NOT age! [See Chapter 36 for details!]

Deacidification of the body "terrain" through increased "bile flow" is absolutely fundamental to female health. Women cannot depend on medical "experts" who base their diagnoses and recommendations on a faulty medical model that **IG-NORES** liver "function"—the **"KEY"** ingredient of female terrain management. When "experts" suffer and die from the very same ailments as their patients, something is wrong!

Female cancer is NOT "genetic"—and it is totally "avoidable" if correct protocols are followed.

Osteoporosis: A "Female" Issue!

Osteoporosis (reduced bone density; honeycombing of the bones) involves vascularization and "invasion!" of bone by blood vessels for the "express" purpose of **WITHDRAWING** minerals "stored" in bone tissue. **"Vascularization"** precedes **BOTH** bone formation and bone dismantling. Osteoporosis is a **symptomatic** "effect"—**NOT** the cause of loss of bone density. The condition has **NOTHING** to do with dietary "calcium" intake or blood calcium levels. Fact is, women with elevated blood calcium levels are "at risk" for a heart attack **FAR** more than women who do **NOT** take "calcium" supplements. [The problem here is the skewing of the calcium : magnesium ratio and "precipitation" of **excess** minerals that clog the arteries.] Osteoporosis is very closely linked to hormone imbalances—and the accumulation of **EXCESS** tissue acids in "both" structural and soluble forms. Thyroid is also an osteoporosis "factor"—as is the **"inability"** to maintain therapeutic levels of Vitamin-C in the "blood!"

Women need **therapeutic** "blood" levels of Vitamin-C for collagen, bone and connective tissue formation or they **CANNOT** reverse osteoporosis and restore their beauty. Traditional Vitamin-C forms like pills, powders and even foods will **NEVER** achieve therapeutic blood levels. Osteoporosis is both **preventable** and **reversable** if the individual is patient and willing to walk the line. [The *Young Again! Protocol*™ calls for the use of L_sP_cC™ to achieve the effect women so badly need. See Chapter 38 *MoonShine* for details!]

First comes damage control. Then comes the rebuilding process. Aging "reversal" is the final step.

Youthful Body & Vanity Issues

The body is composed of **connective, epithelial, muscular** and **nerve** tissues in dozens of forms and combinations that are designed to serve a particular purpose.

Connective tissue performs the functions of binding, supporting and interfacing other tissues. Skin is a "connective" tissue and includes outer dermal surfaces and **sub**cutaneous layers that are served by blood and lymph capillary systems.

The basement membranes of the skin—and the fatty tissues beneath them—is where the body stores **excess** "soluble" acid waste that could have and should exit the body via "bileflow" every day. Storage of cellular waste occurs by **"default"** when **acidic** waste fluids in tissue spaces **FAILS** to be picked-up by the lymphatic system. "Resident" fluid tissue waste is called "amyloid" fluid—and it is very **acid** and produces "cross-linking" of the skin's **COLLAGEN** fibers. Wrinkled leathery skin is the aging "effect!"

[SOC™ lotion softens and breaks cross-linking of the outer skin. SOC™ capsules work from the "inside" by increasing blood and nerve flow into injured, scarred and aged skin which speeds regeneration! VZ II™ "digests" **STRUCTURAL** *"waste" called amyloid plaque and scar tissue. Racemized™ Skin Creme stimulates formation of "new" skin. L_sP_cC™ causes the body to manufacture massive amounts of "new" collagen by delivering Vitamin-C directly into the blood stream* **AS IF** *it was administered by an "IV" needle! When you achieve therapeutic blood levels of Vitamin-C, miracles occur!]*

Venereal Disease • Sexual Excess • Goiter

Sexually transmitted dis-eases (STD's) are on the rise! It is estimated that **3 out of 5** people have it. Monday mornings at the doctor's office provides confirmation of the scale of the problem—a problem that **"transcends"** the issue of "promiscuity" by what it says about people's **"state"** of health. A healthy body terrain does **NOT** contract STD's—or anything else for that matter! Venereal infections occur when the body terrain is **"ripe"** for infection—meaning "acid!" From genital herpes and warts to syphilis, gonorrhea, or chlamydia—the "terrain" **CONTROLS**—and the **liver** control the terrain. *Topical application of MGIW™ Water™ is "useful" for infections of the penis, vagina and vulva. Herpo-Max™ is taken orally to assist and control flare-ups!*

[Your author had a buddy in the army who visited brothels regularly. When asked how many times he had contracted STD, Cal responded "Never! I always take a fresh lemons and wash down immediately afterwards!" The highly acid lemon juice breaks peptide bonds that form protein structures of pathogenic microorganisms. Fine for men but delicate female mucosa cannot tolerate lemon! Women should use diluted raw "apple cider vinegar" and 3% hydrogen peroxide douches "immediately" following unprotected sex.]

Herpes outbreaks are set-off and made worse by stress, chocolate and peanuts. Lysine—a commonly available amino acid—"moderates" outbreaks if taken quickly at outbreak. Herpo-Max™ also works wonders on this "problem"—but ultimately herpes is a **"TERRAIN"** issue!

Sexual excess alters thyroid function as noted by the ancient Hebrews who examined the neck of the newly married bride the morning following the wedding night. A swollen neck was a **SIGN** of marriage consummation and heavy sexual activity. Young adult women who sexually abuse their bodies lose their youthful appearance early and age faster because of stress imposed on their ovaries and thyroid gland. There **is** a "link" between thyroid function and female hormonal balance. Mercury amalgam dental fillings severely depress thyroid function in females of any age.]

A man's inability to get an erection or true frigidity in women is **both** hormone and terrain driven. Poor blood flow, low hydration levels, prostate, thyroid and bowel issues, diabetes, stressed liver and leaky-gut **ALL** play a part.

Soy and canola oils also play a part here. A test lab found that canola oil caused sterility in rabbits, and it definitely messes up milk cows. The book *Our Stolen Future* **EXPOSED** the "zeno" estrogen problem. Soy produces the **very same effects** in women and children as synthetic hormones—and it "damps" thyroid activity, too!

Too frequent pregnancies and prolonged lactation accompanied by a **poor diet** can produce **"goiter"** in women. The female body needs **AT LEAST** two years of rest and nourishment between each child. Iodine may prevent "goiter"—but it does not meet the need for thyroid. [B.T.™ creme meets that need as does HST™ Creme. Woman notice the difference immediately. See the index for more information.]

Blood Sugar Management

Blood-sugar management is a multi-faceted issue that includes dozens of health, diet and lifestyle choices. Fundamental to blood-sugar management is the *Young Again Protocol*™ because it focuses on the "terrain!" And **fundamental** to the terrain is the "liver!" CWD™ is useful for complaints associated with low blood-sugar (moodiness, low energy, weight gain and sleep disorders). PU,™ Gluco Factor-X,™ R/C™ and MZ™ also play a part here. High Enema Therapy™ is **VERY** important to "ongoing" management of the "terrain!"

The goal is always the same: deacidification of the "terrain" and restoration of vital organ function.

Let's Review

The organs burn out when **acid**ification of the terrain occurs. Stress compounds all health and terrain issues. **Excess** manifests as "deficiencies" and dis-ease. Healing "crises" experienced during so called **"cleanses"** are a reflection of the person's toxicity level and their liver's **"INABILITY"** to remove acidic, blood-borne wastes and get them out of the system via increased bile flow and bowel acitivity. **De**acidification lays the foundation for healing and aging reversal. Both involve paying for **past** "choices." The discomfort is "little" compared to the agony of growing old and suffering!The body is a **DYNAMIC** system that succumbs to the process we call aging—by default! Escaping death is not an option Reversing the aging process and enjoying a good life is a matter of choice. **Exercise it!**

A "post-mortem" is a poor way to discover that your "chosen" lifestyle and belief system were defective.

Assist your body—and you will become *Young Again!*

PREVIEW: *Our next chapter discusses HOW the body "manufactures" what it needs by way of the bacteria—and how energy contained in minerals fuels the life process.*

Nano Scale

At "nano scale" matter is so **very** small that things heretofore considered impossible—become very possible!

Source Information Packet
For information, call (800) 659-1882 or (509) 465-4154 or write: John Thomas P.O. Box 1240 Mead Washington 99021-1240 USA fax (509) 466-8103.

It's Your Choice!

You don't have to feel and look "old" and lose control of your life—unless you are **un**willing to take personal responsibility for yourself! The *Young Again Protocol*™ was developed to help people get control of their lives. The programs are **NOT** hard to follow. You do **NOT** have to take time off-work. Suffering and discomfort are **NOT** a problem, considering the "burden" people labor under most days of their lives. Your author knows of **NOTHING** that feels as good as **NOT** having a personal physician and **NOT** having to swallow red, purple, blue and pink "medications" daily! It is a **wonderful** feeling to waken each day and know that **five years from now** you will look and feel better than you did yesterday—and that your tomorrows will be healthy and happy. When you feel "good," you are glad to be alive—and you are a **blessing** to people around you. So **WHAT** is holding you back? **Money?** *The Young Again Protocol*™ can be implemented on a frugal budget! Money is only an excuse—and a bad one at that! **Fear?** You can only **improve** the quality of your life by following the *Young Again Protocol.*™ Fear is just another excuse! An excuse by any other name is still an excuse! Most folks **appreciate** mentoring and guidance in putting their life back together again. If you would like some one-on-one, call and ask for *"Help!"*—and you will receive it **"without"** cost. A consultation is the best way for everybody to find their "comfort" zone and decide if it is possible to implement the ideas and protocols in this book in your life.

Gas-Lady "Gloria"

In March, 1994, in Riverside CA, Gloria R. (age 32) checked into the emergency room—her body a "balloon" and near death. When the doctors and nurses cut her open, her blood turned to white "crystals" as poisonous gas filled the room and some of the medical staff "collapsed"—some in critical condition. Gloria was a customer of my brother. She drank heavily and did drugs. Her body was a "cannister" of *metallic* nitrogen. She could have **spontaneously** burst into **"flames"**—**literally!** Her body was a *"extreme"* example of **ACIDIFICATION!**

Alternative DENTAL Care - At Home!

Take care of your teeth and gums with a Bio-Magnetic™ Irrigator and Oral advantage™. The irrigator manipulates hydrogen ions in water so plaque is **"oxidized"** from the teeth. Oral Advantage™ "neutralizes" oral infections. Do **not** confuse a vibrating tooth brush or a "pic type" squirt-gun with this device! There is no comparison! Your author's teeth are **beautiful** and his gums are **healthy** and his teeth have only been cleaned once in **8 years!** No plaque means no decay or gum disease—and few dental bills. [See pages 79 and 204.]

"False" Readings

The effect of positive energy can **"stir"** the system to the point of illness. This type of reaction is **wrongly** called a "healing crisis." It occurs in people who are very toxic—and who fail to provide a **means** by which acid wastes can **EXIT** their bodies. The body has *innate* intelligence. It **knows** and can **anticipate** the effect of a positive energy substance and protocol. Hence, the *bio-electric* body often **rejects** therapy and supplements that it sorely needs. Sometimes it **"rejects"** because it **"knows"** what it is going to have to go through to heal and that the **"host"** is **NOT** ready or willing to go there.

Often, the body "tricks" its owner by giving **false** muscle tests or false pendulum or vibration chain responses. To be useful, dowsing practices require the novice and professional alike to sharpen their skills and **clear** their minds so "gut" instinct can override personal influence.

Muscle testing is a **"questionable"** practice in the presence of heavy metal contamination of the autonomic nervous system—and skewed "readings" are the result. Muscle testing is highly **"subjective"** and should **NOT** be relied on for diagnosing or prescribing. Better to look for **SIGNS** and rely on **"symptoms"** that are always available if the patient and the practitioner are paying attention and asking enough questions. The information needed is there!

*[Racemized™ products **do not** lend themselves to muscle testing because their energy format is "beyond" the testing dimension.] Initially, people experience a roller-coaster ride on racemized™ products—but as the "terrain" improves, the body settles down and organ function restores itself as the "terrain" improves. First comes damage control. Then comes restoration. Aging reversal is the last step. The reader must think: "Two steps forward; one step backwards!"*

The Pendulum

If you would like to learn how to use a pendulum and vibration chain, order *The Pendulum Kit* and *Vibrations*. They have proven to be the best—and least expensive method to teach people how to "plug into" the *invisible* world of "energy" that is everywhere around us. *The Pendulum Kit* comes complete with a nice bronze pendulum and a beautifully illustrated book, while *Vibrations* comes with a vibration chain. The tools and techniques learned are unique and useful. Dowsing lets people **ACCESS** the big **"internet in the sky"** that has always been there ready and waiting for your inquiry. "Dowsing" is a phenomenon and a GOD-given gift available to anyone desiring to come to grips with the reality of life and energy on planet Earth. [See pages 44-5, 51, 57, 144, 210 and 283.]

18

Biological Alchemy

"Since Einstein, Physics has been relegated to Mathematics, the former having lost all contact with reality. Your magnificent discovery of weak energy transmutations should have marked a scientific turning point, (but instead it) encountered a wall of stupidity."
Ren de Puymorin

...speaking of the work of Professor C. Louis Kervran and his discovery that the motion of life derives from the continuous transformation of one mineral into another or—"transmutation."

"**Alchemy!** *Impossible! This is a good example of just plain old BAD science!*" So ended my official inquiry at the college level—but it did **NOT** end my inquiry!

What sparked the explosive outburst was the trigger word "transmutation"—which means "**alchemy.**" The *attacker* was a superb chemistry instructor who did **not** like the "implications" that your author's questions were raising— like... "*How* do you explain food plants that contain minerals not present in the soil? *How* does the cow produce milk that contains minerals far in excess of her dietary intake? *Where* does the hen get the minerals for her egg shells when they are not in her diet? *Why* does horsetail herb thicken and harden the nails, yet we derive no such benefit from calcium supplements? *How* can organic manganese produce an increase in blood-serum-iron levels when it's not iron? *How* is it that a dried prune has more minerals than a fresh one?" How, indeed? Answers to these questions derive from forgotten geniuses called "wizards"—and compromised and ignored knowledge.

Asking these type of questions is like proclaiming the invention of a perpetual motion machine. They can get a person in a lot of trouble—especially when put to the wrong person.

In our world of neatly packaged chemicals and "defined" laws of chemistry and physics, these questions have no answers. But—make no mistake—these **ARE** valid questions— the kind Professor Kervran liked to ask. The problem isn't the questions posed—but the implications they suggest.

Some people of "science" are intimidated by questions for which they have no answers. Daring to ask them is an assault on "DOGMA"—and enough to get a person branded *"Science heretic!"*—and instant burning at the stake!

Mineral Energy

The "life work" of Professor C. Louis Kervran (1899-1990) has startling implications for the aging-reversal story.

Kervran surmised that the energy *phenomenon* we call LIFE is related to the transformation of one mineral into another. He called this process *"transmutation."* Science calls it alchemy. We will refer to it as "biological alchemy!"

Alter the energy forces within an element and new and different elements manifest—and energy is released! Kervran believed that the energy "released" fueled metabolic processes and was the "life force" of life itself. Transmutation, as he described it, required a change in elemental molecular "structure" at atomic and subatomic levels and the rearrangement of **an**ions and **cat**ions. In other words, COLD fusion!

*[Today, nano technology is a reality and is proving that when elements are scaled down in size, they possess very different "properties." For instance, L_sP_cC™ is nano-scaled Vitamin-C **under** 200 nanometers in size—or about 10,000 molecules to a strand of hair! See Chapter 38 for details.]*

Kervran's discoveries came from **inside** Science's camp. Kervran was a member of both the French and American National Academy of Sciences—the most prestigious watering holes of modern academic science.

Professor Kervran *dared* to ask the right questions. He *sinned* against "science"—and dogma—when he offered God's answer to his fellow man. He broke the rules by **failing** to submit his findings for "peer" review. Great "wizards" have **NO** peers! They see visions of God's handiwork and proclaim the great news—while so-called science curses in **"contempt!"**

Like Copernicus, Kervran's peers *attacked* and *ridiculed* him—as they have done to so many others before him. They "ignored" Kervran—but they could **NOT** deny the **TRUTH** he heralded. When a vessel of **"truth"** is opened—it can **NEVER** again be closed. Truth is a Pandora's Box for those living in ignorance—and especially for individuals who egotistically "flaunt" their prestigious degrees and credentials.

Visions

Kervran surmised that minerals contained concentrated energy forces within their bonds—and his vision of the Creator's handiwork was not unlike that of his contemporary, Dr. Carey Reams. These great men of "science" never met. Each developed his own vision independently. Each spoke of and interpreted the "same" phenomena from their own perspective. Reams called his vision *The Biological Theory of Ionization.* Kervran called his *The Theory of Biological Transmutation.* Both spoke of energy forces that grant permission for life. Both men spoke of energy in terms of a "footprint" or "signature"— the same **phenomenon** described by Schauberger, Tesla, Vincent and Morell and incorporated into the *Young Again Protocol(s)*™ and BFRV™ and MGIW™ water concepts. Reams spoke of positive energy ions called **anions** and negative energy ions called **cations.** Kervran spoke of the rearrangement of energy forces and the rearrangement of these forces at atomic and *subatomic* levels.

Reams spoke of left and right-spin energy and the release of cosmic energy trapped in mineral bonds—ionic bonds! Kervran spoke of mineral **transmutation** in the gut of animals—and in the skin and lymph of Earth—soil and water.

The Sun was a **central** fixture for both men. They saw plants, animals and microbes as **"mediators"** between Sun and Earth. Both men sought to answer the mystery of life and death, health and illness. God answered both men with "living" examples of the benefits of biologically "live" food and biologically friendly water. He answered Reams in English and Kervran in French. Our version will be a translation of both.

Plants • Animals • Microbes
Plants "link" the Sun and animal world to which man's body belongs. Plants "convert" solar energy into carbon sugar molecules with the help of the microbe—bringing energy **into** the Earth—literally! Animals—with the help of microbes— process plant tissue and live off the electron energy released during the digestion process. Animal waste becomes Earth's "skin"—providing for new life—plant, animal and microbe.

Kervran saw mineral energy in a "living" system as *dynamic*—shifting and changing from one element into another. For example, in HEALTHY multiple-stomached ruminants like cows, calcium limestone is "transmutated" into other elements by bacteria to meet the animal's mineral needs. Kervran believed the microbe is the center of the *alchemy* process we call *fusion.* Cold fusion involves the transmutation of one energy field into another—and the release of "energy"— without the big "bang" and heat release of a nuclear event. [Racemized™ sea minerals provide mineral energy.]

Transmutation of mineral energy maintains peak health and provides "life force" in man and animal.

Cows & People
The cow utilizes the transmutation process. She eats plant-life compounds of carbon, hydrogen, sulphur, nitrogen,

sugars, fats, proteins, and minerals—and converts them into *new* and *different* energy forms—like muscle and bone! [Energy is never lost; it only changes form.]

The cow does this by way of enzymes and microbes in her liver and GI tract. The bacteria sharing her system have a *symbiotic* relationship with her. She provides them room and board; they provide her energy and vitality. Without microbes and enzymes, the fantastic biochemical reactions Kervran called *transmutations* **CANNOT** take place. Without microbes, the cow is unable to nourish herself. Without microbes, man grows old and dies early.

The microbe is man's passport to a continued presence on the Earth. However, man's disobedience is causing the microbe to turn against him.

Sick cows have much in common with sick **people**. Both are **UNABLE** to effectively use the transmutation process. Man's state of health or sickness is a reflection of the **"terrain"** and the processes called transmutation and ionization. [Requirements for a healthy life are nutritious, high-energy food, ionic minerals, biologically friendly water, plenty of "sleep," exercise and a low levels of acidic tissue waste.]

Chlorinated water upsets "terrain" balance, causing microbes to **"MORPH"** into *pathogenic* life forms—and an energy **"SHIFT"** accompanied by reduced metabolic activity in the gut and liver. "Raw" tap water with its load of toxic chemicals is one of the primary causes of leaky-gut! Antibiotics cause "MAJOR" intestinal damage by nonselective destruction of friendly bacteria. Poor bile flow is an ongoing terrain issue.

So called "good" bacteria live on right-spin energy. Pathogenic bacteria feed on left-spin energy always present in a toxic terrain. **An**aerobic environments are left-spin environments. **Aerobic** bacteria cannot live in an **an**aerobic environment—and when given no choice, they **forfeit** control, "morph" and attack the host. As always, the "terrain" controls!

Fusion & Fission

Energy—and the manipulation of energy—**governs** body metabolism. Life is an energy tug-of-war between *opposing* energy forces—as illustrated in the aging pyramid on page 198. Transmutation and ionization are energy "manipulations" that can go **either** direction, producing positive and negative energy "shifts" depending on the condition of the "terrain"—reactions that mimic fusion and fission energy shifts.

"Fusion" reactions in a healthy body involve **"controlled"** joining of atoms into larger molecules, tissues and organs. It is the building-up process called "anabolism." **"Uncontrolled"** tissue growth—as with cancer—is "catabolic" in nature and the exact opposite of anabolism. Anabolic activity occurs in highly acidic environments. Healthy fusion reactions occur in the gut, liver and cells of humans, animals, plants and microbes in "controlled" fashion with "predictable" results. Fusion occurs on the Sun's surface, providing Earth and all of Her inhabitants with life-giving "energy!"

"Abnormal" fusion—uncontrolled fusion—is the result of the following: an acidic body terrain, irradiated food, microwaved food and water, prescription and over-the-counter drugs and hormones, radiation therapy, chemotherapy, food laced with additives and analogous hormones, and use of **cordless** and **cellular** phones. [Oxidation and free-radical formation go with uncontrolled fusion reactions and the catabolic process called "aging."]

The Young Again Protocol™ *stops uncontrolled fusion reactions and reverses damage to the "terrain!"*

"Fission" involves the splitting of atoms and molecules. Healthy, "controlled" biological fission activity is what microbes "orchestrate" in a healthy body with a healthy "terrain!" Fission can also be destructive—as in a nuclear "event!" People with cancer are subjected to nuclear "ionizing" that causes healthy tissue to **die** and **turn** cancerous in the process of trying to kill targeted cancerous tissue. Uncontrolled fission and uncontrolled fussion reactions are "birds of a feather." The key concept here is **"control!"**

Skin • Dirt • Soil • Lymph

The Earth has skin. Her skin is called soil. Some folks call soil "dirt." Dirt, however, is *dead* unless it is *energized* with microbes, organic matter and carbon. Microbes *transform* dirt into soil. Soil is biologically "live" dirt. *Soil is alive!*

Water and carbon are the essence of life. Think of water as the Earth's *lymph fluid*—and like our own lymphatic fluids, water is part of the Earth's "energy" communication system. Water transports massive amounts of energy—both good and bad! Soil is an **"energy"** medium. The depth of "healthy" topsoil is a function of carbon, water and microbial activity—and Mother Earth's "aura" is a reflection of these factors.

When Earth becomes stressed, her skin forms boils, her lymph becomes toxic, plants become sick, animals suffer and man experiences dis-ease. The condition of Earth's skin and lymph dictates the quality of life—and which life forms live or die. Life is a microbial event involving transmutation and ionization of mineral energy.

Synchronization

Synchronization is the **end-result** of a chemical reaction. Mix vinegar and baking soda—one acid, the other alkaline—and when the reaction runs its course, two things have transpired. Energy is released in the form of "heat" and *synchronization* occurs between the reactants—meaning the reaction "stops." This example is a simple *inorganic* chemical reaction. The **dynamics** of thousands of reactions in the human body are not quite as simple.

The body's **ability** or **inability** to digest food—potential energy—by **breaking** molecular bonds containing that energy is elemental to health and longevity. Food's energy "footprint" and the state of the "terrain" **govern** the outcome of digestive reactions as much as carbohydrate, protein and fat content.

A dysfunctional liver is the norm in an anaerobic gut and acidic terrain. Healthy food cannot "release" its energy when digestion "stalls." Stalled-out digestion causes food energy to **"synchronize"** by default. High-stress, adverse meal environments only make matters worse!

"Synchronized" energy is energy "on hold!" It is energy that is **NOT** available to the body. People in poor health are in energy **"gridlock"** because their bodies do **NOT** have the ability to respond to or utilize healthy "food." They are **NOT** able to neutralize negative energy forces in control of their terrain. Negative energy environments neutralize healthy "food" energy. Sick bodies and "dis-ease" go with the territory.

DeACIDification of the "terrain" and High Enema Therapy™ are the keys to health and longevity.

When the *bio-electric* body suffers *systemic* synchronization, life becomes impossible! As we approach total synchronization, we lose our "radiance," and our aura dims and fades away until the physical body dies. *"The ghost is gone!"* But synchronized energy "remains" in the form of a cadaver which Earth reclaims. Ashes to ashes! Dust to dust!

Energy is never lost, it merely changes form—including the negative energy of "cancer!" Unless the terrain is "changed," cancer always returns, usually in a different costume and at a different location.

Energy Takeover

Energy is released when chemical bonds are broken. Energy released into a predominantly **anaerobic** environment becomes a negative force—even if the food energy was "positive" in nature. Restated, right-spin energy entering a left-spin "terrain" environment "synchronizes" or it is **hijacked** and used to fuel dis-ease—and that is exactly what cancer does. Cancer "hijacks" energy for its own use!

Cancer lives on negative energy. Manage your TERRAIN and cancer will never become a threat to you.

"Gut" and bowel disorders diminish ionization and transmutation of food mineral energy. A sick liver **automatically** goes with poor digestion—creating the perfect environment for "parasites!" Gas and bloating go with poor digestion, a leaky-gut—and a "terrain" that is out of balance! Cancer **FOLLOWS** years of **abuse** and **neglect!** Cancer "diverts" energy and uses it for evil purposes—like the growth of "tumors" and "masses." People with cancer should **NEVER** be given large amounts of heavy, high-stress, high-protein food. **Moderation** is called for and **viable** digestive "support" is absolutely "critical!" The cancer patient is starving to death **and** unable to process food to obtain nourishment. Whatever food is consumed must "count"—and that is why the emphasis is on Taoist Super Foods under these circumstances. **TIME** is not on the cancer patient's side. Bile flow and lymphatic drainage are marginal—at best! [High Enema Therapy™ and the L/CSF machine are utilized to regain control of the terrain.]

Cancer Plays By A Different Set Of Rules
The rules of life are **different** once a person is under cancer's "pall." Cancer is a **"catabolic"** state and the cancerous person is very fragile. Popular alternative approaches to cancer often fail because the doctor and patient **FAIL** to understand that the rules have **changed!** Clinical nutrition does **NOT** work here! Cancer is like a **"black hole"** drawing in and subverting all *available* energy. It needs energy to grow and spread, and it uses **"biological alchemy"** to release "synchronized" energy to fuel its growth. It is self-perpetuating **UNLESS** the "terrain" is **de**acidified and vital organ function is restored. There will **NEVER** be a "magic bullet" cure for cancer! It is a "terrain" issue that defies medical science's "model." Cancer has but one purpose: rid the Earth of weak organisms.
Cancer is NOT the enemy, but it IS the perfect double agent. First it kills the host. Then it kills itself.
When you are in control of your terrain, **YOU** are in control of **YOUR** life and the *magical* processes that Kervran and Reams "described" so eloquently. Health and vitality are the **"product"** of biological alchemy in a healthy terrain environment—and the process is dependent upon our microbial friends that live in our gut and tissues.
Kervran's and Reams' discoveries "linking" the microbes to the ebb and flow of "life-force" is vital to understanding the process we call "aging." Their discoveries point the way to rejuvenation and good health if we understand the rules of the game and are willing to take personal **responsibility** for ourselves. Only then do we become *Young Again!*

PREVIEW: *Our next chapter is about the gut (small intestine) and E. coli bacteria infections that killed many adults and children during 1993. You will also learn what's behind Montezuma's revenge.*

Squat!

Sit or squat? That is the question. "Natives" squat! And they rarely suffer from bowel disorders. Solution! Use a short 8-10" inch foot stool under your feet when moving your bowels!

The Law

Statutory and common law are not the same. Statutory law is "commercial law;" constitutional law is "common law." Our court system is based on "commercial/maritime" law operating under the UCC (Uniform Commerical Code)—the law of commercial contracts. The "yellow fringed flag" is the flag of "commerce." It is a **"war"** flag and **NOT** the "common law" uS flag of peace. The "peace" flag has not been displayed since before the American civil war when the flag of "war" replaced it. America "officially" went bankrupt in 1933 when Roosevelt called in the gold! At that moment, "people" became commercial "chattel" under a "state of emergency"—**void** of our common law heritage as embodied in the Constitution. Here's proof! When you receive an "offer" in the mail, your name is spelled properly in upper and lower case. After you "apply," your name is in CAPITALS and the fictional "you" is now in "commerce!" Licenses are commercial franchises. Legal process is served upon the **FICTIONAL** "commercial" person who is forced to defend themselves in a "foreign" court under a "foreign" flag. The Social Security System is a commercial system. The "Government" is a commercial entity—a "corporation." We have **NO** constitutional rights—**only** "contract" rights under the UCC that can only be exercised in a UCC court. The "right to...." exists in the "future"—**not** the present. "To" is a future tense preposition. [See pages 168, 229, 292 & 384.]

Flying

To avoid jet lag, sickness and constipation, board the plane with 2 quarts of bottled water and some racemized™ sea minerals and drink a glass of water every "30 minutes!"

Healthy Home Environment

Ozone (O_3) has many forms. **Medical Grade** ozone is useful and beneficial to your health. Use it to rid your home of odors, viruses, molds and pathogenic bacteria in air, carpets and drapes. A medical grade ozone generator is a good way to enjoy a healthy home. Older folks find medical grade ozone **very** beneficial. Protect your family and pet with medical ozone. Environmentally sensitive people get relief when they clear their home's "airspace" of chemical pollutants. One ozone unit treats an entire home and works extremely well with the BFRV™ Air Processor pictured on page 114. [See Pages 132 and 188 for more information on medical grade ozone.]

Cancer "Craps!"

Conventional cancer therapy has more than a little resemblance to the game of "craps." You have stakes—your life. You have rules—*house* rules. You have the dealer—a *house* dealer that wears a white smock and who is controlled by the licensing boards and pharmaceutical industry. You have the *house* support team—they wear uniforms and they have licenses and are trained to do as they have been trained—or as they are told! You have players—who appear to be winning enough to justify your joining the game. You have chips—called insurance, life savings, a farm, a house. You have dice—weighted in the *house's* favor. You have liquor—called radiation and chemotherapy. You have the *house* bouncer—his name is Fear. You have the *house* preacher—his name is Hope. You have odds—the **75%** the house *dealer* gave you during "consultations" prior to joining the game. Games have an end. When you play cancer craps, the game automatically ends when you run out of money or when you die—whichever comes first. The *house* always wins when people play *their* game on *their* turf by *their* rules.

Is there a solution? Yes! **Don't play!** Instead, clean up your body. **LAUGH!** Don't cry "poor me!" Don't dwell on hate, anger and fear. Use your mind to create a new life. Never entertain negative thoughts. Got it? What you say, your body believes! What you think, you get! It took your author 50 years to get this straight—and I am here to tell you that your mind has the ability to create or to destroy! Use it to create a better life and world! **Celebrate!** You're *ALIVE* and if you do what you need to do, you will continue to celebrate life and see your great, great, grandchildren mature—and you will get to experience the many wonders the future holds for those who love life **MORE** than those who fear death. The game of "Cancer Craps" is a "crappy" game!

Lap-Top Computers

Lap-top computers negatively affect the ovaries, prostate and testicles just like a cordless phone affects the brain—and teeth!

High Enema Therapy™ & Bathing Water

"Raw" tap water is **NOT** suitable for doing High (or low) Enema Therapy.™ It damages the delicate intestinal mucosa. Instead, use an **oxidation/reduction** shower filter for "friendly" bathing and therapy water. These filters typically last for 5-8 years. There are no cartridges to change, and they provide full "flow" so you can get "wet!" Your skin and hair will love it, too! [See Pages 163, 203 and 262-3.

Look at all the sick and dying people!

Young Again! Pyramid

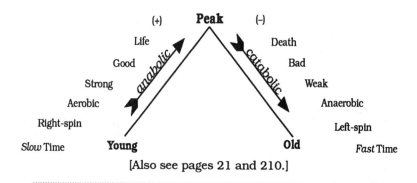

[Also see pages 21 and 210.]

➡ ▢ **Inflammation & Pain**

Pain, inflammation and fever go together. Generally, pain is confirmation of inflammation—but if an infection is brewing you will have fever, too! "Low grade" infections operate "below" radar—like an infected prostate, rotting teeth or inflamed bowel. Pain killing drugs damage the gut lining and should be avoided. The *Young Again*™ solution to these problems is called Inflame Away I & II.™ They are highly effective and gentle, too!

---

pH Scale

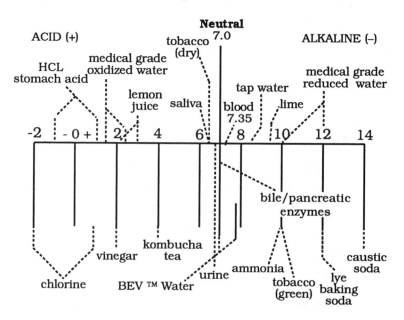

19

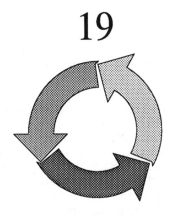

A Tube Within A Tube

Dr. Spot: *"There's always scissors!"*

[Earlier we described some of the characteristics of the integumentary system (skin) as it relates to health. Now, we will consider our "inner" skin and see what part it plays in the process we call aging.]

Man's body is a **TUBE** within a **TUBE**! The skin is our *outer* tube and the mucous membranes form our *inner* tube. The mucous membranes are the soft tissues lining the mouth, nasal passages, respiratory tract, stomach, gut, colon and vagina. The "GI" tract (gasto-intestional tract)—the body's "inner" tube—begins in the mouth and ends at the anus. The vaginal canal and the lungs are **not** part of the GI tract even though they are lined with mucosal tissue. A healthy mucosa is of immense importance to a healthy "terrain!"

The mucous membranes have tremendous significance for the aging and dis-ease story.

The tissues lining the mouth, nasal passages and respiratory tract are classified as *stratified epithelium*. Their job is to **protect** underlying tissues, **secrete** fluids and **transport** waste. The lining of the GI tract is composed of *simple epithelium* whose job it is to **ABSORB** nutrients, **protect** underlying tissues, **SECRETE** mucous and enzymes, and **TRANSPORT** food and waste.

Our **"outer"** tube—the skin—has a combined surface area of about 30,000 square inches. The pores (openings) of the skin are called *stoma*, and there are as many as 3,000 of them per square inch. By comparison, the mucous membranes have an approximate surface area of 18,000,000 (million) square inches or 6,000 times greater than the skin. One inch on the outside equals 6,000 inches on the inside—or a ratio of 1:6,000. **THIS IS IMPORTANT!**

In the healthy person, eating **should** result in "diges-tion," "absorption" and "elimination"—with each and every meal. Food—in and of itself—does **NOT** trigger these very *basic reactions* in the face of a **weakened** "terrain" an **unhealthy** "liver" and **poor** bile-flow. [Intervention using the *Young Again! Protocol(s)* remedies these issues.]

Aging accelerates after age 24—and liver and bile issues create PERFECT conditions for major health problems involving the intestinal mucosa of the "gut!"

All food imposes stress on the body because it must be digested and eliminated. Undigested food putrefies in the gut and fuels parasitic activity, gas and "indigestion" complaints that **ALWAYS** develop into more serious bowel trouble. **Acid Reflux Dis-ease** is the symptomatic "side-effect" of liver, bile flow and bowel issues rolled into one. Acid-reflux is **NOT** a dis-ease—it is a "condition" of the "terrain!"

The longer the transit time from dinner table to toilet, the more health and the "terrain" suffer.

The mucous membranes are a favorite conduit for drug chemotherapy. Medications in the form of suppositories, sublinguals and aerosols are easily absorbed through the mucous membranes of the rectum, vagina and respiratory system. The dosage of "meds" given via the mucosa is always much less than pill or injection dosage. Absorption dynamics and reaction time is much faster, too.

E. coli & The Gut

Nutrient absorption is a function of a healthy mucosal environment in the gut and colon—which is the body's most **"vulnerable"** "terrain." An intestinal infection—as occurs with influenza—causes the natural sloughing action of the mucosa to reach **"avalanche"** proportions.

Normal "sloughing" of intestinal mucosa cells occurs at the rate of approximately **20 million** cells a day. This "sloughing" action is a critically important source of intestinal digestive enzymes. *Pathogenic* infection increases sloughing to such an extent that **digestion** and **absorption** of nutrients and fluids "collapses." The **symptoms** are diarrhea, electrolyte imbalance/,and malnutrition. [Viruses and bacteria attack the liver and "breed" on wastes in the system. "Rubber-legs" and fever are the **"EFFECTS"** of a terrain under siege!]

The infamous **E. coli 0157.H7** bacteria that contami-nated hamburger in the USA in early 1993 produced **severe** sloughing of the intestinal mucosa and "bloody" diarrhea, followed by dehydration, starvation and electrolytic shock in hundreds of children and older people. The young and elderly are vulnerable because of under-developed or fragile immune systems and leaky gut issues.

E. coli 0157.H7 releases an **exo**toxin (*exo*-to export, *toxin*-poison) that destroys the *functional* cells of the liver and kidneys and causes massive cell death. Dead cellular debris **MUST** be removed or gangrene will develop. These conditions overload" the liver—and by default the kidneys—**forcing** the need for emergency kidney dialysis (artificial filtering of the blood) to avoid "septic" shock and toxemia (blood poisoning).

Elderly & Children

The elderly are vulnerable to "pathogenic" bacterial infection because their organs and glands are weak, metabolism is sluggish and their "terrains" are **ACID!** In addition, "ATP" production and reserves are insufficient to fuel recovery.

Children are at the other end of the continuum. They are highly resilient, but their immune systems are not fully developed, and they are often malnourished and toxic because they eat the *usual and customary* American diet. Illness in children **always** involves the **LIVER**—and severe intestinal infections **always** involves **under**hydration and electrolytic imbalance which add additional stress to the terrain.

A stressed "terrain" is a **made-to-order** environment for bacterial infections and viruses, too! Friendly, *non-virulent* strains of E. coli and many other bacteria inhabit the gut and colon. If these "friendly" microbes are eliminated, we die! Overuse of antibiotics reduces their numbers—allowing "non-friendly" life forms to take over. Indiscriminate use of antibiotics, aspirin-type antiinflammatory drugs—plus "flu" vaccinations creates the **"perfect"** conditions for "unfriendly," **virulent** microbes to proliferate and take over the "terrain."

The "terrain" dictates body response. The "terrain" controls the proliferation of pathogenic microbes.

Not Everyone Died

Over a million pounds of E. coli contaminated beef found its way into fast food restaurants—yet only a few hundred people became sick and only six people died. The question is "Why?" The answer is the **"STATE"** of the "terrain" and the vital organs of the sick and dead people. Pathogenic organisms "feed" on negative energy in a **TOXIC, ANAEROBIC** environment, which explains why—in a family with three children all of whom ate contaminated beef—only one child died. No mystery here! The terrain controls! [Contagious diseases throughout history—like bubonic plague, smallpox and typhoid—did **NOT** kill everyone! Those who died had weak livers and waste-filled, higly acid terrains!]

The "terrain" controls sickness and death—or health and vitality. The "terrain" is everything!

These points should raise serious questions about the

"absurdity" of "immunizing" against dis-ease. Remember the "swine flu" **fiasco** in the late 1970's? Or the so-called "Spanish" flu epidemic of 1918 that killed 50,000,000 people worldwide? **Can the reader say "vaccinations?"** It was "government-sponsored" immunizations that created the epidemic and KILLED these people! The history of botched programs by madmen in white smocks with the backing of "government" is something people need to **take-note-of** and **avoid!**]

[The panic seen in the movie Outbreak IS understandable in light of the general level of ignorance regarding contagious dis-ease. Clean-up your act and Ebola plague, Hanta virus, Cryptosporidium bacteria, necrotizing facitis (flesh eating bug) and their likes will pass you by.]

A clean "terrain" is like the blood on the lintel stone over the doorway of the Israelites. Death passes by!

Lack Of Understanding

People of science have difficulty understanding discussions like this because of their training. Scientific thought embraces the "scientific method" and the "Germ Theory." Our discussion does **NOT** fit their **"model"** or false theories, and conflicts with their arrogant *pusillanimous mewings!*

*[Whenever my phone rings and the caller asks "What are your credentials?", I know I have an "expert" on my hands, or someone who wants to defend something. Credentials are for the ego and the licensing boards. Modest professionals have their ego in tow and their ears open for new knowledge. Credentials are "proof" of the ability to regurgitate the "party line!" They are **NOT** indicative of the ability to "think!"]*

Vibrational medicine asks square questions and looks for square answers. It sees health-related problems from an **ENERGY** vantage point. It is **NOT** hindered by the Germ Theory of Disease and other theoretical artifacts! Remember, healthy bodies are nourished bodies; they are clean bodies; they are bodies in good physical condition; they do not support the development of "pathogenic" dis-ease—and they store massive amounts of the energy molecule "ATP" in reserve.

It's The Pits

The small intestine is lined with convoluted folds called *plicae circularis*. These folds are lined with *villi* (little fingers) and *microvilli* (hair-like structures) that increase the surface area of the intestine to 6,000 times that of the outer skin. The microvilli contain the cells that absorb and transport food nutrient energy. The spaces *between* the villi are known as the **Crypts of Lieberkuhn.** The "crypts" are lined with cells that "secrete" digestive enzymes and mucous. But as the "terrain" changes and the body ages, the valleys making up the intestinal "pits" become shallow; the villi and microvilli **"atrophy;"** transit time of food from mouth to anus **slows;** constipation **manifests;** parasites **take-over** and the body turns **acid.** Alterations of the "terrain" take years to fully manifest from **sub**clinical "conditions" to **CLINICAL** dis-ease.

Anaerobic conditions and leaky-gut issues fuel serious changes in the "chemical" make-up of fecal matter interfacing the colon wall. Over time, rubber-like **mucoid** material can accumulate and narrow the lumen (opening) of the colon through which fecal waste passes on the way to the toilet. [Sagged and kinked colons only make matters worse!]

Perhaps the reader can UNDERSTAND why colon cancer is #2 on the list—and a viable threat to everyone!

The colon of a very famous Hollywood cowboy grew to almost 12 inches in diameter at the time of death—yet the lumen was only one inch. The rest was waste matter.

The combined effect of limited digestive and absorptive capability, poor liver function and an acid terrain causes the average person to **forfeit** 75% of their waste-processing capability! The other waste exit portals—lungs, kidneys and skin— were **NEVER** meant to handle the burden and volume imposed upon them when the **liver** is unable to do its job.

A clean bowel and a healthy liver are the difference between youth and vitality vs. old age and death.

*[The **entire** population needs to practice High Enema Therapy™ and get their house in order. Of all the things your author teaches, this procedure is the most important, long term "administrative" tool available to the general public—a procedure that is done at home at little cost. The Young Again™ High Enema Protocol™ is the **fast track** to good health because it increases bile flow and releases the **chocolate pudding** holed-up in the cecum. This is the "stuff" that "fuels" cancer and disease. Your author dumped over 1,600 stones in the early stages of the development of these protocols. Misconceptions and half-truths about High Enema Therapy™ cause people to "avoid" this vitally important health management tool. See pages 163, 203 and 262-3.] The Tissue and Liver Protocol™ package includes a book with "40" full-color pictures of "stuff" that exits people's bodies. Gross? Perhaps! But better to deal with the waste and parasites now "**before**" they get their hooks into you—and you lose control of YOUR life!*

My Story

By 1977, I had reached a plateau in my personal health. I visited a healer who said that I had a blockage in my colon. Subsequent colon therapy confirmed this as I saw hard, compacted fecal material exit my body. The event caused my health to reach **NEW** heights as my body immediately **surged** to a more youthful condition. [**"UNPLUG"** from the "sick-care" system. Your author did it—and so can you!]

A *live testimony* from John Thomas—and you can believe it because your author is **Young Again!**

PREVIEW: *Our next chapter is about YOUR aura. Why do people climb rock mountains? HOW could Jesus pass through the wall of the temple?*

The "Fifth" Horseman

Forget about the four horsemen of the "apocalypse!" It's the **"fifth"** horseman—called **"IGNORANCE"**—that sets the stage for the others. Man's problems will remedy themselves when earth's population dies because of poor **"choices"** in lifestyle!

The *Bio-Magetic*™ Dental Irrigator

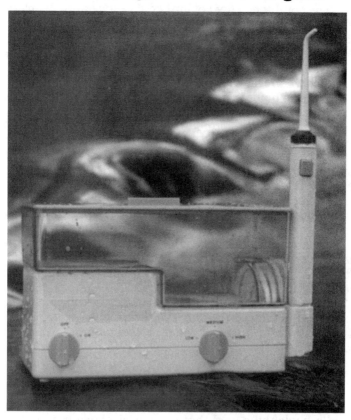

A Highly Effective Dental Appliance
➡ See Oral-Advantage™ pages 149, 187 & 233.]

Oxidation & Aging

Enhanced PAC's prevent uncontrolled cellular oxidation. Uncontrolled oxidation causes the body to "cannibalize" itself. **Oxidation** is another word for **"aging!"** Oxidation, aging and free-radicals have much in common. We ingest large amounts of free-radicals every day. They come from air, water and food. The body also *manufactures* them in the process of *metabolism.* A *free-radical scavenger* is a molecular compound that **neutralizes** free radicals. Free radicals are **highly reactive** molecules that are short or long "electrons"—and set off "chain-style" reactions.

Toxic substances in the body **"morph"** into unpredictable molecules and reactions. Examples are: food additives, fluoride and chlor**amines** (from tap water), soy and canola oils, pesticides, microwaved food and vaccinations.

As we age, the tissues **oxidize** faster and faster. Examples are a massive heart attack and cross-linking of the skin's collagen causing wrinkles and "leathery" skin. The word, **"aging"** sums it up nicely. [SOC™ Lotion and Racemized™ skin creme topically repair damaged skin. SOC™ capsules and VZ™ address wrinkled, scarred and blemished skin—while L$_s$P$_c$C™ accelerates the formation of needed "collagen"—the basis of "young," wrinkle-free skin!]

PAC's prevent rapid oxidation and destructive chain reactions from occurring. PAC's are "proanthrocyanidans" with both **hydro**philic and **hypo**philic qualities in a racemized™ footprint format.

PAC's neutralize waste released into circulation during the **"de**acidification" process of the *Young Again Tissue & Liver Protocol.*™ PAC's minimize acid waste **re**absorption as the waste works its way down 20 feet of intestine on the way to the toilet. Together, PAC's and Yucca Blend™ cause the body to **"release"** stored, "soluble," acid wastes from the tissues.

All dis-ease conditions respond favorably when PAC's are incorporated into the diet. Sickly children and kids with ADD and ADHD show marked improvement when liver function and bile flow gets a boost from PAC'$_s$™and Yucca Blend™. Older folks respond nicely, also.

PAC's are chewable and possess 24,660 activity units per bottle—enough to easily offset the damage done to the liver by drugs and mercury poisoning from those "harmless" amalgam dental fillings. Anyone on medications should use PAC's.

Aging reversal is a very **TALL** order, and the older and sicker you are, the **TALLER** it is! Take PAC's for that added edge—and to protect your liver and rid your body of the "stuff" that drives tissue "oxidation," aging and dis-ease!

The easiest way to minimize oxidative aging is to incorporate the *Young Again Protocol*™ into your daily life. Call and ask for the *Source Packet* and find out how to do it!

"A mind changed against its will is of the same opinion still!"
Unknown

Playing God!

The medical folks and their cronies in the pharmaceutical industry have officially admitted "defeat" in helping women with menstrual difficulties enjoy a *normal* female life. Their latest answer is to **FORCE** the body to **STOP** menstruation altogether. The "pill's" side effects are bad enough—but imagine the implications of this asinine proposal? Madmen in white smocks fixing what God could not. ["Cessation of menses goes with anorexia and bulimia because of "starvation!"] Helping women with menstrual and menopause problems is **not** difficult when the "model" is realistic. The *Young Again Protocol*™ is a simpler path because it puts women in control of their body—and at the same time avoids problems associated with dangerous pharmaceutical drugs prescribed on the basis of a defective "model." The lucky woman doesn't need the medical folks because she looks and feels great!

Cell And Cordless Phones

The side of the skull is "thin"—especially in young people! And because wireless cell phones are part of daily life, your author **STRONGLY** suggests users minimize exposure with a special device that "neutralizes" all wireless phones—and "head-sets," which are 3x more dangerous that the phone! Cordless phones used in the home are equally damaging and should be avoided. A few dollars invested today, is better than a brain tumor or Alzheimers or damaged and destroyed teeth [*Yes* "teeth!] [Please see pages 59, 233 & Chapter 14.]

Heart, Heavy Metals & Chelation

"Chelation" of the blood is **not** to be confused with chelation therapy—**as in cancer!** Chelation employs recognized agents like EDTA that "attach-to" and transport **circulating** heavy metals out of the body. [The medical folks don't like this modality because it **embarrasses** them!] If you have **serious** heart or heavy-metal issues, chelation provides good, short-term relief of **"circulating"** heavy metals. Please **recognize** that metals "bound up" in the tissues are released over many "years!" Follow the *Young Again Protocol*™ "now" and you will never need to do chelation therapy—and you'll greatly improve the quality of your life at the same time, too!

Where Does All That "Stuff" Come From?

About 80% of stool "bulk" is acid waste, dead bacteria and fiber! The body needs 10 years to release and totally clear the "terrain" of both soluble and structural waste. Maintenance of the "terrain" is an **"ongoing"** concept—and well worth the effort!

20

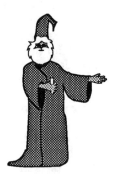

The Aura Effect

"Man's mind stretched to a new idea never
goes back to its original dimension."
Oliver Wendel Holmes

The injury had occurred the night before, but Jerry was not aware of any specific damage. As Jerry and I walked into the shop and began browsing, the lady who owned the shop approached Jerry and said,
"OOOH! You must be hurting pretty bad!"
He looked at her blankly and asked what she meant.
"Oh! Your aura! You have a very BIG hole in it in your groin area. Did you injure yourself?"
Jerry was hurting. He had torn a hernia in the connective tissues of his pelvic region the night before.
What was so intriguing about the encounter was that this lady was a *total stranger!* She knew **nothing** about Jerry, yet she was able to vividly see his **"aura"**—and the hole in it. We had heard of people like this lady, but neither of us had ever met someone with this **"gift"**—or witnessed the phenomenon we had just experienced.

The Glow Of Health
The body has a radiation field surrounding it. This is an established fact. Kirlian photography can capture the aura on a photographic plate—its size, shape and color in direct relation to the overall "condition" of the person's "terrain!"
Jesus was reported to have a *glow* about Him. Whenever He is pictured, the **halo** [Aura effect!] is always seen radiating from His head. The halo and aura are right-spin energy. Many people believe the greater your aura, the more advanced a human being you are. Perhaps. For certain, each of us has an aura—and the greater it is—the **healthier** we are!

When people suffer with dis-ease, the electrical charge of the *bio-electric* body shifts from right-spin "healthy" to one that is left-spin "pathogenic." When we see the sickly pallor of another person, we are taking note of **diminished** "life force" in their **"aura!"** And when that same person returns to a "state" of health, we see it in their pallor and their aura. **"Gut"** instinct plays a very big part in our daily lives. We use it to guide us in dealing with people. The aura is real and has "meaning!"

Energy Drain

Some people are exhausting. I am not speaking of the someone who runs in *hyper drive*—but someone who **"drains"** your energy and leaves you feeling very "tired!" These people are energy black holes and their *presence* is less than refreshing!

Sue operated a massage therapy and iridology clinic for many years. She once commented that certain people drew so much energy from her that she could not work on them. Later, I learned that my wife had ended her friendship with a lady Sue refused to treat. The reason: the lady was *exhausting!*

Sue was an interesting person. She had the uncanny ability to *see* and *feel* things about people who came to her for treatments. They call people like Sue "healer." Sue definitely was a healer. Sue was also a superb organic gardener. Sue had a green thumb and the plants produced abundantly for her. Her plants and soil were "vibrantly" healthy and never required any form of poison to control bugs or weeds.

One day I asked her *"Sue, what is your secret?"* She just smiled. As I came to know her, I realized that she knew how to **speed up** body frequency—through the laying-on of hands. In Sue's case, it was called massage therapy. Sue could **speed-up** the electron flow in the body of the patient to such an extent that the person walked out of her clinic **totally** refreshed and happy to be alive. That is what a "true" body worker does— heals people by manipulating and boosting vital organ energy.

Sue boosted positive energy in the patient by accelerating electron "flow" in the patients **"aura"**—as she "drew off" negative energy. The effect of this energy manipulation was immediately visable in the patients aura and demeanor. Sue had mastered the skill of *energy manipulation.* She realized that **"life"** is a *battleground* of competing energy forces. Sometimes Sue would "shake her hands and arms," walk "barefoot" in grass or sand—or hug a tree barefooted to dissipate negative energy she had "absorbed" from her sick patients.

Energy & Auras

The world is composed of but one thing: **ENERGY!** When energy condenses, science calls it "matter." Matter has three states: gas, liquid and solid. All substances are a variation of energy **density** and vibrational molecular *"frequency!"* Rocks are hard and solid. Skin has texture and can be stretched. Rocks and skin are **not** *really* solids, we just "classify" them as solids. Solids are energy fields joined together in such a way that they take on the shape, feel and smell of something we learn to identify as rock, skin, tomato, etc. All things—**living and non-living**—have an aura. A rock's aura—and the effect it exerts on things near it—can be positive or negative. If the rock's energy state is positive, it will have a therapeutic effect on plants, and visa versa.

Increase electron flow around the nuclei of atoms in a rock—and the rock will change its energy "state!" For example, heat sulphur and it will change from solid to liquid to gas. Water does the same thing when it changes from ice to liquid to steam.

Rocks & Mountains

In the Bible, rocks had significance in matters of health. Rocks have a sacred place in most religions. Rocks are not *live* in the animal sense—but they possess *energy*. Rocks are identified by their energy *footprint* and **signature**.

People like rocks. [Some people like them so much they have a head full of them.] People who climb rock mountains are often asked *"why?"* The answer usually given is *"Because they are there!"* There is a more accurate reason. People climb rocks because the activity is **invigorating**! Climbers absorb fantastic quantities of **ENERGY** from rock mineral formations. Rocks radiate **ENERGY** that "tunes" the climber to Mother Earth's frequency. Climbing rocks is one way for people to tap into nature's energy bank. So is swimming in sea water, walking bare foot in sand and grass, hugging a tree barefoot, or eating food grown on healthy soil.

The human body has the ability to "absorb" or to "donate" energy—regardless if it is positive or negative!

Jesus & The Wall

It is **recorded** in the scriptures that when Jesus was about to be stoned in the Temple, He [passed through the wall and] disappeared, to the frustration of his enemies. As a child, I accepted this story—but I never believed it because anyone with a lick of sense knows you cannot pass *through* a wall.

Today, the story delivers a different message—one that is both factual and explanatory. The Christ possessed the knowledge and ability to **"accelerate"** the flow of electrons in His body and pass through the wall of the temple. By **"speeding up"** His body's electrons to the point of disintegration—much like ice turning to steam! Jesus was able to squeeze "between" the atoms of the stone wall—and vanish! Neither The Christ body nor the wall were solids! Both were composed of energy "particles." Jesus did **not** violate natural law! Rather, He manipulated it!

Life is a **STATEMENT** of positive (+) and negative (–) energy forces. Man gives them different names and classifies them in ways that are more easily understood. For example: good and evil, light and dark, right and wrong, left and right, **YOUNG** and **OLD**—and so on! Life is a mystery of the phenomena we call **ENERGY!** [See page 198 and Chapter 31.]

Reflections

The body's aura is a mirror image of our **"inner state"** of health. We can measure the aura with a pendulum, vibration chain or aurameter—**IF** the person doing the dowsing clears his mind so as not to **interfere** with incoming electrical signals.

The dowsing "trio" teaches the skills of dowsing. [See pages 57, 144, 188, 210 and 283.]

A pendulum is nothing but an antenna that sends **and** receives electrical energy. The "mind" receives the information and "interprets" it. Measuring your body aura establishes a **reference point** that can be used to measure change—or determine the effect a substance is likely to have on the body. The "trick" is "clearing" the mind and asking perceptive questions—questions that produce "vibrational" answers that you can be interpret by **"gut"** instinct!

A pendulum or vibration chain can be used to check food substances, identify left-spin or right-spin apples, carrots, etc. Whatever is being measured is like a radio station transmitting **ENERGY** signals—and the pendulum is the receiving antenna. [A pendulum can also **"transmit"** signals.]

Intuition is a kind of sixth sense that sends and receives energy "signals!" We will discuss this Fourth Dimension concept in Chapter 31.

When aging reverses, the aura "expands" and physical **VITALITY** increases. When "your" aura returns to the energy "state" it was at **before** you "aged," you will be at your **anabolic peak** —as described on pages 21 and 198. In the process, you will discover that the passing of **TIME** actually **"slows"** and eventually **"stops"**—as it has done for your author. When this phenomenon occurs, you have achieved "agelessness" and you are truly *Young Again!*

PREVIEW: *Our next chapter deals with energy and numbers. You will learn that big can mean small and weak can mean strong, and that things are **not** always as they "appear!"*

Life should be a scrapbook of lessons—not mistakes!

"Gauge" Yourself!

Pricking the finger is one way to gauge overall health. If you prick your finger and the blood **fails** to stand-up with a very distinct "pearl"—and instead produces a low-profile crown oozing onto the skin—you *are in trouble!* Blood should be **BRILLIANT** red, never dark! Blood with a *low crown* and dark red in color is in a *pre-cancer* "state." **De**acidification of your body "terrain" is how you reverse aging **"SIGNS!"**

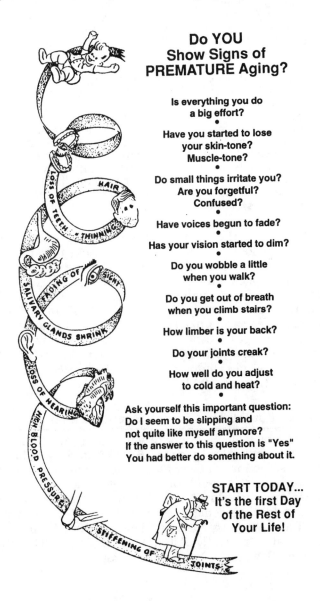

Do YOU Show Signs of PREMATURE Aging?

Is everything you do
a big effort?
•
Have you started to lose
your skin-tone?
Muscle-tone?
•
Do small things irritate you?
Are you forgetful?
Confused?
•
Have voices begun to fade?
Has your vision started to dim?
•
Do you wobble a little
when you walk?
•
Do you get out of breath
when you climb stairs?
•
How limber is your back?
•
Do your joints creak?
•
How well do you adjust
to cold and heat?

Ask yourself this important question:
Do I seem to be slipping and
not quite like myself anymore?
If the answer to this question is "Yes"
You had better do something about it.

START TODAY...
It's the first Day
of the Rest of
Your Life!

Terrain & Hormone "RELATED" Conditions

1. Asthma/emphysema
2. Excess fat/poor figure
3. Thyroid problems
4. Hearing loss
5. Menstrual PMS
6. Prostate trouble
7. Thinning hair
8. Gray hair
9. Cold body/feet/hands
10. Low energy/drive
11. Impotence
12. Bladder/yeast infections
13. Sagging cheeks/neck
14. Skin wrinkles
15. Joint pain/stiff body
16. Female/male cancer
17. Osteoporosis/osteopenia
18. Miscarriage
19. Inability to conceive
20. Cysts on ovaries
21. Loss of physical height
22. Knee/hip problems
23. Low sex drive
24. Painful sex (females)
25. Edema in legs/hands
26. Loss of muscle mass
27. Cellulite (hips/thighs)
28. Irregular menstruation
29. Irritable bowel
30. Fibroid tumors
31. "Overly" tender breasts
32. Endometriosis
33. Depression/gloominess
34. Body painful to touch
35. Nights sweats/hot flashes
36. Loss of muscle tone
37. Arthritis/rheumatism
38. Allergies/sinusitis
39. Sleep/rest issues
40. Gas/bloating after meals
41. Low back pain w/period
42. Menstrual crankiness
43. "Out of control"/anxiety
44. Constipation/hemorrhoids
45. Thinning vaginal walls
46. Dowager Hump/stooped over
47. MS/lupis/fibromyalgia
48. Poor memory/brain fog
49. Degenerative eye problems
50. Low iron, pernicious anemia

Common to the above **SIGNS** and **symptoms** is "hormones," grid-locked "receptors" and an "acid terrain." And central to these is poor **"bile flow"** and a weak "liver!" By following the suggestions in this book and doing the *Young Again Protocol(s)*™ —you will regain control of your life. Restoration of the "terrain" brings hormonal "issues" into perspective and eases fear and anxiety-related stress. Restoration of the **"hormone cycle"** and **"PATIENCE"** allow women to experience the *Vorago*™ *Effect.* [To better understand the Vorago™ **"riddle"** see Chapter 36 *Vorago*™ *Sunrise* and pages 72, 162, 164, 274 and 400.]

Water For Bathing & High Enema Therapy™

Bathe in safe, biologically friendly water using an oxidation/reduction shower filter that goes way **BEYOND** ordinary shower/bath filters. A **"redox"** shower filter makes your skin and hair feel and look healthier—while protecting your liver from chemicals. These are **"full-flow,"** long-lasting filters that do **NOT** require cartridge replacement because there is **NO** cartridge to replace. Filters are inexpensive and easy to install—and provide water that is "perfectly suited" for High Enema Therapy™ and bathing. [See page 60 and Source Page 400.]

21

Carbon
12.01115
C
6

Avogadro's Number

"The health of the people is the foundation upon which their happiness depends."
Benjamin Disraeli

It was a hot August day in 1975—the mercury had reached 95⁰ Fahrenheit. Out of nowhere came what looked to be a "hippie" carrying a clip board. He said, *"I'm from the City of Madison and I'm checking all buildings for proper placement of address numbers—and you don't seem to have any!"*

"Do too!" I retorted.

"Well, I looked and I didn't see any and I want to know what you are going to do about it!" he rattled, as he flashed a copy of the local business ordinance in my face —expecting to cement his authority and intimidate me.

"Do too!" I said again, *"And I can prove it!"*

As we proceeded to the front of the building, I motioned to Dale to follow my new found acquaintance and me.

There we stood! The three of us facing a 4x4 **"blank"** post that formed the door frame—and I said;

"Dale, this fine gentlemen is here from city hall and he says that we are not in compliance with city ordinances regarding having our building properly posted with our street address."

"Right there!" I said. *"See! It says, 505 S. Main.*

The man looked at me and said with a strange look on his face, *"There is no address there! It's blank!"*

"Hmmm!" I buzzed, as I turned to Dale and said,

"Dale, do you see 505 S. Main posted here on this post?" And Dale fired back, *"Sure do! Right there on the post!"*

With that, the man looked at me—then, at Dale—shook his head, ***"gave up"*** and ***"walked away"***—unsure who was nuts—and very unsure about what had just taken place.

Things Not What They Seem

Things are not always what they seem. Sometimes

"nothing" is something. Sometimes something small is really big! Sometimes weak is strong. We cannot always trust our eyes—and sometimes logic does not make sense in the face of conflicting observations and experiences. Sometimes, we must follow our **"instincts"** or be forced to *"walk away!"*
    The man in our story knew when to *walk away.* Science does not. Instead, "science" tries to "make" natural energy **phenomena** comply with its defined **"LAWS"**—and in the process, science completely misses nature's lessons.
    In homeopathy, weak is strong; something that does not exist, does exist; and something that is nothing becomes something.
    These *apparent* "contradictions" cause science and medicine to "ridicule" instead of inquiring with an open mind. They demand scientific **"proof"** backed by a body of **"literature"**—when they should be interested in **"RESULTS!"** They get caught up in **theory** and **method** and forget that their double-blind **"studies"** are riddled with contradictions. [*In the land of the blind, the blind man is king!* Desiderius Erasamus]

Phenomena
    Here are a few examples of electrical phenomena. Let's see if they shed light on the aging process.
    "Biodynamic" agricultural practices *transmute* "energy" in raw cow manure into energy that is immensely more potent and of a very different "nature." Biodynamics calls for a "pinch" of *potentized* horn manure in twenty gallons of high energy water. The energy **from** the potentized substance is **"transferred"** to the water using "convoluted" stirring procedures that **"energize"** and **"concentrate"** ENERGY into the "solution." When applied to acres of dead dirt, the **energized** solution creates an energy **"explosion,"** creating **"soil"** from which life "bursts forth!" Science cannot explain this phenomenon because there is no place for such a phenomenon in its "model." Science is **NOT** interested in **un**scientific results.
    Homeopathic medicine uses the principles of *dilution*, *succussion, resonance* and *transference* to create energy solutions called "remedies" that deal with dis-ease at the Fourth Dimension energy level. For example, add one "drop" of black paint to one gallon of white paint and you have a **MIXTURE** of both colors. The black paint is very "diluted" and exerts **very little** influence on the "white" paint. As more white paint added to the mixture, the "drop" of **black** paint exerts less and less influence on the white paint—but it's still "there!" [This example deals with **"physical"** dilution and the influence of physical black paint on physical white paint.]
    Homeopathic medicine is concerned with the **influence** of **"invisible," "non physical,"** energy forces upon each other

and on the patient and how Fourth Dimension energy manifests itself in the **physical** Third Dimension body.

Potentiation

Homeopathic "remedies" work on the basis of "similars." Homeopathy starts with a substance that has a *similar* vibrational frequency as the dis-ease energy field. The substance is then *diluted*. At each dilution, the remedy is pounded (succussed) so that it will absorb various frequencies (10x, 20x, 50x, 100x, 200x, etc.). This process is called *potentization*—and the remedy is now *"potentized!"* The idea is to create multiple dilutions of different vibrational frequencies that when taken into the body will **"cancel"** the frequency of the targeted [dis-ease or pathogen] energy field. A *potentized* remedy treats the patient at a level that is **beyond** the Third Dimension. In homeopathy, dilution and succussion add **"energy"**—where in our paint example, the black paint became less influential as more white paint was added to the mixture.

Homeopathic remedies are "energetic"—**NOT** physical mixtures. They are energy solutions that produce energy **phenomena** in sick bodies. Remedies are **CONCENTRATED** "energy" derived from the vibrational frequencies of the original "physical" substances. However, the more the remedy is *diluted* and the more it is *succussed*—the more energy the remedy contains and the more effective it becomes. Logic says, a remedy should **NOT** exert any influence because the original substance is weaker—even "non existent!" Energy **transference** and *succussion* pushes the "scientific" mind too far. Logic, however, is faulty here because it is based on Third Dimension physics that does **NOT** apply to Fourth Dimension energy phenomena. Homeopathy **enhances** and **transfers** the the electrical **"signature"** of **NON EXISTANT** physical substances to sick bodies for the purpose of "healing." In homeopathy, something which does **NOT** exist **DOES** exist.

Science does NOT understand homeopathic "principles" because they do NOT fit its "model"—so science ridicules in contempt, instead of acknowledging results!

"MORA" is a spin-off from homeopathy—just as the word processor is a spin-off from the typewriter. MORA electronically *duplicates* energy *signatures* and electronically *transfers* them to the patient instead of giving the patient the actual, physical solution called a "remedy!" The physical remedy is placed into a scanning "well" where the remedy's frequency is **"duplicated"**—much like a computer *scanner* reads a typed page and converts it to codes and signals so the computer can work with it. The **duplicated** frequency is then **"transferred"** to the sick person's body—and healing takes place. The process can be repeated over and over **without**

"consuming" the actual physical "remedy." Homeopathy is **NOT** about "logic!" It is about energy phenomena and results obtained by "altering" energy forces and restoring balance to **BOTH** Third and Fourth Dimensions of the body's "terrain!"

Regardless if a healing modality "fits" accepted medical theory, models, dogma or the LAWS of science— it doesn't matter. The only thing that counts is results!

It's In The Numbers

Amadeo Avogadro (1776-1856) was the Italian chemist who saw big numbers in small things. He developed a method to estimate the number of atoms that exist in a substance by comparing it to a known reference substance whose number of atoms were known—at least, in theory. This reference number is called Avogadro's number or **[N]** in his honor. Like Reams, Pauling, Caisse, Semmelweis, Carson and Gerson, Avogadro was ridiculed by his "peers" for his vision and the **TRUTH** to which he bore witness.

*[Avogadro was a wizard, and wizards don't have peers! But they are surrounded by "bootleggers" who **NEVER** have an original thought and who take credit for others' discoveries.]*

*[Avogadro's reference substance was 12 grams of carbon-12. The carbon atom is extremely **small!** The number of atoms in 12 grams of carbon-12 is extremely **large!** The number of atoms in 12 grams of carbon-12 is estimated to be approximately 602,000,000,000,000,000,000,000 atoms!]*

In homeopathy, the most "powerful" remedy derives from a physical substance that has been **diluted** and **potentized** to a point that **NONE** of the original substance exists. Theoretically and physically speaking—a substance does **NOT** exist once it goes **beyond** Avogadro's number or 22 decimal places. Logic says when a substance ceases to exist—you have reached **NOTHING!** Yet, homeopathic remedies have enormous energy "**footprints**"—considering that they don't exist.

*[A 9x remedy equals 1 part per **billion** (ppb); at 30x it's beyond Avogadro's number with 30 zeros, and so on. Homeovitic remedies are **combinations** of 9x, 20x, 30x, 100x, 200x providing broad spectrum **bioresonance** needed to meet the changing "terrain" requirements of a sick and healing body.]*

Aging & Avogadro's Number

Avogadro's number is **VERY IMPORTANT** to the aging process. If positive energy contained in a highly diluted homeopathic remedy can cause **MASSIVE** change for "good," then negative energy **transference** from a bad lifestyle, food and water should be equally **DISASTROUS** to health and longevity—and it is! The same reasoning holds true for "**negative**" actions and thoughts that spawn effects millions of times greater than the actual event. Like ripples created when a rock is tossed into a pond—negative thoughts and actions produce **exponential** negative "consequences" on health. [Prayer produces similar effects as these concepts.]

Dr. Samuel Hahnemann
Samuel Hahnemann (1755-1843) is considered the father of "modern" homeopathic medicine. He was a brilliant German physician. The electrical phenomenon he discovered is known as the medicine of **"similars"** or homeopathy.

Let's compare homeopathic medicine to allopathic medicine and see if a contrast of the concepts involved will help us understand the aging process.

Allopathic medicine—"Western medicine"—treats disease with drugs and chemicals that are *antagonistic* to the symptoms being treated. Drugs induce a **pathologic** reaction that "stresses" the system with an **opposite-cures-opposite** approach. "Pathologic" reactions induce dis-ease in order to confront the targeted dis-ease—just like "chemotherapy!"

"Medications" are prescribed based on the benefit-to-risk ratio discussed earlier. Pharmacology "recognizes" that all drugs carry **RISK**—and all drugs **DAMAGE** the vital organs. Allopathic medicine attempts to *overpower* dis-ease with drugs that **SHOCK** the body into a condition of **sub**clinical illness. Allopathic medicine uses powerful, left-spin energy drugs as negative energy "bullets" that target the tissues and vital organs to **"FORCE"** a response! Allopathy is the medicine of "opposites" which sheds light on its *dismal* track record!

Homeopathy is the exact **OPPOSITE** of allopathy. Homeopathy uses friendly energy "bullets" with **similar** frequencies to **CANCEL** the energy frequencies of the offending condition. Homeopathy is "legitimate" holistic medicine that says **"Like cures like!"**—without doing damage to the body.

How Homeopathy Was Discovered
Hahnemann was extremely disillusioned with conventional medicine. While treating patients for yellow fever, he discovered that if he gave a healthy person—who did **NOT** have yellow fever—a tea of cinchona bark which was known to be effective against the fever—intermittent fevers would spontaneously develop as if the person had the "condition." [The inner white pulp of **grapefruit** contains **"quinine-like"** factors and should be eaten during bouts with viral infections.]

Hahnemann further discovered that "diluted" substances were more powerful than concentrated ones. He refined his new method of treatment and eventually included emotional and mental disturbances. Remedies were developed by *trial and error* based on their ability to produce a "response" similar to the sick person and was then tested on a "sick" individual to see if it would produce "healing"—as evidenced by a **RETURN** to "health!"

[Present day homeopathic remedies are NOT designed to bring on actual illness or dis-ease in a healthy person. They only cancel offending energy fields existing in the patient.]

Hahnemann experienced much success applying his "remedies"—but noticed their effectiveness increased in direct proportion to **dilution** and **potentization**. In other words, the **MORE** he *diluted* and *succussed* the remedy, the **MORE** effective it was on the patient! His findings were in serious **CONFLICT** with the orthodox medical dogma of his day. The conflict continues to this day!

*[Dosage-related effects—as practiced in modern pharmacokinetics—the study of the dynamics of chemical drugs in the body—looks at the action of drugs on body metabolism with emphasis on **time** required for absorption, **duration** of action, means of **distribution** and **excretion** from the body. These "factors" determine "activity level"—meaning "saturation level" of the drug in the blood and tissues. Allopathic medicine is acutely AWARE of the problems related to drug usage. It walks a tight-rope between short-term "benefits" and short-term "damage" to the vital organs. Long-term damage is SELDOM an issue because it is very hard to prove! New names for strange, new "symptoms" and "dis-eases" are constantly being "conjured up" as a "cover" for long-term damage!]*

Hahnemann got wonderful results using remedies that "exceeded" Avogadro's number. His findings conflict with Newtonian physics which states *"Where there is an action, there is an equal and opposite reaction!"* Accepted "laws" are the basis of our modern-day chemotherapy mentality. Pharmacology and medical science rely on **"saturation effect"** to produce a "measurable" level of drug "activity!" Medical science uses a "sledge hammer" approach based on "opposites," whereas homeopathy uses gentle remedies based on "similars!" [Much **acrimony** exists between these competing medical approaches. It's easy to see **WHY** mainstream doctors *"Just don't get it!"}*

Allopathic medicine **burdens** the body with drugs to a point **BEYOND** what the kidneys, liver, lungs and skin can "excrete"—forcing the body "by default" to respond to "drugs" while the "terrain" weakens! The damage done to the *bio-electric* body varies by **type** and **quantity** of drugs used and **duration** of use. [The "effects" of long-term drug use enhances the "warnings and contra indictions" described in the "fine print" of drug literature and television "warnings!"]

Homeopathy is the modality of **"preference"** for patients and physicians interested in "healing." Remedies address the *subtle-energy* level where dis-ease has its "roots!"

Homeopathy & Agriculture

Modern agriculture uses **SUPER-POTENTIZED** poisons to try to stop insects and weeds. Until recently, large amounts of poison was used. Now very "small" amounts of poison are mixed with large amounts of water. Agricultural and pharmaceutical companies have **"cloned"** Hahnemann's principles of **dilution, potentiation** and **transference** and turned them to **EVIL** purposes. The "ungodly" do the devil's dirty work! *[Your author encourages the reader to plant a garden. Home-grown food makes up for a plethora of poor choices and mistakes in personal lifestyle. Live, fresh food is a gift from God. It causes the cells to resonate "healthy!"]*

Think Small

Americans think **"BIG!"** Big cars, big houses, big meals, big surgeries—and big bottles of medications! People complain and feel cheated when they pay a lot of money for a small bottle of pills that they would be better of without!

In health-related matters, we must learn to think **"small"** in terms of the **HUGE** side-effects created by tiny amounts of "medications" taken in pursuit of a "fix!" We must come to **understand** that the "terrain" is altered by **BOTH** positive and negative energy forces—and that "tiny" amounts of toxic substances produce **BIG** responses with **LONG-TERM** effects on health and longevity.

We are surrounded by "toxic" substances. The prudent person who thinks in terms of the effects of Avogadro's number, stands the best chance of becoming *Young Again!*

PREVIEW: *Our next chapter looks at our multi-dimensional body. It looks at the "terrain" of the bio-electric body and reconsiders Pasteur's obsession with "bugs" and the Germ Theory of Dis-ease.*

Only Two Choices!

Each day of our lives, the body has **only** two choices for dealing with "waste!" Either send **"soluble" acid wastes** down the toilet in the "bile" produced by the liver—or store those **"soluble" acid wastes** in body fat beneath the skin. If the liver is "sick" and can't do its job—or the biliary ducts and gallbladder are "gummed up"—the body will **STORE** the waste "by default!" **Removal** of "soluble" acid wastes is the purpose of the *Young Again (Tissue and Liver) Protocol*™. Removal of **"structural"** acid waste is a very different matter—and a totally **NEW** concept, as you will discover in Chapter 36 *SilkWorm Blues]*

➥ **Please Note:** The BFRV™ trademark replaces the *"abandoned"* BEV acronym, *DUE TO ongoing infringement and "bootlegging"* by individual(s) offering water processing equipment under the "pretense" their equipment fulfills the "terrain" management **CONCEPTS** of the *Young Again Protocol.*™

Medical Grade Ionized Water™

Medical Grade Ionized Water™ is a special class of *therapeutic* water used in special Japanese clinics to treat a complete list of serious medical disorders. In Japan, expensive **clinical** equipment is used to make this water. [A scaled-down, unit is used to make this water in the home—with all of the relevant qualities and benefits to go with it.]

Medical Grade Ionized Water™ is **NOT** about making "high-alkaline" water. MGIW™ is made from BFRV™ water and racemized™ sea minerals that supply **needed** electrons for energy **"transference!"** Raw tap water and common filtered waters are **NEVER** used to create MGIW™ water.

Water pH (acidity/alkalinity)—by itself—has *nothing* to do with the healing qualities of MGIW™ water. Rather, it's the "ORP" (oxidation/reduction potential) that does the "magic!"

Dis-ease has its roots at the cellular level where MGIW™ water™ does its magic. The benefits of high ORP water derive from a combination of purity, ORP and resistivity. Highly *reduced* acid water and highly *oxidized* alkaline waters have pH values of 1.5-2.4 and 10.5-12, respectively—and ORP potentials of -900 and +1200, respectively. "Tiny" highly-**charged** water molecules easily cross cell membranes for delivery of electrons to the mitochondria that make the body's high-energy molecule."ATP!" [See chart on page 306.]

Oxidized water is used for infections, douches, oral and genital herpes and warts—and for beautiful facial skin. **Reduced** water is drunk and **de**acidifies the "terrain!"

MGIW™ water offers major health advantages **not** available by other means. The fundamental "rules" of water call for avoidance of raw tap water, and drinking enough "body-friendly" water and racemized sea mineral electrolytes daily. MGIW™ water is used where added benefit is desired or needed and should be considered **"frosting"** on the cake. MGIW™ water does **NOT** replace the fundamental rules of water previously mentioned. MGIW™ is recommended where **TERRAIN** management fundamentals have been addressed or where *"Time is of essence!"* [The *Young Again (Tissue & Liver and High Enema Therapy™) Protocols*™ restore the "terrain!"]

➥ **See pages 107-110 and diagram on page 306.**

22

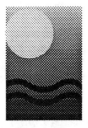

Change The Terrain

"No tree has branches foolish enough to fight among themselves." "Watashi Wa"

The great French bacteriologist, Pasteur, said *"Le microbe c'est tout! **The microbe is everything!"** A contemporary, Claude Bernard retorted, "Le microbe c'est rien. Le terrain c'est tout! The microbe, that's nothing! It is the terrain that's everything!"*

When we look **beyond** the microbe, we see that they are only participants in a grand scheme. Microbes take their cues from the body's "terrain." Microbes cannot prosper unless the **"terrain"** is conducive to their growth. The word **"microbe"** includes bacteria, virus, fungi, yeast and parasites.

The *terrain* **MUST** concern us—because the *terrain* is eveything! It is the doorway through which dis-ease appears and old age expresses itself. The terrain is *multi-dimensional* and goes **BEYOND** our Third Dimension world.

Multi-Dimensional Body

Humans are *multi-dimensional* creatures that experience life on mental, physical and spiritual planes—but life *"extends"* beyond these. We learn early to perceive and interpret our world in physical terms and geometric concepts we call length, width and height—the First, Second and Third Dimensions. But there are other dimensions—**higher dimensions**—we experience from time-to-time like intuition, telepathy, dowsing and maybe even the ability to see holes in another person's aura as discussed in Chapter 20—things that belong to the 4th Dimension and beyond.

Aging & The Fourth Dimension

The higher dimensions are **"invisible"** to all but a few souls. Aging occurs in the **"higher"** realms before it is experienced and seen in the Third Dimension world of the "mirror!" Vitality and health are **controlled** by the energy forces of **BOTH** the Third and Fourth Dimensions. Anything that impacts the Fourth Dimension electric body affects the Third Dimension physical body and visa-versa.

Health and dis-ease are expressions of the ongoing "energy" tug-of-war raging between the invisible Fourth Dimension world and Third Dimension physical reality!

When we die, the tug-of-war is over. The negative energy forces won! Simultaneous with death, vital force (spirit) leaves the body. We *"give up the ghost!"* The spirit returns from whence it came. It returns to a *higher* energy level, perhaps the Fourth Dimension. Maybe higher. No one knows for sure. Call it heaven, hell, hereafter. Suit yourself!

The Fourth Dimension body goes by different names like—**subtle energy, soul, astral, spirit, invisible, bio-electric, etheric, Chi, Qi and Prana.** All of these names refer to the same thing based on different belief systems.

Our Fourth Dimension **"existence"** is invisible. Some folks try to deny its existence—but doing so does **NOT** change the reality of it or alter its influence on our earthly journey.

When we attempt to heal the physical body, but ignore the spirit body—healing **"fails!"** If we allow the electric body to become old, the physical body follows suit. If we experience death in the physical realm, but maintain our hold on our spirit, we are **NOT** really dead—and we return to our physical world with tales of **after** death experiences.

When we cannot hold onto "life" on Earth—or when we have served our purpose for being here—"physical" death of the body takes place.

Vantage Point

The "electric" body is an **extension** of the physical body—and the physical body is the **expression** of the electric body. Our multi-dimensional bodies interface dis-ease, health, life and death. Try and become comfortable with these concepts. Understanding them will help the reader better understand our earthly experience. [To get a wonderful overview for this area of thought, read *The Holographic Universe*.]

Long before dis-ease manifests itself in the physical realm, the *bio-electric* body is undergoing **vibrational changes** that set the course for the physical manifestation of illness. This is what Bernard meant when he said *"The terrain is everything!"*

Understanding our earthly dilemma demands that we adopt a vibrational view of health and dis-ease.

In order to understand the forces of aging, one must understand the idea of an "invisible" world of **"antagonistic"** energy forces. We feel the influence of these invisible forces when they appear in our physical, visible world in the form of **SIGNS** confirmed by the doctor's diagnosis.

The "invisible" world is poorly understood—but it is the arena where the **war** between health and dis-ease is fought. The Third Dimention "visible" world "mirrors" with **SIGNS** and **symptoms** the energy war being continually fought in the Fourth Dimension "invisible" realm.

Food Plants & Insects

Chinese **Taoism** teaches that humans are a reflection of the universe and that **all life** in the physical realm is part of the spirit of the Creator. Man has much in common with plants and insects because they also have a **"dual"** existence.

Plants have many functions. Two functions are the production of food energy and the infusion of solar energy into the soil. In the process of synthesizing food molecules, plants take **CARBON** from the atmosphere and **"infuse"** it into Mother Earth's epidermal and dermal skin layers—top soil and sub top soil—through their roots and foliage.

Plants are **"mediators"** of solar energy. They "capture" and use it to construct complex energy molecules. Organic food molecules contain carbon, oxygen, nitrogen, hydrogen, sulphur and "ionic" minerals. Food molecules are biologically active—driving **"anabolic"** activities called **growth** and **repair.** But when forced to undergo negative circumstances using NPK fertilizers and poisons, food energy molecules destroy and weaken whatever is eating it. [See pages 21, 198 and 306.]

The body needs sulphur and carbon in sulfhydryl form to build healthy connective tissue and restore the body. SOC™ capsules supply sulfhydryl molecules.

Energy Mediation & Stress

Plants **"convert"** solar and cosmic energy into new and different "energy" forms like food crops, wood and high-carbon soil. Insects and microbes are the "middlemen!" Plants need the trillions of unpaid workers in the soil—the microbes—to perform the miracle of **"photosynthesis."** Animals eat plants—converting plant solar energy into animal proteins.

Energy is never lost; it merely changes form! This is Second Law of Thermodynamics—and it is true!

Plant is a "living" **antennae!** Plants receive energy by day from the Sun and by night from the cosmos. By day, they convert solar energy into hydrocarbon sugars (*hydro*-water, *carbon*-atomic element #12) with mineral ions and enzymes supplied by soil bacteria. At night, plants use sugar molecules and earth minerals for growth. The "dew point" is the **PEAK** in plant "growth" when daytime-produced sugars are burned and heat is "given-off"— causing condensation and "dew" on plant leaves. [Early Viking adventurers who landed in New England reported "sweet" early morning dew on the blades of grass.]

All life forms—plant, animal and man—require the help of microbes for their continued existence.

Microbes function as "middlemen" between plants and animals. They use carbon sugars produced by plants for sustenance and as an energy source for breaking soil "ionic" mineral bonds and "covalent" bonds in organic matter. Ionic mineral energy in turn fuels plant growth and the production of healthy food that can sustain animals and man.

Plants submit their order for needed "growth" energy at the *root level.* The bacteria receive and fill the order if they and the soil are both in a **POSITIVE** energy "state." Unfilled orders put plants under "stress"—causing an energy shift to the "left." Stress reduces plants vibrational frequency. Stressed plants **"TRANSMIT"** negative energy signals to nature's garbage crew—the insects, fungi, bacteria and viruses—who oblige and "attack" stressed plant life. [Stress has tremendous influence over the "terrain" of humans, animals and plants.]

[Good food and bio-friendly water are stress management tools. So is yoga, deep breathing, prayer, Qi Gong, Tai Chi, walking barefoot in sand or grass, prayer, sleeping under the stars, exercise, laughing, meditation and positive thoughts. The Young Again Protocol™ indirectly deals with "stress" through deacidification and restoration of the "terrain" and by neutralization of the "cortisol effect" that occurs whenever the adrenal glands come under "load."]

Stress seeks a "release"—just as electricity seeks ground. *Stress management is central to "terrain" management which is central to health and longevity.*

The Carbon Connection

Tissue protein like muscle, bone, cartilage, etc. is composed of amino acids **"linked"** together by peptide bonds. **Sulfonyls** are amino acid protein molecules that contain sulphur in their structure. Carbon is #12 on the periodic table of elements. Carbon is **"UNIQUE"** because it **"bonds"** with many different elements and participates in millions of **different** reactions—all of them unique unto themselves. The carbon atom provides the "skeleton" for the synthesis of pesticides and poisons that the experts just "love" to call "organic!" Compounds of organic synthesis are "organic" by definition—but your author would remind the reader they are also "poisons!"

Look at a chemical's molecular "diagram" and you will see the "-R" group [stands for "reactive" group]. This molecular group determines whether a chemical is DDT, or malathion, or dioxin or some so-called "harmless" organic molecule.

Toxic organic compounds are potent, left-spin energy substances that alter the plant's "terrain" and diminishes plant "life-force." Sick, unhealthy crops should never gain entrance to the food chain. Animals and humans that eat poisoned food "suffer!" Sadly, in only a few decades, man-made organic poisons have spoiled life on Earth.

[Poisons are one of the agendas of the yellow fringed flag "interests" and the "corporate" state—an agenda that says "Cheap food at politically popular prices is desirable." The implied threat here says "Cheap food is better than no food!"]

Plants are living miracles. The "experts" tell us plants only need NPK (nitrogen, phosphorous and potassium) to produce "food." There is a **BIG** difference between food that fills the belly and food capable of producing healthy people.

Food is the ultimate tool for people "control." A gut full of poisoned, empty calories **CANNOT** produce or maintain a healthy human being—or a happy nation. Left-spin energy food feeds violent crime! Violent people suffer from conditions of **"EXCESS!"** *Excess* is another way of saying *"out of balance!"* Excess is easy to confirm upon post-mortem examination—but by then it's **too late!** Sick people make for a sick society!

Too soon old, too late smart is a sorry excuse for loss of your most important treasure—your health!

Explosions

Carey Reams did most of his life's work in the agricultural arena. He believed that plants and animals live on the energy "released" when mineral bonds are broken. He referred to these chemical reactions as "explosions!"

Explosions occur when "rain" water chemically "reacts" with soil minerals and acids releasing growth energy! Rain water releases **far more** energy than does irrigation water. When it rains, grass grows and corn jumps! Rain water is biologically **"active"** water. Rain water has a slightly acid pH.

Plants extract carbon from the "air" and secrete carbonic acid (hydrogen+carbon) from their roots to dissolve ionic mineral bonds and free mineral "ions" from soil and rock—with the help of water. Soil bacteria absorb mineral "ions" into their bodies, digest them and release them in a "solution" mixed with carbon sugars as a chemically stable "glue-like" substance that gives healthy, high-carbon "organic" soil its crumbly texture—causing it to flocculate, hold water and not "leach!"

Carbon-rich soil is healthy, active soil with **"anabolic"** characteristics. It's **"live"** because it is high in what Leonard Ridzon called "biogenic" carbon in his book *The Carbon Cycle.* Soil rich in biogenic carbon yields food that is "nourishing!" When plants call for nourishment, healthy soil supplies needed nutrients from nature's pantry in the soil.

The yardstick of measurement for soil fertility is **"cation exchange capacity"** (CEC). "CEC" is a measure of "available" mineral ions bonded to soil "colloids." Ionic mineral ions are held "on" the soil colloid until the plant needs them. If the plant asks for ions different from what is available, the bacteria use the **transmutation process** described in Chapter 18 to **"transmute"** mineral ions to fit the plant "needs!" Transmutation involves "cold" fusion—orchestrated by soil bacteria.

Carbon acts as a "bridge" in cold fusion reactions, in the soil, or in the gut and liver of man and animal. Carbon underwrites health and aging. The body needs biogenic carbon from healthy food—grown on healthy soil—not from useless carbon in white, table sugar ($C_6H_{12}O_6$).

Transmitters & Receivers

Crops grown on biologically "live" soil as nature intended have a healthy "aura"—and radiate "healthy" energy signals. Plants grown with commercial fertilizers and poison sprays radiate signals in the *"I'm sick, come and eat me!"* wave band. Phil Callahan discovered how insects use their antennae to "intercept" distress signals and navigate by them— like a war plane homing in on its target by following the radar beam to the source. Insects eat "sick" plants—but they do **NOT** wage war against "healthy" plants. Insects and microbes comply with nature's mandate to remove the weak from the Earth. In the human arena, acid waste "build-up" stresses the *bio-electric* body and **weakens** vital organ function. The microbes **"identify"** conditions of stress in the human "terrain"— and attack! Microbes know how to read "code" signals that say *"I'm sick; come and do away with me!"*

Insects have antennae on their heads and cilia (tiny hairlike projections) on their body. These structures are "tuned" to pick-up "signals" emanating from stressed crops. Insects know **"exactly"** which plants represent a meal and which ones do not. Different insects are tuned to different frequencies. You won't find Colorado Potato Beetles eating sweet corn. Nature tunes each insect's antenna to its own *"I'm sick, come and eat me!"* frequency. Plant stress signals transmit in the **near** and **far infrared** spectrums of "lightwave" frequency that are neither audible nor visible to humans. [Identifying **SIGNS** and **symptoms** of "stress" and "excess" in plants is similar to reading the signals in human beings. We are discussing energy phenomena here!]

*[Sunlight light contains all "visible" color frequencies and is part of our Third Dimension experience and world. Light is "electrical" in nature—meaning anything electrical is related to sunlight. Color therapy, cold laser therapy and chi gong therapy are applications and variations of **therapeutic** lightwave en-*

ergy used to promote healing. Microwave ovens, radar, x-rays and energy from "wireless" phones are anti-life, electrical energy in "frequencies" that destroy health.]
Dis-ease belongs to the world of invisible electrical energy, be it in plants, animals or humans!

Observations

Insects "gorge" on sick, weak crops. Crops requiring insecticides to fend off insects are unhealthy. The soil is the "terrain" that controls the health of food crops. People who eat poor quality "food" become unhealthy. Unhealthy food energy is "freak" energy that cannot be utilized by the *bio-electric* body. Organic poisons are **potent** negative energy fields. They work like homeopathic "remedies"—but in **REVERSE**—and their effect on people's health is beyond comprehension.

If sick plants attract predatory insects, viruses, bacteria and molds, can we assume that healthy plants repel them? The answer is a big **YES!** A positive energy **terrain** repels disease—and negative energy attracts the same unless the cycle is broken by exercising **"correct" choices.**

[The use of organic poisons on food crops is similar to medical science's insistence on immunization of the population. Sadly, immunizations do NOT produce immunity. See pages 86, 228-9 and 249.]

Brix • Vitality • Pigments

Dr. Carey Reams pioneered the use of the refractometer—aka: "brixmeter"—for measuring the vitality of food crops. This simple, hand-held device is used to measure **"sucrose"** levels in "solution" in the juices of plants. Sucrose is simple sugar. The more sucrose in plant juices, the **MORE** mineral ions present in the food crop. A full array of mineral ions translate as flavor, vitamins, enzymes, keeping quality, health and vitality. Without these qualities "food" is **NOT** really food and results in degenerative dis-ease and a sick people.
Healthy food could remedy the health care crisis—but it would shut down the sick care industry.

A re-fract-o-meter "refracts" sunlight through plant juices placed on a glass slide for this purpose. The "scale" is 0-32 brix; "0" is the bottom and 32 is the top of the scale. The **lower** the number, the **higher** the level of insect infestation and dis-ease in food corps and ornamentals. In the case of sweet corn, nature's garbage crew will devour corn at 10 brix. At 18 brix, the insects will back-off. At 24 brix, they will cease to be a problem. But at 32 brix, corn will grow 16 feet tall and have 3-4 ears per plant. High brix readings means **NO** dis-ease and healthy crops that don't need insecticide poisons.

Plants grown in highly mineralized, high-carbon soil

are "live" and have high brix readings. "Brix" is a unit of measurement. It is also a "marker." The higher the brix reading, the **MORE** nutritious the food and the greater its *"life force."*

When sugar and mineral ion levels are high, plants do **NOT** "transmit" negative energy "distress" signals to insects and microbes in the *"I'm sick; come and eat me!"* frequency. And when insects stop for a bite, they die because insects are **not** equipped to handle high sucrose levels that turn to alcohol in the insects stomach—killing the bug! Natural pest control!

[Alcohol is a toxin (poison). Yet, when a person is sick, it is helpful to take a **hot** *bath with 1 cup of Epsom salt, 1 qt. of 3% hydrogen peroxide and a pulverized ginger root after drinking a "shot glass" of whiskey. The alcohol* **KILLS** *multiplying pathogenic microbes in the "terrain" and* **SHOCKS** *the system. Perform High Enema Therapy™ before the bath. Then, go to bed! In countries where sanitation is a major issue, alcohol is taken with meals as a way to "control" incoming dis-ease organisms.]*

The Rainbow

Sunlight contains all of the colors of the rainbow. Plants "display" the colors of the rainbow in the **"PIGMENTS"** of their leaves and tissues. Pigments are "frozen sunlight.™" Pigments are frozen sunlight "energy!" Frozen sunlight is the basis of racemized™ SunLight™ creme—a transdermal skin creme with "health" benefits for people in general—and women in particular! Women who use it on their breasts daily can stop worrying about going down to a breast condition that begins with the letter "C". SunLight™ Creme is part of the *Young Again (Female) Protocol.™* It is used to create the wonderful **Vorago**™ **effect** in women. See Chapter 36 *Vorago™ SunRise.]*

Insect infestation & Crops

Protein content is another way of gauging "life-force!" Unfortunately, all proteins are not the same. Some proteins are "freak" proteins! Protein content by itself does **NOT** qualify a food crop's energy footprint and signature as "healthy!" **Soy** protein, for example, is a very unhealthy protein. [More later!]

99% of food grown in the uSA is of low brix and low vitality. "Funny" protein food spoils easily and breeds violence in children and adults!

[The "experts" and the chemical companies—along with their "yellow fringed flag" friends—don't like the implications of a healthy population. Sick food, weak minds and violence are part of our obsession with sports. Rome took a similar path **AFTER** *desecrating its "standards"—the equivalent of our flag and flag poles—with "adornments" like the yellow fringe, the ball, the eagle, the spear—adornments seen* **EVERYWHERE** *in the uSA—adornments that take precedence over the flag of*

peace by creating a **BOGUS** *"jurisdiction" and* **meaning;** *adornments that effectively impose "foreign" corporate "state" jurisdiction over Citizens. Please recall these words from the uS Constitution—which is a* **"common law"** *organic document—* **NOT** *a statutory document.* **"No State shall create another "state" from within a state or from a combination of states."** *The "state" referred to by this "prohibition" is a foreign* **"condition"** *that is repugnant to the Constitution and the rights of its citizens. The US Flag of War is the* **ONLY** *flag displayed worldwide, which explains "why" we are in a perpetual* **"state"** *of emergency and* **"state"** *of war. "Their" courts say it is illegal to burn "their" flag! Our politicians have the "Roman Dis-ease" and they catch it from each other! Legacy, ego and "corporate" national interest take precedence over the good of the people. An artificial foreign goverment "condition"—like the U. S. Government—is* **NOT** *the same as the united State of America or its people. The movie "The Last Samurai" hinted at corruption of "national interest" by the yellow fringed flag forces. Those "interests" control the food supply and the sick-care industry. Poor-quality food is "perfect" for perpetuating a* **militaristic** *society that does as it is told. The Supreme Court—a "maritime" court over the "District of Columbia"—operates under the same "flag" and only pretends to "rule" on constitutional issues just like federal courts and lower petit courts. [For a better understanding of these issues, see pages 168, 196, 361 and 384.]*

   The U S flag of "WAR" has an aspect ratio of 1:1.7 as opposed to the US Flag of Peace on the front cover of this book whose ratio is 1:1.9.

   Civilizations deteriorate because nature's dietary laws are ignored. Sick food and water spawns social excess. Birth defects are part of the "terrain" story and are linked to poisoned food and water. The pregnant woman's liver—and her unborn baby—labor under dietary and environmental imposed stress.

   "In a nation whose legions once commanded the known world, the people cry but for two things: bread and more games." -Pliny

Eat Your Vaccinations, Dear!

   Inferior food with short shelf life is behind the drive to "irradiate" the food supply and genetically manipulate food crops. Madmen scientists are now gene-splicing dis-ease pathogens into plant DNA in an effort to produce "immunity!"

   [If historical myth has any substance, your author would remind the reader that Atlantis and its people were destroyed for genetic cruelties and cross breeding of life forms. Genesis says "Kind begets kind." Prior to the Israelites taking of the "promised land," they cleansed that land of genetically cross bred "giants"—the descendants of the "nephelim." Your author "pre-

dicts" that eating genetically manipulated food will weaken the population and that our offspring will experience gross pathologies with no hope of cure. Darwin's "survival of the fittest" will take on new meaning.]

We are breaking the rules when we cross species lines. Cross breeding of species produces offspring whose vibrational **signatures** and DNA are "freak!"

[We are making another mistake by classifying animal fats and plant-derived "liquid" oils together—as "lipids"—just because they have similar characteristics. The difference between them is immense and **"central"** to health and longevity. Fats are "solid" at room temperature, oils are not. Fats are the basis of our hormones. Butter and lard are fats, oils are not. Animal fat from healthy animals is important to good health.]

Parenteral Nutrition

Food energy is metabolized into the glucose sugar molecule in the **"LIVER!"** Glucose fuels ATP production via the Krebs Cycle in the electron transport chain of the mitochondria that live in our cells. ATP is our energy molecule—and the **end product** of the food we eat. Glucose is **stored** in the liver and muscles as "glycogen." Lactic acid accumulation—and sore muscles from strenuous activity—are byproducts of poor liver function and incomplete burning of the glucose sugar molecule in the **absence** of cellular oxygen.

It is standard medical procedure to add minerals and vitamins to glucose solutions for people on any form of "parenteral" nutrition—nutrition administered by any method other than by mouth—such as intravenously or using a feed tube inserted directly into the stomach or small intestine.

Parenteral nutrition is a "pathetic" way to keep someone alive. It's a glimpse of the **FUTURE** for those who "think" they can **IGNORE** nature's laws—or who think they can "buy" good health via the sick-care system. The Young Again! Protocol(s)™ return "control" of the terrain to the individual.

The Terrain Of Weeds

Weeds are a yardstick of soil fertility and health. They tell a story—and their presence holds meaning. The popular definition of a weed is "something growing out of place"—but the definition is based on ignorance. Weeds grow where they choose because they have a job to do. Their job is to *absorb* negative energy and restore soil energy and balance.

Weeds—like bacteria and viruses—only grow where the "TERRAIN" is to their liking!

[We bought a home with a large yard infested with quack grass. The neighbors laughed when we said we would get rid of the quack grass and have a nice garden. They stopped *laughing when we shared beautiful vegetables with them. Change the soils TERRAIN—and no more quack grass! Quack grass grows on soil that is low in organic matter with a high pH, an unbalanced decay system, and an **excess** of aluminum. So we "hand" dug, shook and piled the quack grass. We then built four or five compost piles around the garden site using organic matter of all types —including quack grass, leaves, grass clippings—plus chicken manure as a "starter," granite dust, gypsum, soft rock phosphate, and red wigglers (worms). We turned the piles biweekly. After two months, we spread the finished compost and dug it into the top four inches of soil. After this process, we could NOT get quack grass to grow. The reason? We changed the **TERRAIN** of the soil. We helped Mother Earth energize her "skin." Every weed has a place and a time. Change the soil environment and weeds will cease to be a problem. Some weeds grow where crops can't grow; some weeds grow with food crops. Weeds provide balance.]*

Your author remembers a story an acquaintance told how the pioneers abused the soil as they came west. They found virgin soils high in life-giving energy and nutrients. They would move on as soon as the soil had "burned itself out." Later—after the deserted farm had sat for 8 or 10 years—Tex's father would buy the farm for next to nothing and presto, the soil produced crops! Tex's father understood that weeds play a very important part in life on this planet. Weeds **ONLY** proliferate when the *terrain* dictates their presence. Sick soils produce "sick" food and noxious weeds. We should not be surprised when people who eat "sick" food grown on "sick" soil become "sick" people! [The "terrain" controls!]

Weeds, insects, bacteria and viruses are our friends. Understand them and you will enjoy a better life.

Hybrid Food

The advent of the hybrid seed has particular significance for the health-minded person. The hybrid was heralded as a wonderful thing. Bigger crops, sweeter corn, better germination and more control at harvest. Some of these things are true, but there are serious trade-offs—like unbalanced enzymes and vitamins, "freak" proteins and poor mineral uptake.

*["**Hybrid**" crops withstand NPK salt fertilizers and poisons used to "force" food crops to produce on sick soils. Hybrid seeds came into "fashion" because seed companies could "**patent**" them. The farmer—ever dependent on bank loans— was "persuaded"to use these new seeds. In the words of one farmer, "We traded open-pollinated seed left over from the past harvest—which was a FREE gift from God—for these damnable hybrids that we have to buy every year!"]*

Powerful commercial interests operating behind the

"yellow fringed flag" took control of the people's food supply. High-vitality food from healthy soil was traded for empty calories and poisoned crops from sick soil. The Earth and her inhabitants are now paying the price.

The "ag" schools and government "experts" said "Hybrids are the wave of the future!" And a poor future it has turned out to be.

Native Wisdom

We live in a world beset with conflict. The four corners of the square are at odds with each other. Philosophy, science, law and religion have lost their moorings. The people gyrate from pole to pole—confused, mad, frustrated, depressed, violent—at odds with their world and themselves. They need wisdom and guidance. My friend comes from the Lakota nation of American Indians. His native name is *Watashi Wa* which translates "*I am here*" I am glad he is. Watashi Wa offered some Lakota wisdom that health-minded people need to incorporate into their lives. "*No tree has branches that fight among themselves.*" We cannot enjoy good health or fulfill our destinies when we are at odds with ourselves and the world. [The symbol shown here reflects the dilemma mankind faces.

Hybrid Inferiority

When we eat food grown from hybrid seeds, we are eating food that is genetically weak. Hybrids do **NOT** reproduce true to their own kind. They *defy* the ultimate test of viability for any living thing: offspring that duplicate the parents. Hybrid seeds are **"freak"** offspring of controlled breeding techniques and they are inferior. Their energy **"signature"** is left-spin! Hybrid food is **INFERIOR** food and should be avoided. Food crops grown from hybrid seed play into the hands of the yellow fringed flag "devils" who **CONTROL** commodity prices and markets—and the food supply of the whole world. Remember these points when experts in the "media" **HYPE** the wonders of genetically engineered crops and irradiated food. Behind the rhetoric, you will find sick food, human suffering and sick "violence" prone societies.

Food is a gift from God. It is NOT a plaything!

Eat nutritious, healthy, food and drink biologically friendly water. Do these things and you will enjoy health and vitality as you become *Young Again!*

PREVIEW: *Our next chapter is about "OBESITY." Learn the "real" reason for obesity. Whether you are thin or not, the chapter contains VALUABLE information that you will need to understand the remainder of this book.*

Learn At Home

Would "you" like to **"learn"** human anatomy, physiology and microbiology? These subjects are easily learned by **"coloring"** by the numbers using illustrated **"plates"** supported by clear, concise text—done at your own speed! [See pages 274 & 400.]

Gums & Teeth

Bleeding and infected gums are **NO** small matter—and neither are cavities and loose and dying teeth. If you wish to deal with these issues and save yourself a lot of misery and expense, use the BioMagnetic Dental Irrigator™ and Oral Advantage™. [See pages 51, 93, 118, 149, 187 and 204.]

Magnetic Health

Depolarization of body tissues and the "terrain" is an "ongoing" issue. It occurs daily, when people are exposed to extraneous microwave signals, 110 v. electrical "energy" grids, fluorescent lights and computers—all of which are present everywhere in the world in which we live.

Wireless phones account for **MASSIVE** amounts of extreme low-frequency radiation that interferes with cellular balance, body physiology, teeth and brain function.

To protect yourself, consider the following:

Super Magnets™ speed cellular activity by stimulating mitochondrial activity and nerve flow while **BOOSTING immune function**. Super Magnets™ are helpful for **carpel tunnel** issues, **sleep** irregularities, and help with **major or minor injuries** —like a bad fall, a mashed finger, broken bones, head injuries, etc. When used **immediately** after an injury, pain and swelling are lessened, blood and lymph flow in and around traumatized tissue increases, and healing occurs faster.

There are **ONLY** a few magnetic products that are worth bothering with—most are useless. The **Super Magnet**™ **pendant** is suspended from the neck directly over the thymus area (breast cleavage area). Medical grade **mattress pads** "repolarize" the entire body during the sleep cycle. To be effective, pads **MUST** possess six characteristics: quantity of magnets, gauss rating, placement, thickness, surface area and polarity direction. **Biogenic**™ **Super Mattress Pads meet ALL six requirements and are "made to order" according to bed size.**

Modern medicine classifies magnetics as *witchcraft*, but users of Biogenic™ magnetic products know better! All energy has [+ -] "polarity!" We are surrounded by a sea of energy. Energy management is part of "terrain" management. [See pages 49, 81 and 144.]

Source Information Packet
For information, call (800) 659-1882 or (509) 465-4154 or write: **John Thomas P.O. Box 1240 Mead Washington 99021-1240 USA fax (509) 466-8103.**

High Enema Therapy™

High Enema Therapy™ speeds **de**acidification of the tissues, blood and lymph. This wonderfully simple and low-cost procedure is a "given" in the battle to get well, stay well and stop the aging clock. Terrain management does **NOT** get more **basic** than this. Many people are **unjustifiably** *squeamish* on this subject. Your author has taught thousands of people the correct procedures. People who practice the protocol "see" their lives transformed. The *Young Again (High EnemaTherapy™) Protocol™* only sounds like a "pain-in-the-butt!" It is very easy to do. The wise person practices **"prevention"** and heads off trouble before dis-ease announces itself. Why wait for the doctor's diagnosis when you can **AVOID** your "day of reckoning" for as long as you wish to live a healthy life?

Parasites & Food Poisoning

Parasites are a monumental problem—but parasites are **NOT** the enemy! Rather, they reflect loss of control over the body's "terrain." Let me assure the reader that everyone has parasites. How does your author know? Because every time food or water enters your mouth, parasite eggs and adults come along for the ride. Parasites are part of life! But **IF** the digestive system is working "correctly"—and few are—the **peptide bonds** joining the amino acids comprising protein "life forms" called "parasites" are **broken**—killing parasites and their eggs. Digestion of parasitic life forms is one good reason to use Yucca Blend,™ DiSorb Aid II™ and R/BHCl™ **after** meals. Digestion of food, avoiding a toxic bowel, indigestion, acid-relfux and increased flow of "bile" are a few more reasons. These products work wonders for travelers to India and Mexico, etc. No sickness or diarrhea. If you want to be super safe—in or out of the country—wash your hands, keep the nails short—and have the "waiter" bring a bowel of lemon wedges and eat the "pulp" from 3 wedges each—**BEFORE, DURING and AFTER** meals. [Chew charcoal tablets for food poisoning or "violent" illness following meals. See page 64.]

If friends ask what you are doing, don't spoil their meal with parasite stories. Just tell them "Lemons help digestion and weight control" —and play dumb!

Parasite Purge™ I & II—plus Yucca Blend™—deal with parasites in the brain, heart, lungs, spleen and other "vital" organs while driving intestinal parasites out of the body. It takes 60 days to "clear" the vital organs of parasites and to dismantle and shed the debris that was once "creatures" feeding on acid waste in YOUR body. [See pages 69, 156, 180, 234, 316 and 318.]

23

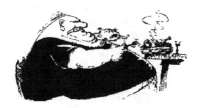

Fat Falstaff

Shakespeare's Prince Hall
to grossly overweight Falstaff:

*"Leave gormandizing; know the grave doth gape?
For thee thrice wider than four other men!"*

*"If you don't want to be obese, change the rules of
the game by changing your "terrain!*
John Thomas

Obesity is the **"curse"** of the industrialized world! We eat the wrong things instead of the right things. We live to eat, when we should eat to live. We eat much, when we could eat little. We dig our grave with our "teeth!"

Obesity is the **"effect"**—not the cause! It has **"NOTH-ING"** to do with genetic inheritance—and **everything** to do with incorrect choices. We are concerned with the **"factors"** that **DRIVE** obesity—and obesity's influence on aging. Pounds and inches "mirror" the internal condition of the "terrain!"

Obesity is dis-ease "in the making" and the harbinger of serious health issues to come. Lifestyle and dietary choices **CONTROL** the obesity story—but insufficient physical acitvity and **"stress"** also play major roles. "Stress" whips the adrenal glands and increases cortisol production. **"Excess"** cortisol upsets hormonal balance and increases the production of "estrogen" by "fat cells" in **BOTH** men and women. **"Excess"** estrogen unbalances the system and increases the production of body fat in a never-ending cycle. [Strangely, when raw **virgin** coconut oil is added to the diet, people lose weight! Healthy fat does **NOT** make people fat!]

Experience teaches that it is easier to take fat off fat people than it is to fatten-up skinny people.

Lack of **physical work** and **load-bearing activity** contribute to connective tissue degeneration by stifling circulation of lymphatic fluids. Exercise is a "tool"—not a goal!

*[At age "61," your author is down to a "33" inch waist.
Before age 55, he had never weighed over 160 pounds—even*

*when in the army! Today [2006] my weight is 175 pounds and muscle mass has increased by two coat sizes while my waistline dropped by "5" inches. The **"strange"** part of my story is that 40% of my dietary caloric intake is fats and oils. I have **boundless** energy and I do **hard physical work** with a shovel and wheel barrow in my 1 acre "garden"—and I am rarely tired even though I work "14-hour" days. [These facts are **SIGNS** and **symptoms** of aging reversal! When you restore your "terrain," obesity and other health issues seem to go "Bye, bye!"]*

The "Condition" Called Obesity

Obesity is a **"condition"** that operates by its own set of rules—like cancer! Usual and customary dietary approachs to obesity **FAIL** because they ignore liver function, stress, leaky-gut, cortisol production, digestion, **de**acidification, hormonal issues, thyroid function, bile flow—and bowel activity. **Ignore** these "terrain" factors—and you will either **become** obese or you will **FAIL** to lose weight and **FAIL** to maintain critical muscle mass. Obesity is the "symptom"—not the cause!

When you **de**acidify the "terrain," restore liver function, boost bile flow and address fundamental issues raised in this book—your body will **"MORPH"** and become a "burner" of **dietary** and **excess** body fat instead of cannibalizing muscle mass in search of needed protein.

The obese body CRAVES nourishment and will "cannibalize" muscle tissue to obtain needed protein "before" it will burn stored body fat.

It takes **"TIME"** and **"PATIENCE"** to restore the terrain and **"train"** the body to become a "fat burner." If correct food ratios are followed **and** the "terrain" is restored—fat will turn into muscle mass. Muscle is a **SIGN** of health—and youth!

Obesity is a "symptomatic" confirmation of metabolic "slow down" and loss of control of the "terrain." Obesity is the most obvious **SIGN** of aging because *"The fat is there!"* Obesity doesn't just "happen!" It is a self-imposed condition underwritten by ignorance, lack of self-love, poor dietary and lifestyle choices—and most importantly, "terrain" issues.

Obesity self-perpetuates through ignorance, reliance on a FAULTY thinking—and social myths.

Bio-junk diets "sabotage" efforts to avoid or control obesity. The obesity "curse" **cannot** be blamed on "genes!" Genes "mirror" dis-ease conditions **AFTER** they occur—and automatically **"SELF-CORRECT"** when the "terrain" is resored. We have the "same" genes as our ancestors. Continued human "existence" proves genetics does **NOT** drive obesity or other health issues. "Entropy" **ONLY** haunts the human condition when control over the "terrain" is forfeited! [See page 306.] Obesity is at "epidemic" levels because of poor choices and plain old ignorance! As body fat increases, vitality and organ function diminishes. Excess body fat is **"confirmation"** of metabolic slowdown and loss of vital organ function. The doctor's diganosis of "dis-ease" is **OFFICIAL** notice that the "terrain" has reached the "tipping point." Let's discuss the genesis of diabetes, as an example.

Diabetes (Type ll) & Auto-Immune Issues

Obesity does **NOT** cause diabetes, but it usually accompanies it—and given enough "TIME" most overweight people become Type ll diabetics. That is the pattern!

"Leaky-gut" heavily influences the terrain and is a **HUGE** contributing factor in **both** obesity and diabetes. Behind a leaky-gut, you will **ALWAYS** find a poorly functioning liver, weak bile-flow and acidification of the "terrain!"

"Leaky gut" is behind virtually every *auto-immune* condition known—and with very few exceptions all major disease conditions are **"autoimmune"** in nature. Old-time healers and health crusaders suspected that the colon was the source of major dis-ease. They were not far off the mark. Liver, bile-flow and leaky gut are **"ground zero"** of dis-ease!

[You author believes that the liver and bile flow are at the core of acidification and terrain issues, and that leaky-gut and colon issues follow in the wake of liver and bile flow issues!]

Autoimmune conditions cause the immune system to **ATTACK** the "host!" Leaky gut allows oversized food and drug molecules **ACCESS** to the blood stream via a "porous" gut wall—something that should **NEVER** occur!

Properly digested food energy goes to the liver for conversion to glucose before distribution to the tissues.

Indiscriminate use of antibiotics and non-steroidal anti-inflammatory drugs—like aspirin and pain killers—destroy the lining of the "gut." [The gut wall must be repaired for the terrain to heal, and that is the purpose of R/C™ and MZ.™]

Wide-spread consumption of "high fructose corn syrup"—especially in the aftermath of antibiotic use—causes intestinal and bowel disorders to grow **"exponentially!"** Yeast infections in women are "symptomatic" of a very **ACID** terrain and a gut that is in horrible shape. [Women who eat "raw," non pasteurized sauerkraut two times a day find wonderful relief!]

It should **NOT** surprise anyone that the **SAME** 75% of the "population" that is obese also suffers from leaky-gut issues and auto-immune "conditions"—and they will statistically succumb to diabetes, too! Diabetes is a leaky gut, auto-immune-driven condition—but not everyone with a leakygut becomes a diabetic. Diabetes will reach **"EPIDEMIC"** levels among the baby boomers who refuse to exercise "choice!"

Insulin does NOT cure diabetes—but it eventually

kills the diabetic while "managing" the symptoms.

Better you **NEVER** reach the point where you have to use insulin in **any** form! Diabetes is reversible—**BUT** it is a tricky and difficult condition to address when someone is already using insulin. Of the four major dis-ease conditions that accelerate aging and early death [heart attack/stroke, cancer, arthritis and diabetes], diabetes is by far the most difficult to reverse because there are so many conflicting "terrain" issues. However, diabetes is totally **"AVOIDABLE!"**

Dietary choice—and the ability or inability to fully digest food—exerts huge influence over the diabetic's "terrain." Leaky-gut issues play an equally important part in the acidification of the "terrain!" Acid waste that cannot be removed from the system because of a faulty liver and poor bile flow are **stored** in the body fat beneath the skin.

Production and accumulation of acid wastes goes with excess body fat. Everyone who is fat is "acid"—but everyone who is "acid" is not necessarily fat.

The fat body is "burdened" and has **LIMITED** ability to restore itself. When body fat levels rise, metabolic rate "slows" and there is less energy available to do the job. Hence, the fat person gets fatter and recovery becomes ever more difficult.

For many people, obesity **CONTROLS** every aspect of their daily life—as well as their self esteem. Obese people are picked-on from kindergarten forward. Children and people are cruel! Obesity precipitates the development of a **"defensive"** attitude—the fat person's version of "short man" syndrome. Obese and short people understandably tend to **OVER** compensate with a very noticeable "chip" on their shoulder. As Mick Jaeger sang, *"I can't get no satisfaction!"*

There is one acceptable solution for the obese person: change the "terrain" and change the rules!

Get Out Of Jail • Permanent Parole

Obesity is a vicious cycle. The obese person knows that things are "different" for them. Both the game **and** the rules are not the same as for "regular" people. The obese person **MUST** learn to think in terms of "jail!" Self-imposed "jail" as a result of plain old ignorance reinforced by medical and social "myth" about obesity and its causes. Central to obesity is a highly acid, waste filled "terrain;" out-of-balance hormones; "starvation" on a full-belly; and a body that needs a "jump start!"

The purpose of the *Young again! (Tissue and Liver) Protocol*™ is to get the obese person's metabolism "out of jail!" And once "free," the fat person is placed on **"permanent"** parole with the practice of High [and low] Enema Therapy™ for the **remainder** of their life. Those who "backslide" go back to jail—and lose their $200 as in the game of Monopoly!

Deacidfication of the fat person's body creates a roller coaster effect which should be both expected and welcomed! Healing occur when toxic waste energy is released from the fatty **sub**cutaneous tissues into the **blood and lymphatic systems**—and again when waste-laden bile flows into the **intestines**. The "mission" of terrain restoration **CANNOT** occur unless bile wastes "physically" reach the toilet bowl! The gallbladder is a **"RESERVOIR"** for bile which it "dumps" into the small intestine two inches **below** the stomach—or about 20 feet **UP** from the anus. Sluggish bowels set the stage of bile "reabsorption" through a leaky-gut wall. Bowel activity is a multi faceted issue! [See page 150.]

Eat Less • Live Longer

Little food is required to maintain good health **IF** the food is of high vitality and digestion goes to completion. Ultimately food heals the body and restores health—but only if the "terrain" can respond. So-called "organic" food—by itself—is **NOT** enough to restore the terrain because the "rules" change when puberty "peaks" at age "25"—and again after age "40" when menopause and andropause manifest. [Obesity issues "compound" the aging story outlined so far.]

Fresh beet and carrot juices are very helpful for the obese person **IF** used in "moderation!" These juices are the "blood" of plants. They are the plants' "life-force"—and are an **"ABSOLUTELY"**essential source of potassium. Potassium drives sodium **OUT** of the cells. [Fresh vegetable juices increase bile flow. Fresh, raw, organic vegetables, healthy proteins and dietary fats go with god health. A raw egg blended in juice is a wonderful source of protein. Eat lots of "free range" eggs in any form!]

Avoid over-cooked food. Eat one third of your food RAW! "Chew" your food—and avoid liquids with meals. Drink plenty of water between meals and you will secrete enough saliva to begin the digestion process in the mouth.

It has been demonstrated over and over again that animals live longer when food intake is reduced to 75% of "optimum" intake level. To reduce food intake and not feel hungry, nourishment and fat intake are **"critical."** When food intake is reduced, the choice of food had better be nourishing!

Sabotage & Body Instinct

The body has *innate intelligence*. It is intuitively smart. It knows what to do to keep itself alive. It can withstand horrendous abuse—and survive—but it can't do it forever. Eventually, the system "overloads" and the body dies!

Turning on the body's fat-burning "pathways" requires **ENERGY**—and effort! The body cannot heal or rejuvenate without sufficient food energy."Digestion" of food must go to completion or food and supplements revert to "liability" status. [DisorbAid ll™ and R/BHCl™ solve digestion issues.]

In the "obese" body, the most nutritious food can become a liability unless "terrain" issues are addressed and liver and bile-flow functions are restored! The obese person must truly desire healing **or** there will be a mind-body tug of war! Obesity is always accompanied by "bowel" issues. So-called "regular" bowel activity doesn't mean "bile" is flowing sufficiently heavy enough to keep the terrain from going into **acid**-waste overload. Bowel issues and colon cancer are a problem for everyone—sooner or later—and obesity definitely makes matters worse!

Fat bodies are sick bodies—and sick bodies often REJECT nourishing food because they can't process it!

Kindling Wood & Fat

Once the *Young Again Protocol*™ is begun, the body will accept high-quality proteins, **complex** carbohydrates, healthy fats and fresh vegetable juices. These foods can sustain a person for many hours. [Fresh beet and carrot juice and a few **SUPER FOODS** sustain your author all day. The **"pigments"** in the juice are the plant's "blood!"]

People confuse complex carbohydrates with worthless starches and sugars found in processed foods. They are **NOT** the same! The body needs complex carbohydrates to oxidize fat. *Complex carbohydrates are to fat-burning what kindling wood is to a wood log.*

In other words, the body can't "burn" fat without something to "kindle" it—and keep it going. Healthy bodies obtain up to "40%" of energy needs from the burning of fat. The **LAST** energy source the unhealthy body will "tap" is "stored" body fat. The fat body draws on muscle-tissue protein **BEFORE** it taps fat reserves. The body will **NOT** release "toxic" waste stored in body fat **unless** it is certain the "waste" can be **safely** moved **OUT** of the body. [The purpose of the *Young Again Protocol*™ is to "create" the conditions for waste **release** and **transport**—and to **MINIMIZE** stress on the vital organs.

Oxidation Of Fat

Aerobic exercise activates fat-burning enzymes. Exercise should demand 60—80% of the maximum heart rate (MHR) for a minimum of twelve minutes—causing the **liver** to produce enzymes that oxidize **small** amounts of fat during exercise and **LARGE** amounts **throughout** the day. Exercise and fat-burning go together—**NOT** because exercise burns fatbut because exercise increases metabolic activity and circulation of blood and lymphatic fluids that transport acidic, waste-laden, amyloid fluid from the tissues.

Exercise should NEVER be used to "offset" poor choices in food, water and lifestyle.

Basal Metabolism

Basal metabolism refers to the **minimum** energy requirements necessary to maintain "life." Basal metabolic rate is usually measured upon waking from sleep, before pulse and temperature rise or the emotions become stirred. Nutritional needs—as reflected in charts and graphs dealing with height, weight and activity—are based on basal metabolic rate.

Total "caloric" intake can be misleading. For example, your author is 5' 11" tall with a 33" waist at 175 pounds. According to the "experts," my body needs approximately 2200 (K)calories a day based on my *activity* level. This is my total daily energy requirement. [Caloric intake is always based on carbohydrate, protein and fat intake.]

Of the 2,200 (K)calories needed, 80% is used to meet **"minimum"** physiologic needs like heart, temperature, breathing, peristalsis, mental processes, etc. If 12 minutes of "brisk" aerobic exercise is added to my daily routine, my energy needs **only** increase by 300 (K)calories. And if those (K)calories are **not** added to my dietary intake, my body will **"WITHDRAW"** them from my fat "reserves" by **burning** excess fat—**PROVIDING** my diet is sound and my "terrain" can respond.

Acid waste management is CENTRAL to weight control and aging reversal. Waste management is the key to a long and healthy life.

One reason fat people "stay" fat is that their bodies are "programmed" **NOT** to lose weight. Terrain management requires **patience** because weight-reduction and health restoration are **one-day-at-a-time** projects. The fat person needs the **same** type of focus—and patience—as cancer patients. Deacidificaion **precedes** fat reduction!

Deacidification is basic to losing weight—and so is "training" the body to function as a "fat burner!"

Thermogenic Supplements

Thermogenic supplements (*thermo*-heat; *gen*-production of, *ic*-pertaining to) help the body to burn fat. Certain herbs like Guarana, when "complexed" with a full array of other ingredients, work well. Cayenne pepper is a **superb** thermogenic supplement with "many" benefits and no downside issues. Most thermogenics work best when taken shortly before food. Enhanced PAC's™ assist thermogenic supplementation by boosting liver function. So does "14 day" Kombucha tea and Yucca Herbal Blend.™ Flushing **sludge** and **stones** from the liver and gall bladder **dramatically** affects metabolic rate and "terrain" response. Hydration is crucial to waste movement. [Men should try to drink 1 gallon of healthy water daily; women, 3/4 gallon daily. Put racemized™ sea minerals in **"every"** glass of water—regardless of the type of water drunk—to maintain body fluid "electrolyte" levels at peak levels.]

Oxygen • Exercise • Salt

Fat will **NOT** "burn" [Think, "oxidize!"] unless oxygen is present. Insufficient tissue oxygen means no oxidation. High ORP, Medical Grade Ionized Water™ and aerobic exercise supply oxygen to the mitochondria in the cells for the production of ATP. Fat is oxidized in the **LIVER** if fat-burning enzymes are present in sufficient quantity.

Obese people find it difficult to get their bodies moving—especially aerobically!

Use exercise equipment that does not jar the joints. Start slow. Each day increase time. Exercise to **circulate** waste, **NOT** burn fat. Follow the Young Again™ Protocol.™ Follow a daily routine! Get **OFF** "salt" and **all** prepared foods. **Avoid** restaurant food. **Avoid** "MSG" (monosodium glutamate) also called **"hydrolized vegetable protein."** MSG is an— "excitotoxin! [The best choices of granular table salt is Celtic™ salt, Redmond™ salt, and Real™ salt. Find them on the net.]

Common table salt and so-called "sea salt" contain 98% sodium. Health type salts contain only 35% sodium and 65% trace minerals. [Racemized™ liquid sea minerals are 99.5% trace mineral **ions** with very little sodium. They are used in drinking water to boost nerve activity and blood flow.]

Racemized™ sea minerals reduce the Rouleau effect and increase waste movement. [See pages 136 & 177.]

Obesity, high blood pressure and elevated sodium levels often go together. Low blood fluid volume from insufficient water intake is **OFTEN** the cause of elevated blood pressure. Stagnant amyloid waste in the tissues accumulates excess water—which is why obese people are often **"edematous!"** Exercise increases fluid movement and removal of blood borne waste by the liver. Liver waste is called "**bile**" and is stored in the gallbladder. Increased bile flow is **"CRITICAL"** to fat metabolism aid digestion. Bile activates the bowels. [Yucca Herbal Blend™ works as a "solvent" by increasing bile flow for faster removal of **waste** from the "terrain."]

Address the fundamentals and obesity goes away. Obesity "mirrors" the condition of the "terrain."

Excess sodium does not accumulate in the cells— **"providing"** plenty of *organic potassium* is made available to the body on a daily basis. To repeat, fresh vegetable juice is the **BEST** source of potassium. Potassium pills are useless—and

explain why people who take diuretics and potassium pills generally go "downhill!" Potassium is **NOT** "stored" and must be resupplied each and every day! When the "terrain" is unbalanced and dietary intake of potassium is insufficient, the body is forced to **withdraw** potassium ions from "inside" the cells in exchange for sodium ions. Elevated sodium ion levels "inside" the cells is spelled "**DEATH!**" Cellular mitochondria multiply and produce the ATP energy molecule in a potassium-"**rich**" environment. ATP production has huge implications for fat metabolism by liver cells called "hepatocytes."
The obese body needs ATP to POWER the transformation to a slim, muscular and healthy body.

Fats • Proteins • Allergies
Fats and "**essential**" **fatty acids** are central to healthy body metabolism. In fact, life—and hormonal production—is **impossible** without essential fatty acids. Fats [and oils] should comprise about "40%" of dietary "caloric" intake. Do **NOT** be afraid of naturally saturated fats like coconut oil and animal fats—they are very good for you. Butter and olive oil are fine. **Avoid** margarine, soy and canola oils. **Avoid** flax oil; it is **EXTREMELY** unstable; grinding causes rancidity. [See page 270.] Rancid oils are **EXTREMELY** toxic [Essential fatty acid supplementation is accomplished using R/EFA™.]
Cholesterol is essential for sexual hormone production and healthy cellular metabolism.
[In John Noble's classic I was A Slave In Russia, Noble told how when he was in the Soviet gulag prison system (1945-1954), human slaves were given a thimble full of sunflower oil each day. Without it, the prisoners would die!]
Without sufficient intake of dietary fats, energy pathways shut down and life becomes difficult. Fat-free diets are DESTROYING women's health.
[Proteins should be carefully scrutinized as to quality, quantity and source. Healthy dietary "proteins" are **critical** *to healing. Eat only "free-range" beef and chicken. Lamb can only be raised "free range!" Avoid cheese.* **NEVER** *eat "junk" proteins—like TVP (textured vegetable protein). [When you get to the "hereafter" and you look in God's recipe book for healthy living, you will* **NOT** *find recipes calling for TVP, tofu or soy and canola oils!]* **Egg protein***—from "healthy" chickens—is the most complete, least expensive and readily available dietary protein.* **Soy protein is bad news!** *[R/HCl™ insures that proteins are broken down in the "stomach;" DiSorb Aid II™ works in the "gut!"]*
Poor protein digestion and leaky-gut issues result in mucous congestion and auto-immune-type dis-eases.
Food allergies, asthma, earache and sinus troubles are "red flags" that the body is **TOXIC** and overloaded with mucous

and serious **terrain** clean-up is needed. [MX™ is a modified DNA used to to break up mucous and cause it to "flow!" High Enema Therapy™ is of pivotal importance in dislodging mucous congestion throughout the entire body. **"Wet-hot"** and **"wet-cold"** therapy also works wonders! [See page 399.]

Healthy food is a powerful gift from God. Prepared foods are a good way to experience "hell" on earth!

[Super foods are powerful, right-spin energy foods. Racemized™ Algae enhances fat metabolism, boosts energy and remedies anema/low blood iron when used with racemized™ liver capsules and Cobo-12™ creme. Harmonic™ Pollen and Harmonic™ Royal Jelly from northern British Columbia are pure, raw "low-stress" foods with huge energy footprints for easy "digestion." Your author uses both these "super" foods for maximum nourishment and for hormonal benefits.]

Water & Obesity

Water is "central" to the obesity story because water is central to all metabolic functions. The three variables of water consumption are: quantity, frequency and the "nature" of the water. Because the obese body is more heavily "burdened," **all** systems work **"overtime"** at a reduced metabolic rate for lack of available energy; joints are strained; liver function is marginal; bile-flow is insufficient; the heart is overworked; and lymphatic drainage is poor. *"I rest my case!"*

[The path to youth and vitality is difficult even for "normal" body types. For the obese person, it is better to go slow for reasons of safety—and compassion! The Young Again Protocol™ is adjusted to meet individual needs.]

Magnetic Sponge

BFRV™ and Medical Grade high ORP waters functon like magnetic sponges in "liquid" form. These waters bond to toxic wastes and carry them **OUT** of the system. In the process, the water "excites" cell chemistry and stimulates metabolic activity and increased production of the ATP energy molecule— all of which boost fat metabolism and terrain restoration.

*[BFRV™ is a **proprietary** water concept that fulfills the requirements of the Young Again Protocol.™ BFRV™ is the **"foundation"** water for the creation of Medical Grade Ionized Water™ (MGIW™). which has therapeutic qualities that dwarf and defy conventional viewpoints about "water!" Detractors "attack" these **esoteric** concepts **and** your author because they do **NOT** understand the concepts under discussion. They "think" in Third Dimension terms and fail to realize that there is more to "water" than hardware and filters. Water is a "living" substance! People who drink BFRV™ and MGIW™ water know it and benefit accordingly.]*

➡ **Please Note:** The BFRV™ trademark replaces the *"aban-doned"* BEV acronym, *DUE TO ongoing infringement and "bootlegging"* by individual(s) offering water processing equipment under the "pretense" their equipment fulfills the "terrain" managment **CONCEPTS** of the *Young Again Protocol.*™

Fat & Chain Reactions

Metabolism is a "process" involving the vital organs and a continuous series of biochemical reactions that "stall out" when the body is missing needed raw materials to function—or if under stress and systemic **"excess."**

When metabolism slows, aging accelerates. The body has only "3" choices when dealing with **TOXIC substances**—regardless of their source. It can try to dismantle (oxidize) them; it can try to expel them from the system; or—by default—it will store them in body fat made for this purpose.

"Bio-junk" diets and "raw" tap water contain **radiomimetic** chemicals that "mimic" hormones. These chemicals are potent and the body isolates and stores them in the fat to protect itself. Weak livers and poor bile-flow are typical of a sick "terrain" that has no choice but to store "freak" molecules instead of excreting them. [The *Young Again (Tissue and Liver) Protocol*™ moves toxic substances out of the body in the bile.]

*[It is common for the liver and gallbladder to be "loaded" with **pellets** and **stones,** sludge and **scar-tissue** that limit bile flow. This is what your author means when he speaks of clogged and congested biliary ducts in the liver that results in poor bile flow! A healthy liver processes 90% of the body's waste. Bile that **FAILS** to exit the system turns the terrain into a very acidic environment and severely burdens the kidneys.]*

The body uses fatty tissue to store its metabolic waste. Body fat level should be about 20%.

Feel Worse First!

During the early stages of the **de**acidification process, expect to feel worse **BEFORE** feeling better. It's two steps forward; one step backwards! A response of any type indicates "action!" High [and low] Enema Therapy™ speeds the flow of waste from the body. The *Young Again (Tissue & Liver) Protocol*™ gets the process going—but it is **NOT** like typical "cleanses" because it causes the body to release "soluble" acid wastes locked up in the body fat so it cannot "circulate!" Getting the body to let go of highly toxic waste is a very **TALL** order—and the only way the body will cooperate is to make provision for **"safe"** processing of the waste. During the two months the protocol is followed, you lead a **normal** life and eat a **normal** diet. Purges are done one week apart. First come green stones followed by brown, black and red. The *Young Again Protocol*™ definitely works! It offers obese, sick and dying people an opportunity to **"change"** the direction of their lives—**NOT** by addressing dis-ease—but by changing the "terrain!"

Diuretics & Weight Control

AVOID pharmaceutical diuretics (water pills) to reduce weight! Diuretics destroy celluralr potassium levels. Potassium pills do **NOT** replenish lost potassium! Potassium loss promotes sodium invasion of the cells and shuts down mitochondria production of ATP. Potassium from fresh vegetable juices drives **OUT** intercellular sodium from inside the cells. **Edema** is confirmation of excess sodium and amyloid waste. [Water-Out™ is a safe, short term answer for serious edema, if fresh vegetable juice is taken at the same time.]

Obese people get to play by the same rules as everyone else—AFTER they restore their "terrains!"

When the obese person becomes "thin," no one needs to tell him or her that they **ARE** *Young Again!*

PREVIEW: *Our next chapter deals with the relationship between lightning, energy, vitality and BROWN FAT!*

"Nothing transforms a person as much as changing from a negative to a positive attitude." Paul C. Bragg

---

Are You Feeling Overwhelmed?

Making the transition from the "normal" good old American diet to a healthy one can be challenging. New ways to healthfully prepare food and new types of strange foods are challenging for conventional cooks. The person eating these "strange" new foods often does **not** appreciate "tampering!" Go slow. Think simple. Good food is easy to prepare because you don't have to do much to prepare it. Invest in a good cook book like *Nourishing Traditions.* Visit health food stores or food co-ops and buy a supply of **basic** food staples. Mix them *among* your regular food dishes on the dinner table. **AVOID** soy, canola oil and tofu. Do **NOT** buy prepared foods; they are a guaranteed ticket to the grave. Convert your family one step at a time using mainstay dishes. Make your changes slowly! [Food is one of the four "joys" of the human experience. [Sex, family and friends and having a good "bowel movement" are the other three joys of life. Make them count!]

"If we eat wrongly, no doctor can cure us. If we eat rightly, no doctor is needed." Victor Rocine

Iron & Disease

Dietary iron is **NOT** the same as **"heme"** iron—the latter being the type of iron found in the blood. Heme iron is central to a healthy condition and a high metabolic rate. Heme iron is the oxygen-carrying protein molecule in blood called **"heme**oglobin." Elemental iron—as in iron compounds—is an **oxidizer**—and plays havoc in the body by fueling the production of "free radicals." Iron supplements are **bad** because they supply pathogenic bacteria with iron metabolites! Pathogenic organisms "feed on" iron metabolites, producing toxins that **weaken** the body and **hammer** the immune system. Iron compounds serve as a breeding ground and fuel for pathogenic microbes and parasites. The healthy body does **NOT** need "iron" supplements—and the unhealthy body becomes ever more sick by taking them.

The best way to increase the production of **"heme"** iron is by using racemized™ algae and racemized,™ predigested, liver capsules along with Cobo-12™ creme. Racemized™ R/C™ and PAC's neutralize elemental iron "free radical" oxidation of healthy tissue and blood. Avoid iron pills!

Breast Implants: Silicone or Soy?

Thousands of women suffer from the toxic side effects of silicone breast implants because they trusted the "experts" who told them they are "safe."

Implants *leak!* There are **NO** exceptions! Silicone is **"thixotrophic"**—meaning it bonds to blood and lymphatic plasma proteins and "migrates"—putting **severe** stress on the immune system. Restoration of the "terrain" is critically important for women with implants. [SunLight™ Creme **protects** breast tissue and keeps it "healthy!"]

The latest in "safe" breast implants is "soy oil." Soy oil is an industrial oil. Avoid it in your food—and don't be foolish enough to implant it into your breasts.

The silicone problem can be safely managed—but women must learn to think and act "outside the box" to avoid the problems associated with it. [SOC™ **scavenges** stray silicone and heavy metals and carries them **OUT** of the body. VZ II™ *"eats"* amyloid plaque and scar tissue. L_sP_cC™ sppeds formation of healthy, new collagen. [See pages 60, 127, 149, 152, 162, 177, 205, 247 and Chapters 36, and 37.]

Acne!

Problem: bowels, liver, hormones, leaky-gut and diet. Acne is acne whether in a teenager or an adult. **Solution:** change the *terrain* by following the *Young Again Protocol(s)*.™ Specifically, use Yucca Blend,™ Inflame Away II,™ DiSorb Aid II,™ and simple 1-bag enemas am and pm. [Acne is the **SIGN**—it is **NOT** the cause—nor it is **NOT** a skin infection issue either!]

Old Body.....New Body?

We are "supposed" to regenerate a **NEW** body every 7 years. But as we age the process **"slows,"** taking up to 15 years to get a "new body." The problem is that your "new" body can take so long to develop that it is **"worn out"** and in worse shape than was your present body when you began the process years earlier. The difference between the two is called **"aging!"**

If you want to *speed* the aging *reversal* process and have a *younger, stronger* and *better* body than the one you traded in, implement the ideas in this book—along with some GH_3+ and Kombucha tea while you are at it. GH_3+™ has a rejuvenatory effect on all body tissues.

And so does L_sP_cC™ and Skin And Body Toner™. They cause the skin to take on a youthful appearance. Liver spots fade away. Hair color slowly returns. [At 61 years of age, your author's hair is *jet black*—and he does NOT **use shoe polish** to color it, either! He regrew a full head of his own hair, too!]

Facial blemishes from acne call for R/Skin Creme™ and SOC™ Lotion. "Terrain" issues dictate how fast each person's body responds to different health challenges.

A youthful appearance is PRICELESS! It translates into a good job, respect and high self esteem.

R/EFA*—The Rest Of The Story!

Essential fatty acids (EFA) are fundamental to good health—that's why they are called "essential." Formulation and rancidity are critical issues. Freshness, light-proof encapsulation, a "black" bottle and racemization™ of the formula's footprint are also part of the story. 75% of brain tissue is composed of fatty acids. Alzheimers is a "brain" deterioration issue—and it takes three women for every man. Children with learning problems respond nicely to R/EFA™ and PAC.™

Nerve Synapses & Schwann's Cells

A "dashed" line resembles a nerve **axon.** Schwann's cells heavily populate the "synapses" ["gaps!"] controlling nerve signal transmission along the axon. Aging and hormone "issues" cripple Schwann's cell activity, causing the neurilemma [myelin sheath] to deteriorate. Nerve-related conditions like MS, Lupus, Fibromyalgia, Peripheral Neuropathy and Shingles are preventable and can be corrected with direct "personal" intervention by the individual who follows the *Young Again Protocol*™. Start now and **avoid** the misery later!

"The difference between an old man and an old gentleman is the way he dresses and looks."

Vaccinations & Agents!

Vaccinations are part of "life." They are so **pervasive** that health-minded people had best "tune in" to the Jeckyl-and-Hyde nature of vaccines if they hope to enjoy a long and healthy life—and avoid seeing innocent children harmed!

Vaccines **"supposedly"** cause antibody formation against "future" exposure to contagious **"agents!"** Introduction by needle of **pathogenic** "agents" in a serum of **foreign** protein is the methodology used.

Immunity and antibodies are desirable, but the long-term **effects** of vaccinations are not! Immune system response to **artificial** exposure to foreign "agents" via vaccination **forces** the body to **react** out of self-preservation to the **"invading"** organisms and carrier proteins. [An "agent" represents a foreign entity that does **NOT** have you or your child's best interest in mind. That entity is the medical system!]

Natural, cell-mediated immunity is *different* from vaccination *induced* attempts to *force* antibody formation and immunity. Vaccinations set up "resident" enemy troops throughout the body. Later, when we are weak or old, the foreign troops bring about insurrection from **"within!"**

Vaccines create electrical *static* because their **signature** is *foreign* to the body. Their vibrational frequency interferes with health and longevity by creating "disharmony" at the *subtle-energy* level of our being.

If you have been vaccinated, it's **VERY** important that you **REVERSE** the process and eliminate foreign protein energy fields from your system. If these substances are not **neutralized** and **driven** from the body, they will **eventually** manifest as chronic, degenerative dis-ease.

The best way to deal with vaccination-induced foreign "agents" is to **"erase"** their **signatures** using full spectrum, **homeovitic** remedies. [See page 250, next.]

"Immunizations" sound great—but the side effects can be **"heart breaking"**—especially in children whose immune systems are under developed. Always **buffer** vaccinations to avoid **DEATH**, autism, hearing loss and Type 1 (childhood) diabetes in your child. Parents **MUST** think *outside the box.* **NEVER** attempt to "inform" bureaucrats and medical lackeys about the dangers of vaccinations. These people are "agents" of foreign "interests!" *Do not cast your pearls before swine!*

"Ask" for guidance "before" your child is vaccinated. Parents should avoid vaccinations before age 2 and preferably **NOT** until "4" years of age. For **documentation** on the dangers of immunizations, contact the National Vaccine Information center, 512 Maple Ave. West #206, Vienna, VA 22180, and New Atlantean Press, Box 9638, Santa Fe NM 87504.

Knowledge dispels ignorance and fear, so learn what you need to know before you need to know it.

Adam blamed Eve; Eve blamed the Serpent; etc!

Homeopathy & Homeovitics

"Homeopathy is wholly capable of satisfying the therapeutic demands of this age better than any other system or school of medicine."

Charles F. Menninger, M.D.

Homeovitic detoxification is a *crucial* step in the treatment of dis-ease and chronic health conditions.

Homeopathy teaches that *symptoms* of disease are a *natural* part of the healing process and that their expression should be *encouraged* rather than **suppressed!**

Homeovitic remedies restore the body's vibratory frequency. They are **NOT** drugs. Some remedies are very specific; others are very general. Some treat substance problems, while others treat emotional problems. Homeo**vitic** remedies are **NOT** available in health stores—and are **SUPERIOR** to common homeopathics.

Homeovitic remedies have an energy *footprint* that is similar to that of the offending substance. If the body is sick, a healthy *systemic* frequency must be reestablished. Homeovitic remedies provide complementary *biogenic* and *nutritional* support—and are *vitalized* to 9x, 20x, 30x, 100x, and 200x mixed, multiple frequencies so they can "adjust" as the terrain *shifts* as healing progresses.

Potentiation (elevation of potential energy) makes a substance more powerful than normal. ***Succussion*** (pounding of a substance to elevate frequency) and ***dilution*** (thinning of the remedy) are employed to bring about ***resonance*** and ***transference***—processes that involve the manipulation of Hertz rate, making homeovitics **SUPERIOR** to common remedies.

Vitalization enhances the energy *footprint* of a substance by a stepwise series of dilutions + succussions designed to increase ***resonance*** (vibrational frequency) so energy can be transferred from the "vitalized" substance to a less active substance—as in a sick body! [See Chapter 21 *Avogadro's Number.*]

Transfer of resonance to toxins occurs when the vitalized substance (vitic) is similar (homeo) to the lesser active substance. Thus, all ***vitalized*** substances obey the law of similars (homeovitic) which says *"Like is cured by like!"*

"The cause is the cure!" is even more specific. For instance, the use of the mercury "footprint" in its *vitalized* form removes mercury energies from the body through ***resonance*** and ***transference***. **Transference** of energy from the *vitalized* substance to offending substance speeds healing and eases stress on the body's vital energy reserves.

Homeovitic remedies are "mixed" *multiple* potency solutions providing *biogenic* support and cellular rejuvenation by dealing with **underlying** health issues at the ***subtle energy* level.**

Homeovitic remedies are very effective and are generally used **LATE** in the *Young Again Protocol*™—where they will render the **maximum benefit** to the user.

[Ask for the homeovitic information available through the Source Packet. See Chapter 21 *Avogadro's Number* for a fuller discussion of these **"esoteric"** concepts.]

Your Electrical "grid!"

Loss of potassium from the cells and invasion of sodium into the cells causes your electrical "grid" to shut down! Your only defense is to juice vegetables daily!

24

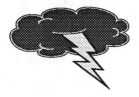

Brown Fat

"Where I am, death is not. Where death is, I am not."
Epicurus

In 1976, Peking, China, (now Beijing) suffered a massive man-made earthquake that killed 650,000 people. The events prior to its occurrence were exactly in line with the predictions of the electrical wizard, Nicola Tesla (1865-1942). Tesla said earthquakes could be **created** by manipulating massive amounts of electrical ENERGY!

Tesla predicted a highly charged ionic atmosphere would be exhibited. Buildings and objects may have an iridescent blue-green glow surrounding them. Multi-colored lightning—red, blue, and gold—may be seen in the early morning sky around the epicenter for hours **prior** to the event. The earthquake would be the **EFFECT** of a massive electrical energy discharge, not the cause. [Some of effects were demonstrated in the movie *Under Siege Two! Dark Territory!*]

Lightning seen in the sky and the electrical phenomenon of the *bio-electric* body are **expressions** of electrical phenomena. There is no essential difference between them! [In 1898 Dr. Enderlein said the is **NO** difference between plants and animals—and he was correct!. See page 139, Chapter 14.]

The physical body is **"condensed"** energy that we can see and touch. The **"physical"** body belongs to the Third Dimension world where "condensed" sunlight energy takes physical form. The *bio-electric* body, however, belongs to the "invisible" world of the Fourth Dimension—as does our "aura" which is a "generated" electrical field radiating from the physical body. Energy that is "generated" must have a source— meaning, something has to generate it. We are interested in the body's source of "generated" energy because production and use of biological energy **defines** the process called "aging!"

The body's bio-electric energy field—the aura—is only one version of bio-electric lightning!

Bio-electric Lightning!

Animals produce electrical discharges similar to lightning. For example, electric eels and electric rays—creatures of the ocean—release enough electricity to light the dark at night and even kill a man. The Portuguese Man o' War—a jelly fish and a mass of mere transparent protoplasm—can kill any living thing coming within the grasp of its umbrella of tentacles. It kills with a **MASSIVE** discharge of bio-electric *lightning.*

Consider the electrical spectacular that occurs when human sperm enters the ovum at fertilization, releasing over 480,000 volts of electricity. [Yes! 480,000 volts!]

The electrical "discharge" coagulates the ovum's outer surface, preventing penetration by other sperm. This massive electrical event is the beginning of a new "life!" Death is a similar—but opposite—electrical event where "spirit" energy exits the body and returns from whence it came. Think of death as metabolic "synchronicity."

[While we are on this earth, it behooves us to understand the **SOURCE** *of the bio-electric lightning that keeps us alive. Understanding it is the key to becoming Young Again!]*

The Body "Electric"

The body is a flesh-and-blood electrical **storage** battery and power **generation** system in one. Peak health depends on the *bio-electric* body's ability to generate and store electrical **ENERGY!** We are dependent on **fuel** source and a **storage** and **transmission** system to distribute our energy—and a method to **control** its ebb and flow. Every aspect of daily life "mirrors" the electrical nature of our "terrain!"

We "draw" on our energy reserves as needed—and we recharge and replenish them by eating food and through sleep and "terran" **de**acidification. Failure to restore electrical balance causes partial or total energy "synchronization." A completely **de**composed corpse is an example of energy synchronization. Aging is the abbreviated version—the *crock-pot* version—and is confirmation of **diminished** electrical "vitality." Aging is slow death.

"Terrain" issues, diminished vital organ function and subnormal ATP production are key aging factors!

The Mitochondria

The **mitochondria** are "bacteria" inhabiting the cells of all mammals. In humans, there are about 10,000 mitochondria in every cell. They were first observed through the microscope around the year 1800. However, they were not officially identified as "living" organisms—capable of independent existence and given a name—until approximately 1935.

The *mitochondria* derive their name from the Greek *mitos*—a thread, and *chondros*—a grain. These root words describe their shape—"not" their function. Originally, the mitochondria were "thought" to be artifacts (waste) or organelles (tiny bodies) within the cells. Later, it was discovered that they are our **SOURCE** of *bio-electric lightning!* Life is **impossible** without the mitochondria. They process our glucose sugars and produce the *life-force* energy molecule **"adenosine triphosphate" (ATP).** Glucose is our energy "fuel!" It is stored in the liver and muscles as glycogen. When energy is needed, the cells convert glycogen to glucose and the mitochondria "burn" the sugars—**by way of the Krebs Cycle and glycolysis**—and create the "ATP" molecule.

Conversion of carbohydrates, fats and proteins into *glucose energy* takes place in the liver. Aerobic exercise [external respiration] utilizes the lungs to supply oxygen to the liver's functional cells—the *hepatocytes*—for production of enzymes necessary for food energy **conversion** into glucose. "Internal" **cellular** respiration is accomplished with the help of our bacterial friends—the mitochondria.

Mitochondria Control Aging

The mitochondria are **both** power generators and storage batteries and are referred to as the **power house** of the cell because they convert energy into metabolic "electricity."

The mitochondria replicate (reproduce) on their own. This is important! They are **NOT** dependent on the host even though they reside in our cells and are influenced by the body terrain environment. They have their own DNA code. [Please think of DNA as cellular programming *software*, genetic instructions and a road map all in one.]

Mitochondrial activity drives "anabolism"—the growth and repair process. Anabolism is a youthful condition and the opposite of "catabolism."

As we age, anabolism gives way to catabolism. When we reach our *anabolic peak,* growth and repair of body tissue slows. Energy production slows. Hormone production slows. Health and vitality diminishes—and aging begins!

Mitochondrial ATP is the right-spin, positive energy that keeps us **"alive!"** Diminished mitochondrial activity is what is seen in the mirror. When ATP energy production levels fall short of our minimum requirements—we die!

Growth Plates

Medical science's *dividing line* between youth and old age is based on long-bone extension. When the growth plates—between the diaphysis (shank of the long bones) and the epiphysis (end of the long bones) "close," science says we cross the threshold into that *twilight zone* between youth and old age known as the "middle years." Whatever growth—or the lack thereof—"occurring" **prior** to growth plate closure is considered to be a "done deal" because we have "officially" stopped growing. This event occurs between ages "18" and "22."

*[Your author's right knee was operated on 25 years ago at age "36"—and it gave him fits until age 52 when it began to "regenerate!" At age "61" there is **no trace** of surgical intervention and I have no limitations. How regeneration was accomplished is the theme and basis of this book—and the development of the Young Again Protocol(s).™]*

*[Science's definition of aging focuses on the extension of long bones. **Our** definition focuses on the body's shift from anabolism to catabolism—which can be accelerated or reversed, at will! Our focus is on **perpetual growth and repair** of body tissues—**instead** of long-bone extension. We are concerned with those "factors" that control aging and reversal!]*

When the mitochondria fail to produce adequate ATP to meet the body's needs for growth and repair, we age! Aging is the passing of *bio-electric* **TIME.** Our friends, the mitochondria, control **TIME.** [See Chapter 31 *Time & Space.*]

We must learn HOW to assist the mitochondria if we want to reverse aging and stop the passing of TIME.

The Sweat Zones

The sweat zones of the body are areas of heat production and waste energy release. Concentrations of mitochondria in the sweat zones confirm the relationship between mitochondrial activity and **ENERGY** management. These zones also reflect heavy lymphatic fluid activity.

The lymphatic system is cancer's electrical highway. The lymph nodes are power stations and they are heavily concentrated in the sweat zones of the body.

The lymphatic system's job is multiple in nature. It includes tissue and cellular waste management and **circulation** of tissue and amyloid fluids and serum plasma proteins to the blood stream. The lymphatic system is the body's **PRIMARY** protein "communication" system. Lymph nodes **retain** toxic energy and releases it later, when the body can handle it. [Swollen tonsils are a good example. Body hair is found in areas of high lymphatic activity and toxicity—like the groin, arm pits, chest and head.]

The purpose of body hair is to siphon off and release toxic energy stored in the fat layer below the skin.

Hair Analysis

Hair analysis measures **"excess"** waste in the body—but it is a **"past tense"** measure and should **NOT** be relied upon or used as a basis for diagnosis of a dis-ease "condition!" Hair analysis is **NOT** a measure of deficiencies as commonly believed. We do **NOT** suffer from deficiencies—only from conditions of **"EXCESS"** that produce **SIGNS** and **symptoms** that we think of as "deficiencies." For example, hair is analyzed and found to contain mercury which may be coming from the amalgam fillings in the teeth or from the diet. Whatever the source, the person is **"excreting"** mercury ions—via the hair. That's good! [The body is releasing a highly toxic metal whose presence in any amount is **"excess!"**] Now, let's say hair analysis shows "no" mercury even though there are mercury fillings in the teeth? What does this mean? It means the person's skin and hair [hair being an extension of skin] either isn't working as it should or the person's body will **NOT** release the mercury from storage for fear of doing serious damage. We should assume dangerous levels of mercury are building up in the body tissues—instead of exiting through the bile, urine, bowel and hair/skin. To repeat, there is **NO SUCH THING** as a deficiency dis-ease!

Using hair analysis and live blood cell microscopy to "diagnose" and "prescribe" is questionable, considering the nature of **SIGNS** and symptoms of **"excess!"** These approaches are tools of "observation" only. [The basis of the problem here is a defective medical model and failure to "think!"]

Hair and live blood cell analysis are tools of observation that hint at conditions within the "terrain!"

Dr. Guenther Enderlein's ground breaking microscopic work a century ago proved there is **no** such thing as deficiency dis-ease—only conditions of **excess!** Thinking in terms of deficiencies is as **backward** as believing in the germ theory of disease—and vaccination-induced "immunity."

Healthy, fast-growing, naturally colored hair is good whether it be leg, arm pit, groin, full body (not women) or on top of the head! Hairy men have a "hairy edge" over "smoothies!" Male body hair is an "advantage!" The liver controls all issues of hair, "terrain" and skin. Hair is an "extension" of the skin and loss of hair is a **"SIGN"** of aging and "thyroid" issues.

Healthy hair is affected by BROWN fat levels, mitochondrial activity and deacidification of the terrain!

Insects • Birds • Sperm

Insects and birds have heavy concentrations of mitochondria in the muscles responsible for flight because that is where the ATP energy molecule is needed, stored and used.

Human sperm makes the long trip into the woman's fallopian tubes to fertilize the ovum with power **generated** by the mitochondria. The base of the sperm's tail is heavily laden with mitochondria. When sperm fertilizes the egg (ovum), the electrical **discharge** of 480,000 volts of electricity comes from **both** the sperm and the ovum. Both are "energy" bodies—one is **HUGE** the other is **miniscule**.

The electrical discharge the **ovum** generates is only 0.19 volts. The discharge by the sperm is 25,263,157 times **GREATER** than that of the ovum—a huge difference! There is a **massive** difference in physical size between the sperm and ovum. The volume of the ovum is 1,760,000³ microns; and the sperm 21³ microns. When we divide the size of the ovum by the size of the sperm, we find that the egg is 83,809 times **GREATER**! These differences in **physical size** and **electrical potential** generates the release of the 480,000 volts called *bio-electric lightning!*

At Birth
Mitochondrial count—and their activity level at birth—is very high, as is the level of **BROWN FAT** which we will discuss shortly. Brown fat is one reason why children and "young" people are warm blooded and older people—whose metabolism is slowing—are cold! [In women, "coldness" is one of **"8"** symptoms indicating a sluggish thryroid condition. The other **"7" symptoms** are: dry, wrinkled skin, thin/falling hair, sore joints, low energy, diminished muscle mass, excess fat, and "brain fog" and memory complaints.

The mitochondria produce the huge amounts of energy children require to grow to adulthood in a few short years. The ability of children and teens to stay warm—even when subjected to cold conditions—says a lot about **"brown fat"** levels.

As we grow, we experience the ebb and flow of energy called **health and dis-ease.** By the time we reach adulthood, the growth plates in the long-bones have closed and we reach our maximum physical height. Once we cross the "threshold" of our anabolic peak, we experience an energy shift as we begin the *descent* into old age. [See diagrams on pages 21 and 198.]

If we are willing to take responsibility for our lives, we can recapture our anabolic peak, reopen the puberty window, and watch aging reverse itself!

As the *bio-electric* body becomes "acid" and hormonally unbalanced, mitochondrial production of ATP falls. Next, mitochondrial replication falls. Then, ATP reserves fall as **BROWN FAT** levels "shrink," dis-ease manifests—and the doctor gets to provide a "diagnosis!"

Sleep • Detoxification • Illness
Sleep is a **"critical"** aspect of the aging reversal process. Rest gives the *bio-electric* body a chance to recover and heal. During the **"sleep cycle,"** ATP energy **must** be **AVAILABLE** or healing and regeneration will stall out! Sleep doesn't come in a bottle—and lack of it is worse than eating "sugar! Illness like flu, hepatitis, and cancer—means there is **insuffi-**

cient "available" ATP and **too much** acid waste to allow **NORMAL** activities of growth and repair.

Infants and sick people need additional sleep because their bodies are growing and in need of repair.
When we **FORCE** the body to work under conditions of high **"stress"**—we "squander" **BOTH** production and use of mitochondrial ATP that should be used for **de**toxification and healing. Mitochondrial activity requires **sleep** and **lifting** the burden of excess waste from the "terrain!" The best way to **"lift"** the waste burden is through HET (High Enema Therapy™). HET, sleep and fresh vegetable juices are the "perfect" combination to increase mitochondrial activity and numbers for increase ATP production and build ATP reserves.

*[Mitochondrial replication means the doubling of DNA and genetic material —so two bacteria are created out of one. This process is called **mitosis**.]*
When mitochondrial activity is **unable** to return to peak levels, we break through a **TIME** "barrier" and experience an aging **"plateau."** [All of us have seen parents and friends jerk-and-slide their way "down" the catabolic side of the aging pyramid shown on pages 21 and 198.]

Aging accelerates in direct relationship to mitochondrial slowdown, build-up of acid wastes in the tissues, hormonal shortfalls and loss of liver function.

Sodium & Waste

Aging, toxicity and catabolism are "peas in a pod." Toxic substances come in many forms and **EXCESS** sodium chloride (table salt) is one of them. Sodium is of particular **importance** to our discussion of the mitochondria. Even "moderate" levels of sodium have the characteristics of a **poison** and a **preservative** because it **SHUTS DOWN"** the mitochondrial-orchestrated electrical **"GRID!"** Sodium ions must not be allowed to overrun and unbalance the blood and lymph "tissue fluids!"

*[Blood "circulates" because we have a heart to pump it! Blood fluid volume is composed of water, **plasma proteins**, mineral electrolytes and cellular waste. Lymphatic fluids circulates by way of the lymphatic system—which does **NOT** have a heart and depends on physical movement and exercise. Blood and lymphatic "tissues" are **NOT** sterile as taught in medical schools—and the **ONLY** way these tissues are cleared of waste and debris is by liver "filtration" [90%] and the kidney "filtration" [10%]. They are dynamic, **organism-bearing** tissues that are easily altered by diet and stress. [Elimination of **"Rouleau"** from blood as shown on page 136] is accomplished by manipulating the electrical **"charge"** on red blood corpuscles so they will not "clump." [Racemized™ sea mineral ions in drinking water is the very best tool for this task.]*

It is **impossible** to get too little sodium in the diet. And yet most people suffer from symptoms of blood electrolyte "imbalance." Heart attack, heat stroke and heat exhaustion are good examples of the problem. Conventional medical thought calls for increased sodium intake in hot weather—but this approach ignores electrolytic "balance" and mitochondrial slow-down in production of the energy molecule "ATP!"

The bio-electric body needs a broad-based dietary intake of "electrolytes" each and every day!

Sometimes sodium can save a life when faced with heat stroke or heat exhaustion [They are **not** the same thing!]—but sodium will **NOT** stop a heart attack. Racemized™ sea minerals can both stop and prevent **"electrolyte-driven"** heart attack—and if introduced into the person's system at the time of the event or immediately thereafter, they minimize the damage!

Under **"normal"** conditions, all but a very tiny "fraction" of sodium ions are **"OUTSIDE"** cell membranes in the amyloid fluid **between** the cells. Potassium lines the **"INSIDE"** of cell membranes. A healthy body maintains a balanced **RATIO** of sodium to potassium. When we eat devitalized and processed foods, we ingest **excess** sodium in the face of **INSUFFICIENT** potassium and upset ratio balance.

Potassium **must** be supplied **"DAILY!"** It **cannot** be "stored." The more sodium consumed and the more acid waste that accumulates, the greater the **"out flow"** of potassium ions **from** the cells. Loss of potassium fuels the aging process.

The BIG Shift!

With the exception of one electron in the outer valence shell, potassium and sodium are "twins!" Under normal conditions, few sodium ions (Na^+) are allowed inside the cells. Excess sodium ions gain entrance to the cells as potassium ions (K^+) are given-up by the cells for use elsewhere in the body. This **"one-for-one"** exchange occurs in the face of **EXCESS** sodium and a potassium **shortfall!** [Fresh vegetable juices are the very best source of "usable" potassium!]

Sodium and potassium ions **BOTH** carry a (+) charge and are very close in size—so it is **easy** for sodium to go into the cell as the potassium comes out when the body "steals" potassium from the cells to meet its needs. The problem is that the "reverse" exchange requires more time and effort to turn around. [Normally, the body makes use of the *process* called *biological alchemy* [See Chapter 18.] to meet its mineral ion needs—but this process **"collapses"** in a highly acid environment that by definition is in a condition of **"excess!"**

When Na^+ ions invade the cells, mitochondrial activity *slows,* vitality *wanes* and dis-ease *follows* as acidification accelerates and the "ATP-driven" electrical grid **shuts down!** It is under these conditions that "**cannibalization**" of muscle mass occurs as the body attempts to meet its **protein** needs. This process of "debilitation" is **obvious** in very sick and older people. It is **less obvious** in people who—for the moment—are doing fine, but who **FAIL** to understand the aging "process" and how to care for themselves before crisis stikes!

*[Older people—and people suffering from degenerative dis-ease—build-up **MASSIVE** amounts of acid waste in their tissues. Edema manifests when turgor is lost. Turgor is resistance of the skin to "deformation." Edema is a waterlogged condition of the extremities (hands, legs, ankles, and feet)].*

Serious health "conditions" develop over many years and few people see'em coming—or act to prevent it!

Edema • Salt • Hair

Edema is **more** than water retention. It is a **SIGN** of excess **amyloid** fluid in the tissues, excess sodium levels, a weak heart and kidney problems. [Obesity is another dynamic that only makes matters worse. Interestingly, when obese people "dump" tissue-bound acid waste, they drop weight, too!]

Allopathic medicine relies on diuretics to force **excess** fluids from the tissues. In the process, potassium loss increases and the body is forced to **cannibalize** muscle protein and **deplete** fat stores. When the body runs out of reserves, the person's weight **evaporates** overnight—leaving skin and bones! [Avoid using pharmaceutical "diuretics" (aka "water pills!") It is better and safer to drink "fresh" vegatable juices. [Aspar-Max™ and Water Out™ are both safe and useful adjuncts here.]

[As waste and acidity levels "increase"—body hair disappears as seen in elderly and dying people. Hairless legs, fungus under the toe nails, and feet irregularities are SIGNS of high toxicity, sodium overload and potassium depletion.]

Hair is crucial to deacidification of the "terain!" Lost hair regrows if the Young Again Protocol™ is followed—and lots of patience is exercised.

"Stop" using "common" table salt at the dinner table to avoid sodium overload. Use less salt than recipes call for by dissolving a "pinch" in a bit of water and add to the recipe. Better still, use home-grown food. It doesn't need salt because it is loaded with "mineral ions!" Salt's effects are **"insidious"**—and cancer **LOVES** high-sodium environments. They **"surround"** themselves in sodium-saturated tissue. [Sodium doesn't cause cancer, but it does go with the territory!]

Cancers are strong, sodium-saturated energy fields. Cancer TUMORS "import" and "condense" toxic energy. Cancer MASSES export negative energy. [See page 307.]

Sodium invasion of the cells is the equivalent of shutting down power in "Jurassic Park!" When the power goes off, nature's dinosaurs—the cancer viruses—**"ACTIVATE"** and **pirate** your very own energy to take **control** of DNA and RNA cellular "software" and multiply exponentially (2, 4, 8, 16, 32, 64,128, 256, etc.). [Never forget, cancer's job is to **eliminate** the weak from the Earth. We "go down" because we are "weak!"]

Viruses gain entrance and proliferate in our cells when our electrical defenses have been "sabotaged!"

*[BFRV™ and Medical Grade Ionized Water(s)™ with racemized™ sea mineral ions speed **deacidification**. They are **PERFECT carrier solvents** due to their ORP potential and ability to "transport" excess sodium **OUT** of the cells and body.]*

Sodium must be DRIVEN OUT of the cells in the presence of HIGH potassium ion levels.

*[As cellular sodium is replaced by potassium, the mitochondria come back to life, multiply and produce ATP! A balanced sodium : potassium ratio allows the cells to reestablish membrane "polarity." **Repolarization** must occur **before** mitochondrial ATP production can significantly "elevate.]*

Brown Fat & The Mitochondria

Brown fat has a great deal to do with vitality and rejuvenation—and it explanis **why** some people are fat, skinny, sick, energetic, long lived, etc.

Officially, brown fat is called *brown adipose tissue* (BAT). BAT was only recently discovered—and it is "brown" because of the **extremely heavy concentrations** of mitochondria. BAT is extremely biologically active tissue. Except for the word **"fat,"** BAT has **NO** resemblance in **appearance or function** to its shirt-tale relative white adipose tissue (WAT) that is thought of when we hear the words "fat" and "obesity!"

Officially, BAT is responsible for **"non-shivering thermogenesis"**—the generation of heat in the absence of shivering. Shivering is a normal body response and part of the "heat-production process" under **cold** and **high stress** conditions—as occurs after a serious automobile accident.

BAT has a massive blood supply compared to WAT, but WAT should **not** be thought of as "stagnant" tissue. It also is heavily vascularized and subject to constant remodeling. ["Cellulite" is **very** stagnant and **highly** toxic waste tissue that is hard to break-down without the body roller. See index.]

Babies have higher concentrations of BAT than do adults. People who live and work in cold climates have more BAT than people in warm climates. Japanese women skin divers have very high concentrations of BAT and are able to bear frigid ocean water for hours at a time. [The more BAT, the higher the producton of the ATP energy molecule.]

Healthy people have more BAT than do sick people. Thin people have more BAT than fat people. The more BAT

you have, the more muscle mass and energy you will have. BAT and WAT are "terrain" issues of the opposite type.

To better understand BAT, let's review the physiological process called **thermogenic hyperphagia** *(thermo*-heat; *genic*-pertaining to the production of; *hyper*-above normal; *phagia*-that which eats. People who are **subclinically** sick or who suffer with degenerative dis-ease have **low** concentrations of BAT! Obese people do **not** have enough BAT. As WAT increases in a person's body, BAT decreases. When we reach our **anabolic** peak, BAT loss accelerates, obesity becomes an issue, vitality wanes—and aging accelerates. This downward spiral **BEGINS** around age 24—and is **very obvious** in young people today!

In industrial societies, BAT loss among women is epidemic—and accelerates the onset of menopause! **P**remenopausal **"symptoms"** are now appearing "20" years **before** official onset of menopause and are now **"rampant"** in women who are only in their late twenties and early thirties.

SIGNS and symptoms of aging develop in direct relationship to loss of BAT, hormonal imbalance and acidification of the "terrain!"

[Racemized™ hormone precursors encourage BAT formation and help reverse menopausal and andropausal complaints by reopening the puberty window. The Young Again Protocol(s)™ help the body restore a youthful metabolism. Use of the L/CSF™ machine and the Lymphatic Body Roller™—for breaking down cellulite—are also part of the BAT story.]

Subjecting the body to cold is **VERY** beneficial. Swim regularly in a cold pool, ocean, or lake—preferably after steambathing or hot-tubbing. Never "plunge" into cold water as this can cause drowning due to the "gasp" reflex! Do yard work and take walks during the cold months dressed "lightly" to encourage BAT formation and strengthen the immune system. Finish a hot bath or shower with a "quick" **ice cold** shower!

Your author's favorite cold therapy is a work out on a Nordic Trac™ aerobic exerciser OUTSIDE in boxer shorts! "COLD" stimulates mental focus, breaks up congestion, and increases blood and lymph flow.

[Gluco Factor-X™ and CWD™ stimulate BAT activity, as does B.T. Thyroid™ Creme, Skin & Body Toner,™ HST™ Creme and racemized™ hGH precursor.]

Increase your brown fat levels in your body to restore yourself to your **former** anabolic peak. [See pages 21 and 198.] When you reach that peak, you are *Young Again!*

PREVIEW: *Our next chapter is going to SHOCK you! You are going to learn WHY men and women are going bald—and **what** can be done about it! You are also going to discover the relationship between certain cooking oils and the HIV/AIDS virus.*

High Enema Therapy™ "Myths"

People have *misconceptions* and *hang-ups* about High Enema Therapy™ (HET). Your author decided to challenge "health" experts about all their crazy ideas. Here is what your author discovered about HET. An enema is **not** a colonic—and neither is 5 gallons of water! HET does **not** cause dependency. HET does **not** steal friendly flora from the colon. HET does **not** cause loss of electrolytes. HET does **not** cause constipation. Lastly, the purpose of High Enema Therapy™ is **not** to clean the colon. The reader will find the pieces of the HET "riddle" sewn into the fabric of this book. And if the reader would like to know "**why**" everybody's future had **BETTER** include High (and low) Enema Therapy,™ your author will be happy to field your questions and help you connect the dots outlined in the book. When your life is on the line, you will do **whatever** it takes to restore your terrain and regain control of your "terrain"—or you will die! It is a matter of choice—and far too many people choose "**NOT**" to "live!"

Sandra says *"It's time to stop hanging onto your crap!"*

Medical Studies & "Your" Life

People rely on the advice of their practitioner. Practitioners, in turn, *foolishly* rely on the *credibility* of medical studies to guide them. Most medical studies are flawed. For the patient, *bogus* medical studies mean the difference between life and death at worst—or pain and suffering at best. For the patient, flawed studies are a **"disaster!"** Before me is a news article captioned *"Fraud Mars Breast Cancer Research."* Investigators found more than a **DECADE** of fraudulent breast cancer research—including the use of mammograms that damages women's breast tissue and "spreads" cancer! These reports are frightening, but the **"message"** is clear. Your **MUST** learn to think for yourself because you **cannot** rely on scientific "studies" and "experts" to save you. Hopefully, that is why you are reading this book. And please, don't fall into the trap of conjuring reasons why the *Young Again! Protocol(s)* will not work for you. **If you want your "life back" be willing to do what needs to be done! Excuses don't wash!** Health and longevity are gifts we experience in the **"wake"** of personal responsibility and informed action. So get to work and experience the miracle of "rejuvenation" in your life—as your author did in his life. It feels wonderful to be age "19" at age "61!"

P.S. Readers are best served if they "consult" **before** deciding on a course of action. There are "no" fees of any kind—and what you will learn from your author will astound you!

25

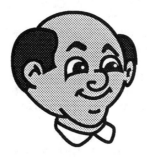

Bald Heads & Oils

"Hair on my legs, hair on my chest, but no hair on my head?"
Uncle Ross

Balding is a **SIGN** of premature aging—and so is thinning hair! Balding is **loathed** by men, yet it is accepted as inevitable if it "runs" in the family. The **"experts"** tell us balding is a genetic trait—but they are **wrong!** Balding is neither inevitable, nor genetic, nor is it permanent. Balding **"mirrors"** liver function, bile flow, systemic **"excess,"** digestive issues, hormones, thyroid, electrolyte levels—and poor diet.

Hair follicles go dormant in a toxic scalp—and they come back to life if stimulated and given the opportunity!

Scalp toxicity and hair follicle dormancy are also linked to consumption of certain dietary oils. Eat the oils the experts recommend and you will likely go bald or develop thin hair—as well as succumb to degenerative "conditions" like arthritis, gout, heart problems, stroke, cancer and prostate trouble.

Almost *everything* the public has been taught about dietary oils and fats—isn't so! We have been manipulated and lied to. It's time to wake up!

A Short History Of Oils

Beginning in the 1930's, cotton seed oil became the primary "liquid" dietary oil substitute for fats like butter and lard. During WW ll, cotton seed oil was **hydrogenated** to create a butter substitute that was **SOLID** at room temperature. They called it **oleo**margarine; margarine or *oleo* for short. War mentality caused the public to "accept" oleo and by the 50's—when your author was growing up—margarine was considered an *acceptable* butter substitute. By the early 1960's, Americans experienced another fundamental **"shift"** in the "type" of dietary oils and fats they were eating. But this time, the move was even further away from "solid" fats like butter, lard and coconut—to so-called "healthy" oils and "lighter" margarines.

While the media and the *experts* vilified butter and lard, the Cholesterol **"THEORY"** of Cardiovascular Dis-ease became the new scientific "buzz" within the halls of academia. The spill-over effect engulfed the populace with fear and almost total rejection of butter, lard and eggs. Later, new cliches and buzz words were added to the American vocabulary—like "unsaturated" and "poly unsaturated." Corn and safflower oils replaced cotton seed oil for those with finer tastes and fatter wallets. Oleo was history and margarine was coming into its hey-day. Few people ate butter. Lard was only for the poor.

By the late 1960's, SOY BEAN oil began to appear on supermarket shelves and in thousands of *processed* foods. Cotton seed, corn and safflower oils were still in wide use, but there was a new focus—health! Soy bean oil became **SYNONYMOUS** with **"health"**and the health food "movement!"

The shift away from natural fats—like butter, lard and and coconut oil—to liquid and hydrogenated margarines, coupled with chlorination and fluoridation of public water supplies, sparked a dramatic increase in heart dis-ease.

The experts **"blamed"** saturated fats and cholesterol for the rise in cardiovascular problems and the increase in degenerative dis-ease—while they **"ignored"** the dietary problems inherent in **"processed"** foods as they repeatedly uttered the mantra *"Balding is a genetic problem!"* [In the process, they indicted God for constructing a faulty human model.]

*[The experts like to razzle dazzle us with scientific hocus pocus. They control the flow of information in schools and the media so the "folks" never make the connection between cause and effect on hundreds of health issues. Balding is just one of these issues. **LOOK** at all the (young) folks with balding heads and thinning hair. **IGNORE** the experts!]*

With the advent of the "new, healtheir" healthier oils and soft margarines, **balding** and **thinning** hair increased in both sexes, young and old. The only person who noticed that something was **WRONG** was an agronomist named Dr. Carey Reams. His was a voice "crying in the wilderness."

Please acquaint yourself with the following terms so we may continue our story with better understanding.

Arteriosclerosis—abnormal hardening of the walls of the arterioles (small arteries) due to fibrous thickening of the connective tissues of the artery wall, plus hyalinization and infiltration of lipids (fats) into the intima (innermost wall).

Atherosclerosis—a form of simple intimal arteriosclerosis with atheromatous deposits within and beneath the intima (inner wall) of the arteries.

Atheromatous deposits—the fatty *degeneration* of the

artery walls with infiltration by lipids (fats)—as in arteriosclerosis. Cellular debris, waste and "excess" calcium deposits are usually involved in the deposition process.

Intima—the innermost layer of the three layers composing the artery wall. [The "media" is the middle wall and the third outer wall is made of connective tissue.]

Hyalin—a glassy, clear, "abnormal" substance in body tissues; degenerative in "excess;" forerunner to formation of scar tissue; major component of amyloid plaque that forms when amyloid fluid "morphs" into structural amyloid plaque.

Amyloid plaque and amyloid fluid—excess tissue waste that "drives" aging and the pathological "dis-ease!" Amyloid plaque is **"STRUCTURAL," "non soluble"** waste tissue formed when amyloid fluid "morhps" from fluid to structural "state." Amyloid fluid is acid-laden tissue fluid that was **NOT** picked-up by the lymphatic capillaries and circulated to the blood and **OUT** of the body by way of the liver, bile, gallbladder and bowels. Amyloid fluid is **"soluble"** acidic waste in "liquid" state—and provides the perfect "substrate" [Think breeding ground!] for viruses, bacteria, fungi and yeast. Amyloid **"defines"** the aging and is always part of degenerative pathological dis-ease regardless of an individual's age.

Hyalinization—the "transitory" process by which tissues age; involves stagnant, semi-fluid tissue waste composed of albumin, hyaluranic acid, minerals and waste in a "gelatinous" state preceding metamorphosis into "structural" amyloid plaque; process of invasion of soft and connective tissue cellular spaces; a degenerative process.

Plaque—cholesterol containing material deposited into the intima and/or media of the arteries; atheromatous deposits of hyalin; degenerative in nature; hyalinization.

The Soy Connection

Dr. Carey Reams often commented on the rise in "balding"—but it was my friend, Tom Mahoney, who provided the clue that solved the puzzle. It was an **"agricultural"** clue.

Tom talked of a strange family of plants called **"Fabales."** He observed that if cattle or sheep were allowed to graze on soy for a *sufficient* length of time, their health would suffer and their hair would **thin** and **fall out.**

Tom's observations were the "clue" your author needed to solve Dr. Carey Reams' 30-year-old observation. Reams was sure there was a **"link"** between the dietary ingestion of soy, balding, degenerative dis-ease and aging.

Soy & PHG

Soybean oil and soybean curd (tofu) contain a toxic biochemical called **phyto-hema-glutinin** or PHG for short.

Dissected, the word looks like this: *phyt(e)*-that which comes from plants), *hem(e)*-blood, *glutinin*-a vegetable protein "glue."
  PHG is a large protein molecule that has proven to be specific in its ability to agglutinate human blood.
  [Agglutination means to "glue;" to cause to "adhere;" to "clot!" The **Rouleau Effect** *pictured on page 136 shows red blood corpuscles "clinging" to each other—slowing blood flow and waste removal. Soy is rich in PHG and promotes "Rouleau!"]*
  PHG causes blood to **thicken** and circulation to **slow** and take on **"clotting"** qualities. It combines with blood-borne impurities forming "plaques" in the very fine capillaries of the posterior eye, ears—and scalp! PHG **"MAGNIFIES,"** Rouleau affects 95% of the population—and PHG **magnifies** the effect. PHG "numbs" the immune system's T cells and negatively impacts the central and peripheral nervous systems.
  PHG kills rats, DEAD! It is poisonous to all living things. As with any systemic poison, **quantity** consumed, **length** of exposure and **individual** predisposition dictate why some people's bodies tolerate soy oil and proteins even though both are bad for you and "cumulative" in their effects!
  Soy has hormonal overtones that "mimic" **SYNTHETIC** estrogens! Soy ingestion is a **MAJOR** problem for children and women. Soy causes **MAJOR** thyroid problems in females—and particularly in females burdened by **"MERCURY"** poisoning leaching from **so-called** "silver" amalgam dental fillings that their **"CULPABLE"** dentist kindly forgot to mention! Soy's hormonal influence on developing children is downright "scary!" Soy **alters** vital organ function!
  Soy products are promoted as **"THE"** answer to the problems of world hunger by the "cartels!" Unfortunately, those "touting" soy falsehoods are as ignorant as their target audience—or **just maybe** they are bought and paid for stooges of "industry" and yellow-fringed flag "corporate" government. [Inability to think "outside the box," the desire for peer "acceptance" and "inflated" egos are very effective social "girdles!"]
  Remember this rule: If the media touts it, and the government supports it, and industry pushes it and everyone nags you to do it, IGNORE IT!

Soy & Digestion
  Soy interferes with digestion! Soy beans produce gas and upset body chemistry. Peanuts are another *famous* member of the Fabale family of plants—and many people cannot digest peanut products. Peanuts contain very little PHG in comparison to soy. Other Fabale family foods are garbanzo beans (chic peas), fava beans, lentils, and mung beans, but these contain *almost* **no** PHG. Two Fabale legumes that cause serious long-term problems for *grazing* animals are clover and

alfalfa. In the field, they can be deadly toxic and cause bloating in ruminants. Cows, horses and sheep thrive on grasses which contain **"growth"** energy proteins, mineral ions and balanced sugars. Grasses have a different "spin" on their nutrient molecules than do legumes like alfalfa, clover and soy. Soy PHG **"reacts"** with circulating minerals and dissolved blood gases like chlorine and fluorine—forming **"sludge"** in the blood circulatory system that oddly resembles bath tub scum—similar to the scum and bath tub ring when using Grandma's lye soap in hard water. [See Chapter 15.]

*[Municipalities use chemicals like sodium hypo-chlorite (sodium hydroxide + chlorine) to treat public water supplies. Sodium hydroxide (lye) is what Grandma used to make her lye soap. It is extremely alkaline (pH 12). Chlorine is extremely acidic (-2 and +2 pH) and is used to kill bacteria. Hydroxide is used to raise pH so the acidic water will not kill you. **Haloge-**nated (chlorinated and fluoridated) tap water "reacts" with dietary oils and other circulating wastes and forms "plagues." [Plaques can be "digested" and removed from the body by using VZ™ and following the Young Again Protocol.™]*

Anatomy & Physiology 101
Lipids [oils and fats] are absorbed by a different mechanism and pathway than are carbohydrates and proteins. Lipids are absorbed through the gut wall by **"special"** lymphatic capillaries that feed into the portal vein that feeds **directly** into the **"LIVER!"** This is very **IMPORTANT!**

*[Portal **vein** blood feeding the liver is 50% venus (non-oxygenated) and 50% arterial ("oxygenated") blood—where hepatic **artery** blood feeding the liver is 100% oxygenated blood. Blood **returning** to the heart is oxygen-poor and circulates through the lungs before returning to the left side of the heart for distribution to the body. Venus blood is dark red; arterial blood is bright red!]*

*[The lymphatic system drains the tissues of highly "acid" amyloid fluid. Lymph fluids join the blood supply at the left subclavian vein which flows into the superior vena cava **vein** returning venus blood to the right side of the heart. Returning "venus blood"—**rich in acid wastes from the tissues**—combines with PHG and inorganic minerals and forms "athero-sclerotic plaques" in the artery walls. The mechanics of the process provide the reader a "clue" about **"clogged"** heart muscle arteries and "by-pass" surgery. Readers who would like to learn more can do it by "coloring!" See pages 233 and 274.]*

*[The heart pumps **deoxygenated** blood to the lungs for "oxygenation" **AND** "transference" of waste energy through "respiration" before it is returned to the left side of the heart for distribution to the body. Only **AFTER** "oxygenated" blood re-*

turns to the heart is it sent to the liver for cleaning by way of the portal **vein**—*the same vein that transports dietary lipids to the liver from the intestine.* *["Clogged" heart muscle arteries occlude because blood "feeding" the heart muscle is loaded with toxic, acid waste. Portal blood is a 50/50 mixture of waste-laden oxygenated blood and* **deoxygenated** *blood.]*

Approximately, "40%" of blood leaving the heart feeds the head [ears, eyes and brain] via the **carotid** arteries—and in frigid conditions, approximately 40% of body heat is "lost" through the head! These are the arteries on both sides of the esophagus that are usually involved in "stroke."

Electrically charged waste "precipitates" called "plaque" collect on arterial walls similarly to minerals in water pipes! Plaque slows blood flow, raises blood pressure—and hinders oxygen delivery. Plaque causes the lining of the arteries to harden, deteriorate—and form "clots!" When plaque "breaks loose," it migrates into the neck or the brain, blocking blood and oxygen flow. The event is called "stroke." If the oxygen supply to the heart becomes severely limited due to plaque formation, it is called "heart attack." However, heart attack is more often an **"electrolyte"** event from a shortfall of "magnesium" ions! [The *Young Again* solution is called racemized™ sea minerals and are used in every glass of water every day!]

[Thick, waste-laden blood clogs the VERY FINE blood capillaries feeding the posterior eye, ears and scalp. Conditions like macular degeneration, retinitis, glaucoma, tinnitis, balding and thinning hair and deafness are all **"terrain"** *issues involving "heavy" blood and a waste-filled body. The Young Again Protocol(s) were developed for these "conditions!" Yucca Blend,™ VZ II™ and L_sP_cC™ work well is patience is exercised.]*

Deterioration of the eyes and ears—along with snoring and sinus congestion—are terrain issues.

Alfalfa Sprouts

Alfalfa is a legume of the family "fabale." Alfalfa sprouts are a popular vegetarian delight—but there is a caveat that comes with them. Alfalfa **sprouts** contain powerful *phytotoxins* and are detrimental to people with weak immune systems. In dry leaf form, as used in food supplements, alfalfa does not pose a problem. But "fresh" alfalfa sprouts should be avoided like the plague! Cancer patients should **NEVER** eat **alfalfa "sprouts"** because the phytotoxins in them **depress** immune function and create **"EXCESS"** that fuels cancer. Clover and mustard sprouts should also be avoided. Other popular sprouts are fine.

Occasional sickness means your immune system is functioning and your body KNOWS when things are out of balance. Occasional illness is a good sign.

The Hormone Connection

Soy has hormonal **"overtones!"** Growth and "regeneration" is hormone-driven and hormonal **"confusion"** skews the process. Recall how children "bolt" into adulthood in just a few years. We are talking male and female sexual hormones—as well as thyroid, adrenal and growth hormone. These hormones influence aging and regeneration—and all of them are **"orchestrated"** by the **"LIVER"**—which also controls "bile flow" and the bowels.

Aging is only given the title of "dis-ease" after the doctor provides a "label" based on SIGNS!

Hair and nails are *extensions* of **"skin."** Hair follicles are heavy energy feeders. They have their roots in the fatty tissues beneath the skin. Hair requires a plentiful blood supply and good lymph circulation—and the condition of one's "hair" is a direct reflection of "stored" acid waste in the subcutaneous tissues. Poor, slow-growing hair—along with balding and graying—is really "one" issue! Hair mirrors the internal health of the body from the "outside!" Teeth and gums provide the **"EARLIEST"** of "clues" about acidification of the "terrain!" [Joint problems, Alzheimers, sexual disfunction, bowel problems, and sleep disorders tell their own "stories!"]

More Information On Soy

Soy beans are *unlike* other beans. Soy is a *toxic* plant! It is one of two **toxic** seed-oil plants grown for their **"industrial"** oils. Insects seldom touch soy. Soybean plants—and canola, too—thrive on toxic soil and air. Soy proteins have a powerful left-spin and should never be consumed. Soybean plants absorb and store toxic energy in their **"oil!"**

Few people know that soybeans were genetically altered in the middle 1950's with that "harmless" process called **"irradiation!"** This was done to **INCREASE** soy-bean oil content and to create a plant that would *prosper* on toxic soils.

Powerful **"interests"** made sure "corporate" government funded soy research. These same "interests" promote vaccinations and tout the Cholesterol and Germ Theories. Industry needed an industrial oil crop that would prosper on "negative" energy soils treated with synthetic salt fertilizers and poisonous sprays. [The soy cartel is **NOT** concerned about the long-term effects of soy on people.]

Soy oil is an "industrial" oil that is being peddled as a food oil. Soy protein is the waste spin-off.

Soy Baby Formula • State of Israel

The toxic nature of soy has been known for a long time—and yet soy oil is added to **THOUSANDS** of **processed** foods. Soy is now substituted for dairy products which have their own share of problems. Soy infant formulas are **VERY BAD** for baby! Soy's "hormonal" influence on sexual hormones and thyroid development—especially in females regardless of age—is well documented. In August, 2005, **Israel "WARNED"** its citizens to **AVOID** soy products! [Breast milk is #1; goat milk is #2—or "make" your own formula using the recipe on page 382.]

*[Flax oil is good but "very" **UNSTABLE!** Grinding turns oil "rancid!" Instead, buy "fresh" seed; put one teaspoon of seed in a glass of water; cover with saran; refrigerate overnight; warm and drink in morning. Do **NOT** use after 12 hours! See page 243.]*

Soy and Canola oil make excellent substrates for synthetic diesel fuel—but they are NOT food oils!

*[Peanut oil is an interesting oil. Edgar Cayce said it was a good massage oil for the skin—and it is! But when ingested it causes problems. Epsom salts is another example. They are great in bath water—but are extremely **TOXIC** if taken orally as misguided health gurus recomend for so-called "cleanses!"]*

The best liquid dietary "oil" to use is **OLIVE OIL!** Oils are liquid at room temperature. Fats—like butter, lard and coconut are solid. Olive oil is the product of a **fruit**—as is coconut oil. If olive oil was good enough for Jesus, it's good enough for you and me! Nut oils and sesame oil are fine, too. Flax oil is **highly** unstable and is best **AVOIDED,** due to issues of rancidity. Avoid corn, safflower, and cotton seed oils, too.

Tofu is a **very** popular food among vegetarians. Tofu is the protein and fat curd of the soybean. It is rich in PHG and is therefore toxic. If you make Tofu a regular part of your diet, long-term health will **suffer** and you will grow **OLD** and see your connective tissues **breakdown!** Tofu should **NEVER** be eaten by recovering cancer patients! [Please note: 99% of vitamin E capsules use soy oil as the carrier.]

People ask *"But what about soy protein?"* My answer is "avoid it" like the plague! Soy protein has a left spin; it's the wrong **"kind"** of protein. Scientists tell us *"Protein is protein!"*—but they also tell us *"Sugar is sugar!"* So why differentiate their chemical structure with names like maltose, fructose, sucrose, lactose and invert? They say *"The body doesn't know the difference!"*—but it does! As for the latest, "popular" granulated artificial sweetener that is *"Made from xxxxx so it tastes [and cooks] like xxxxx!"* and is supposedly "better" and "safer" than xxxxx —**AVOID IT!** Figure it out! **Chlorine**—a **"halogen"** gas—is used to alter the molecular structure of sugar—creating a Frankenstein! Want proof? Go to Dr. Mercola.com and check it out for yourself! [See Chapter 16.]

All substances have an energy "signature"—including proteins. Soy protein is extremely difficult to digest because it contains large quantities of trypsin, a harmful substance that inhibits digestion and enlarges the pancreas. Foods high in trypsin fuel cancer, too! Soy is also high in phytates, which are salts of phytic acid. Phytates cause widespread mineral imbalances, and soy has the **highest** phytate content of **any food plant EVER studied!** Vegetarians who consume soy and tofu eventually experience degeneration of the connective tissues and the build-up of **excesses** in the system. Phytates deprive the body of zinc which the body uses to ward off diabetes—and strengthens the immune system. Soy produces connective tissue disorders in laboratory mice and in children—affecting bones, cartilage, muscles, tendons, ligaments, skin and the myelin sheath protecting nerve fibers.

Soy is an **"antigen"** and is extremely antagonistic to the "terrain." Food **"allergies"** go with acid-waste overload, poor liver function, leaky gut, use of antibiotics and *non steroidal* anti-inflammatory drugs like aspirin. Allergies are "terrain" issues. Allergenic foods—like soy—are "antigens!"

Debating The Issues!
Your author is fully aware that his views are totally contrary to what the **experts** have to say about just about everything! A week doesn't pass that some new "study" or MLM marketing scheme lands on my desk with a note asking me to debate the issues regarding soy. **Sorry! There is nothing to debate!** Believe the experts if you wish! In the end, I can assure you the scoffers will be "dead" right!

Rotenone • Fish • Insects • Soy
Rotenone is used by organic gardeners as a "natural" organic pesticide. It is also used for poisoning unwanted fish species in lakes throughout North America. **Rotenone comes from the *soybean!* *Roten*** is Japanese for *derris*. It means to destroy, to tear apart. "Derris" is the specie name for the soybean within the family Fabale. Home gardeners have been told by the **"experts"** that rotenone is great stuff. However, if you read the label, you will be warned against breathing the dust.

When inhaled, rotenone is absorbed through the mucous membranes. These membranes are a direct conduit into the blood and lymph and provide easy access to the body's **IMMUNE** system. A breath of rotenone dust is a direct shot at the central and peripheral nervous systems. It is the **glycosides** in the rotenone that brings on **paralysis** of the muscles.

*[We can LEARN from watching an insect that has been dusted with rotenone. Insects react to rotenone in a matter of seconds with TOTAL paralysis! This **harmless** (?) stuff from SOYBEANS shuts down the insect's nervous system and breathing muscles. Soy does the same thing to people—but it does it a day at a time over many years!]*

In lakes, rotenone causes a complex *series* of metabolic

reactions that **"prevent"** fish from extracting **ENERGY** from nutrients! **Rotenone can kill ALL the fish in a lake with an application as small as 1 part per million (ppm)!** One-half pound of rotenone is equivalent to 60,000 ppm. One-half pound equals 8 ounces or 7,500 ppm per ounce. The *experts* tell us that it would take **1 ounce** of rotenone to kill a 150 pound man. If 1 ppm can kill all the fish in a lake, do you think it would require a concentration that is 7,499 times greater to kill a human being? It "appears" that the expert's calculations as to what is a "safe" amount of this **poison** the human body can handle is "off" a bit. Mind you, the experts don't know or care what is a safe amount. These are the same "experts" Rachel Carson struggled against in her effort to warn mankind of the inherent danger of pesticides. Read *Silent Spring* and *Our Stolen Future.* [When you ingest soy, you are ingesting PHG—which "gums" your blood and puts your IMMUNE and NERVOUS systems under severe stress. Avoid all soy!]

Sweet Proteins

Glycine is an amino acid. It is one of approximately 23 amino acids that form larger molecules called "proteins." Sow peas (soy beans) are extremely rich in glycine containing proteins because they were *irradiated* and *genetically engineered* to produce high-glycine proteins for the production of "glycerol!" Industry **isolates** glycine through a process called "hydrolysis." The product is a glycocide concentrate called **glycine-max!** Liquid glycerol is extremely sweet and syrupy. ["Organic" soy comes from irradiated seed, also!]

The **"-ol"** on a chemical name means the molecule is an "alcoh**ol**." Alcohols are excellent "non-polar" solvents. Glycerol **dissolves** fatty substances like our cellular membranes and attacks the myelin sheath on nerve fibers. [Nitro**glycerine**—as in "TNT" (dynamite)—is made from glycerol!]

Glycine-max glycerol is used as a solvent and as a plasticizer in the manufacture of hundreds of plastics.

Subject soy oil to "heat" in the presence of organic compounds like those in our blood and "sticky" resins form. Sticky blood slows capillary blood flow. The body stores these resins in the soft tissues and **fat** under the skin. Blood-vessel degeneration and plaque formation are part of this scenario.

Glycosides • Opium • Morphine • Atropine

Glycosides—like rotenone from soybeans—cause physiologic reactions in humans and animals. *Morphine* and *atropine* are examples of drugs that contain high concentrations of glycosides. **Morphine** comes from opium and alters the **central nervous system** affecting muscle control, pupil dilation—and is extremely reactive in the body. **Atropine** comes from the belladonna family of plants. It alters response to electrical signals and causes paralysis of the **"parasympathetic"** nervous system—the part of our nervous system over which we have **NO** direct control—like the heart, breathing muscles and intestinal peristalsis. *Digitalis* is a glycoside that comes from Foxglove. Plant-produced **morphine, atropine,** and **digitalis** are very effective and have few side effects. **"Synthetic"** glycosides have been **"substituted"** for the real thing with serious side effects for patients. And the experts say there is no difference between *real* and *synthesized* compounds. Really?

Soy & Dog Food

In front of me is a label from a can of a well-known brand of dog food. From 1993-1998, you could find it on supermarket shelves. It says **"Soy FREE • Highly Digestible."**

The implications of the words on the label and those on TV ads (January 6, 1994) indicate that there is a serious problem with soy protein in dog food. Some dog food manufactures tout *digestibility* because they **REMOVED** soy from their products. Manufacturers are "close-mouthed" about the **long-term** *degenerative* effects of soy on dogs. They are afraid of retaliation by the soy cartel and their bureaucratic thugs.

The dog-food and grazing-animal connection confirms the problem of soy oil and soy protein in **HUMAN** metabolism. Soy causes serious degenerative problems in humans—but it is **NOT** being taken out of our food. Instead, the experts "tout" soy as a "perfect" food—and "wonder stories" accompany the introduction of some new soy "miracle" product!

[If soy is toxic to dogs (carnivores) and grazing animals (herbivores), what do you think it does to human beings (omnivores) who are a little of both? Maybe people should decide what pedigree they would like to be so they can qualify for soy-free, highly digestible food—arf, arf!]

Conclusion

We **know** the cumulative effects of soybean oil, canola oil, tofu, and alfalfa sprouts on humans and animals—and on blood, the central and peripheral nervous systems, the immune system—and how they "block" hormone receptors.

Please **do not** call your author and demand "documentation!" There is plenty of valid information available for those who can **"think"** without the blessings of higher authority.

Ignore the experts and you stand a much better chance of becoming *Young Again!*

PREVIEW: *In our next chapter, you will learn about the connection between blindness, glaucoma, and canola oil.*

Home Smart vs. School Smart

The very best way to learn anatomy/physiology and microbiology is by "coloring!" You can learn these difficult subjects easily at home! [See Pages 233, 267 and Source Page 400.]

The Misery Index

Joint and back pain "limit" one's life! Here are some helpful hints to ease the misery: L_sP_cC,™ VZ,™ R/J Factors 1 & 11™ and Skin & Body Toner.™ Add High (and low) Enema Therapy™ and **de**acidification of the terrain using the *Young Again! (Tissue and Liver) Protocol*™ and you have the recipe!

The Vorago™ Effect

"Lucky" is the woman who can "freeze" the magic of youth as described in the *Vorago Effect.*™ See Chapter 35 and pages 72, 164, 212 and 274 to learn more!

Bone Density

Bone-density tests don't offer any solutions—except the usual misguided advice to take "calcium"—so why bother with them? Better to read and "understand" this book and know "why" and "how" osteoporosis develops. Then the reader can ignore and escape the experts in the "sick-care" system!

War Games

Gulf War veterans were "ordered" to take a drug called Pyridostigmine Bromide (PB) every day. This drug interferes with *acetylcholinesterase*—an enzyme that is critical to nerve synapse function (nerve signal transmission). **The side effects were known and predictable!** PB produces the symptoms being experienced by Gulf War veterans. The question is, **who** ordered its use and **why?** The answer is: "the experts!" **When** will these same experts tell the public about the terminal side effects our—**Iraq War**—soldiers will experience from spent uranium ammunition? Uranium **"atomizes"** as bullets leave the gun barrel. Spent uranium dust is extremely **HEAVY** and radioactive, too! Can you guess what happens when it is inhaled into the lungs? **NEVER** trust the experts and their cronies because they all work for and are paid by the yellow fringed flag folks who foment wars, manipulate our money, control information flow and *"Kill us, unforgiven!"* [See Chapter 40.] **IF** the body is given the opportunity, and provided protection, it will release toxic substances from the organs and tissues. Otherwise, the body **WILL NOT** release the stuff for fear of harm! Opportunity and protection is what the *Young Again Protocol(s)*™ are about. If toxic materials are not flushed from the body, aging and dis-ease result. It is a matter of **choice!** Hopefully, the reader will make good choices!

Hair Growth

"B" vitamins and thyroid function are CRITICAL to maintaining a full heal of hair. Hair is an extension of "skin"—and skin is a reflection of the "terrain"—so "hair" is a **"HEALTH"** issue! Typically, 95% of B-vitamins are lost and destroyed in the GI tract—so a different "mechanism" and "pathway" has been discovered that avoids destruction and loss of the "B's. Now, up to 100% "absorption" is possible by encapsulating the "B's" in phospha-tidyl-choline [a "fatty" acid jelly] at nanoscale. The jelly delivers the "B's" directly to the blood stream with **equal** benefits to an "IV" needle! The benefits for the scalp and hairplus increased **ENERGY** is "awesome!" [HST™ creme provides direct stimulation to "dormant" hair follicles—offering a totally novel approach to hair regrowth and hair maintenance!

War In The Marketplace

People resist "change"—especially on "volatile" issues like war! But if an enemy can be "created," resistance "vanishes" quickly! **And so it is with issues of "health!"** After 20 years of mental "softening," the memory fades—as does people's "resistance," making the metamorphosis complete! The soy and canola oil cartels **"created"** hostility towards butter, coconut oil and lard—while simultaneously creating **demand** for **"industrial"** oils—like soy and canola—marketed as "healthy" food oils, making the metamorphosis complete! [Your author refers the reader to Sun Tzu's 6th century B.C. book *The Art Of War*, summarized as follows: *Outline an agenda, disseminate disinformation and misinformation, create confusion and dissension, raise an army of experts, use subversion, quote statistics, and finally create fear. Fear leads to panic, and panic to victory.*] Sun Tzu was correct! The game is called **divide and conquer!** It's simple. It works. His book was the official training manual during the rise of the Soviet empire. **Notice** what the experts preach. **See** which way the masses are moving. *Tune into* what the media is pushing. **Now! Go the other way as you spread the word! Few things are what they appear!**

The "250" Club

The "250" Club is open to anyone who would like to live 250 vibrant, healthy years. The club will serve as a role model for society and a tool for teaching children to live in harmony with God and nature. Think of the suffering and strife that could be eliminated through the transfer of "knowledge" to our great grand children. Life on Earth might even become a joy. The club has no meetings or dues. We lead by example!

Before

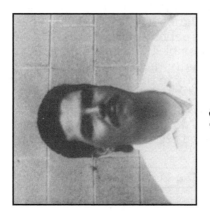

After

Glen Roundtree is living proof of the effectiveness of Harmonic™ Silver Water on severe burns. His face healed "scar free," but his hands and arms are scarred where he was treated by allopathic doctors using conventional therapy.

Harmonic™ Silver Water is "tuned" to hertz frequencies that complement the bio-electric body. It goes beyond common colloidal silvers that are based on PPM (parts per million). This Fourth Dimension product uses the homeopathic principles of *resonance* and *transference* to promote healing. Everyone should have a bottle on hand. Great for colds and flu and dozens of other uses.

26

Blindness & Oils

"Since the days of revelation, the same four corrupting errors have been made over and over again: submission to faulty and unworthy authority; submission to what was customary to believe; submission to prejudices of the mob; and worst of all, concealment of ignorance by a false show of unheld knowledge, for no other reason than pride."
Roger Bacon

Each year, millions of people lose their vision to "conditions" like glaucoma and macular degeneration—conditions the **"experts"** call dis-ease! Atrophy (deterioration) of the optic nerve and macula **always** involve inflammation and deterioration—and both of them have a common cause, too!

For years, the *experts* have told the public that **glaucoma** results from fluid pressure build-up in the eye. By definition, **macular degeneration** means deterioration of the "macula" which is the "yellow spot" in the back of the eye where visual images are received and sent to the brain for recognition. **Retinitis** means inflammation of the retina. [Supposedly, these conditions have different causes, but the experts can't tell you what the causes are—only the **"symptoms!"** Their *theories* about the etiology (causes) of eye degeneration are based on a *faulty* medical model.]

[These days "enlightened" experts admit they were **wrong** *about glaucoma—and to save face, they have birthed a "new" theory that says glaucoma is the result of a deficiency of oxygen to the eye! This is true! But their explanation does* **NOT** *explain why there is an oxygen problem. Sadly, they don't know what to do about it, either! They just don't get it!]*

Causes of Eye Deterioration
Eye deterioration results from insufficient blood flow **INTO** the posterior eye and insufficient waste and lymph flow **OUT** of the posterior eye. Build up of cellular waste "marginalizes" nerve" activity. Loss of vision is the result!

Stagnant acid waste forms amyolid tissue, then scar tissue—and eventually blindness results.

Dietary habits play a big role in development of all disease—including vision problems. By the time the problem manifests, all the doctor can do is look for **"SIGNS"**—so he can conjure a "diagnosis" and design a "treatment" plan to deal with the symptoms—while **"ignoring"** the cause(s).

Eye problems are summed up in a two words. **"TERRAIN"** and **"LIVER."** Hormones, leaky gut, stress and dietary "oils" also also have a part in eye "dis-ease." Oils like canola and soy affect blood agglutination. Agglutination (clumping) of red blood corpuscles affects eye health. Behind **EACH** eye is **"80" MILES** of blood capillaries that "service" the posterior eye. Agglutinated blood cannot freely circulate in the extremely fine capillaries of the posterior eye causing an oxygen and nutrient **"deficit"** that shuts down mitochondrial production of ATP.

Waste buildup in the tissues of the eye creates the perfect environment for diminished vision and cataracts.

Invasion of the body's terrain—by yeast—is a major health issue. Yeast is **NOT** the cause of dis-ease—but it is a **"symptom!"** Yeast overgrowth goes with eye, ear and sinus problems by **feeding** on stagnant waste lodged in the tissues of the head. Congestion is the "effect" of microbial **OVERGROWTH** in the **"stagnant"** fluid wastes of the head and chest. Stagnant fluid waste eventually **"MORPHS"** into **"STRUCTURAL"** matter called "amyloid plaque!" The body has **"no mechanism"** to rid itself of "non-soluble," "structural" waste— and that is the reason people "age!" [The *Young Again*™ solution is to **"EAT"** structural amyloid plaque and scar tissue and return it to "liquid" state for removal from the body by the lymphatic system. Racemized VZ™ does the job!]

Eye "floaters" are symptomatic of YEAST overgrowth—and an acid, waste-filled terrain!

Canola of Rape?

Loss of vision is a **known** characteristic side effect of rape oil—but deterioration takes years to manifest. Rape oil *antagonizes* the central and peripheral nervous systems.

The name *"canola" masked* the introduction of **rape oil** to America. **Canola** is a "coined" word that appeared out of nowhere! The flip side of the canola coin reads **"RAPE!"** Of course, canola sounds much nicer than "rape!" Canola oil comes from rape seed—which is part of the Mustard family of plants. Rape is the **MOST** toxic of all so-called food oils. Rape is a toxic plant and insects don't like rape because it is poisonous to all but a few of them.

Rape seed oil is a hundred times more toxic than soy oil. Rape oil is an industrial oil—NOT a food oil.

Canola oil is a *semi-drying* oil that is used as a lubricant, fuel, soap and synthetic rubber base—and as an illuminant for the slick color pages you see in magazines. Canola is an **industrial** oil. It does **NOT** belong in the body! Canola oil—like soy oil and soy protein—has some interesting characteristics *and* effects on living systems. For example, it forms latex-like substances that "clog" the system and **agglutinate** red blood corpuscles just like soy—only much worse!

Rape oil stresses the terrain and contributes to development of dis-ease in ANIMALS—and humans!

Rape oil was in widespread use in animal feeds in England and Europe between 1986 and 1991 when it was thrown out. Do you remember reading about the cows, pigs and sheep that went **"blind"** and crazy and attacked people?

*[Not long after the first edition of this book appeared, a woman called from Chicago to say that she was in England when Mad Cow Disease was at its peak. She told me she witnessed a news report on television that told people not to panic if they had been using rape oil in their diet and were over 65 years of age because the effects take **at least** ten years to manifest—and in all likelihood most of these people would be dead by then anyway. Interesting!]*

"Experts" *blamed* erratic animal behavior on a viral disease called *scrapie*. However, when rape oil was removed from animal feed, scrapie disappeared. A thoughtful reader sent your author an in depth study of the affects of Canola on dairy cattle in Canada. The results were **NOT** good! Today, Americans are using rape (canola) oil . Now, canola oil is our problem! Canola is widely used in thousands of processed foods—with the **blessings** of government "watchdog" agencies, of course.

Officially, canola oil is known as "LEAR" oil. The acronym stands for *low erucic acid rape.* Experts in industry like to tell the story of how canola was developed in Canada—and that it is safe to eat. They admit it was developed from the rape seed, but through **"genetic engineering"** [Think, irradiation!] it is no longer rape—but instead, "canola!" Experts love to talk about canola's "qualities"—like its unsaturated structure, and wonderful digestibility, and fatty acid makeup. They malign naturally saturated oils and fats like coconut and butter—and come to the rescue with canola oil. They even tell us how Asia has warmly embraced canola due to its distinctive flavor. [Isn't it wonderful how multinational oil cartels "help" third world people? Doesn't this story remind you of the introduction of microwave ovens and margarine and.......?]

An "earthy" old west expression sums up industry flim-flam accompanying the "smoke and mirror" introduction of rape oil into the diets of unsuspecting people world-wide. That expression is *"Horse Shit & Gun Smoke!"* The word *canola* provided a perfect "warm fuzzy" marketing "cover" for food cartel "interests" at work behind the scenes!

Chemical Warfare

The chemical warfare agent "MUSTARD GAS" is derived from rape oil. This is the chemical agent responsible for blistering the lungs and skin of hundreds of thousands of solders and civilians during WW I. Reports from the French indicate mustard gas was used during the Gulf War.

Between 1950 and 1953, white mustard seed (rape seed) was *irradiated* in Sweden to increase seed production and oil content. *Irradiation* is the same process the *experts* are using to make "our" food **"safe"** to eat. Today 2006, genetically engineered fruits and vegetables have innocent things like hepatitis-B spliced into their DNA. This is a good example of misuse of technology and abuse of public trust by powerful interests and "watchdog" bureaucratic agencies.

*[Canola oil contains large amounts of **iso-thio-cyanates** which are **"cyanide-containing"** compounds. Cyanide **INHIB- ITS** mitochondrial production of ATP—the energy molecule fueling body metabolism and "life!"]*

Canola Oil & Body Metabolism

In biochemistry, substances that *bind* metabolic enzymes and *block* their activity in the body are called "inhibitors." Throughout this book, your author has used terms like "bio-junk diet," "toxic and acid waste," "negative, left-spin energy," "drugs," etc. to describe **unfriendly** energy fields.

Unfriendly substances in canola and soy oils fuel the formation of **covalent bonds.** Generally, covalent bonds are *irreversible* and—once formed—**CANNOT** be broken by **normal** metabolic reactions. This is particularly true of hormone analogs contained in birth control pills, estrogen replacements and *anabolic* steroids. Zeno estrogen analogs are ubiquitous and unavoidable because they are everywhere in the environment. The question is *"What do we do about them?"*

The Young Again Protocol*™ *reverses systemic damage from hormone analogs and restores the terrain.

Consider the pesticide **"malathion."** It binds to the active site of the enzyme *acetylcholinesterase* and stops this enzyme from doing what it is supposed to do—which is to split acetylcholine into choline and acetate. Malathion is the so-called "harmless" pesticide used on the Med Fly and every living thing in California in 1991 and again in 1994 and in Texas in 1995. Malathion is an **"organophosphate."**

Nerve Function & Organophosphates

Acetycholine is critical to **NERVE impulse transmission.** When inhibited, nerve synapses do not function normally and the muscles do not respond. For example, think of a garage door opener. If no signal is sent, the door does **not** open. In the case of the body, the hand or leg does **not** respond. Perhaps you have noticed the tremendous increase in disorders like Systemic Lupus, Multiple Sclerosis, Cerebral Palsy, Restless Legs Syndrome and Peripheral Neuropathy in recent years. Soy and canola oils are "players" in the development of these "conditions"—as are **organophosphate** insecticides and zeno estrogen hormone analogs.

Acetylcholinesterase inhibitors cause paralysis of the striated (skeletal) muscles—and spasms of the muscles of the respiratory system.

That is **"why"** malathion and its derivatives are the pesticides of choice by the "experts!" They kill insects by causing **muscle paralysis**—just like *rotenone* from soybeans. [See Chapter 25!] If malathion inhibits insect *metabolism*, do you think it might also inhibit human metabolism, too?

Agents *orange* and *blue* were the herbicides used in Vietnam to defoliate jungle cover. Both are organophosphate compounds. Vietnam vets and the Vietnamese people **"know"** first-hand about them! Government "experts" who okayed their use and chemical companies that manufactured them "later" admitted to their toxic effects on **PEOPLE** and the **environment!** Present-day "stooges" in academia and government continue to **"abba dabba"** the public with stories of "safe" science and "cheap" food through the use of poisons.

Canola oil is rich in glycosides. Glycosides cause serious problems in the human body by blocking enzyme function and locking up nerve and hormone receptors.

Glycosides interfere with body biochemistry of humans and animals. Consider the effects of a rattlesnake bite. Glycosides in the venom **inhibit** muscle enzymes and cause instant immobilization and tissue necrosis. Insect and animal venom are *unfriendly* "proteins." How the body responds to **foreign** proteins determines life, death, dis-ease—whether it be a vaccination, snake bite, insect or spider bite. The response is determined by the condition of the LIVER and the TERRAIN!

Canola Oil • HIV & AIDS

Canola glycosides depress the immune system, causing the **white blood cell defense system**—the T-cells—to go into a stupor! Glycosides **ALTER** the body's "terrain." Alcohol and glycoside "-R" groups in Canola **alter** immune system response. [Fluoride, immunizations, antibiotics, **artificial sweetners,** food additives and bio-junk diets play complementary roles in immune system malfunction and collapse!]

[An *"alcohol" is a chemistry term referring to a molecule with an alcohol "reactive" group attached to the organic molecule. The "-R" group is what gives organic compounds their individual "personality"—good and bad! Canola alcohol and glycoside molecules have personalities that are "unfriendly" as well as* **"unpredictable"** *when turned loose in* **"living"** *sys-*

tems. The same thing can be said of organophosphate molecules in pesticides and herbicides.]

When medical experts check your blood for the presence of the HIV virus, they are **NOT** seeing what is really going on in the body's "terrain." If the white blood cell count is normal, they will tell you that you do **NOT** have "HIV." What they don't see is that the T-cells are in a *stupor* and unable to respond and defend the "terrain"—creating an *opportunistic* situation that allows microbial life forms in blood and lymph to go **"undetected"** and **"MORPH"**—bypassing immune system "T" cell defenses—and get a foothold. As Claude Barnard said *"The terrain is everything!"* —and it is!

The microbe is NOT the cause of dis-ease, but the microbe does take advantage of a toxic "terrain!"

Once inside the cells, viruses like HIV take over RNA and DNA and **"hijack"** production of mitochondrial ATP "energy" for their own use. Quietly, viruses **"replicate"** and one day—BANG!—you wake up and you are dying of AIDS. [In actuality, you don't die from AIDS—but from conditions like pneumonia, hepatitis, etc. that manifest in a weakened and defensless "terrain!" The acronym "AIDS" stands for Acquired Immune Deficiency Syndrome.]

AIDS & Green Monkeys

In his earth-shaking book, *AIDS The End of Civilization,* Dr. William Campbell Douglass asked *"Do you really think some Green Monkey all of a sudden bit some guy in the ass and presto AIDS was all over the world?"*

Dr. Douglass was commenting on the "hype" that the Centers for Disease Control in Atlanta was "peddling" to the public about the AIDS virus—"HIV." Douglass' book tells the "whole" story of the development of HIV at the Ft. Detrick, Maryland, military installation. His story is well documented and confirms the theme of the futuristic movies *Outbreak* and *The Twelve Monkeys* which your author recommends! [In 2006, the big scare is "bird flu!" If an epidemic does "erupt," you can bet it will be because of the "vaccinations" that preceded it—just like the so-called Spanish influenza epidemic in 1918.]

Lorenzo's Oil

The movie, *Lorenzo's Oil,* offers another good example of how far off course medical science has strayed and how muddled is the scientific mind. Early on in the movie, the experts said the problem with the dying child was **not** in the math (body pH). They were wrong. The dying boy had an extremely **ACID** terrain! He was so **"acid"** that the myelin sheath covering his nerve fibers was "dissolving"—causing his system to collapse. He was given **OLIVE** oil to cause massive "bile

flow!" The oil *shocked* his body into a **LESS** acid condition. Lorenzo's oil was not rape oil—as the "experts" calimed!
The situation today regarding degenerative nerve disorders is exactly the same issue! An ACID terrain!

Connect The Dots.....

By now, it should be obvious to the reader that an **acid** terrain, marginal liver function and poor bile flow are major health issues—and that there is a direct link between dis-ease and **processed** foods containing substances that **"CONFUSE"** the body and weaken the immune system. Each of us **MUST** take **control** of our life and personal responsibility for our health if we hope to avert or remedy serious dis-ease and early death. **We are "on our own!"** So why allow yourself to become entangled in the "sick care" system?
The "health care" industry is an oxymoron. It protects its health and economic interests—not yours!
When you understand the rules of the game—health, aging reversal and longevity take on a different connotation. Replace ignorance with knowledge based on a realistic "model," and you will be on your way to becoming *Young Again!*

PREVIEW: *Our next chapter looks at the connection between onions, the liver and aging.*

Overdrive!

"Stress" of any type puts the adrenal glands into **"overdrive"** through increased cortisol production. Elevated cortisol levels ravage health and hormones—especially in women. PU™ gets you **OUT** of "overdrive" so the body can settle, repair and heal.

Hang & Stretch

It's important to hang and "s-t-r-e-t-c-h" every day. Hang by your ankles using a floatation table—and by your hands using a simple trapeze or chin-up bar. Hanging by your hands allows lymph nodes in the under-arm and breast/chest area to "drain!" Lymphatic drainage in the chest area is **extremely** important and a good way to avoid breast cancer! The shoulders are a problem area for women, so go easy, ladies!

Vibrations!

Learn to use a vibration chain for determining energy "spin," drawing away pain from points of injury or inflammation—and to locate and eliminate noxious electrical energy fields in your home. *Vibrations* is a book worth owning and the perfect member of a trilogy that includes the *Pendulum Kit* and *Map Dowsing.* (See Pages 57, 144, 188 and 210.)

Comfrey Greens

In the good old days—before the Feds decided to save us from the evils of comfrey—it could be found in health stores. Today if you want comfrey, you have to grow it yourself or have someone grow it for you. And if you are smart that is exactly what you will do! Comfrey "pops up" in early Spring. Eaten like spinach, the leaves and blossoms are at their very best! Steam until wilted, yet bright green in color. Add a little olive oil and lemon, apple cider or wine vinegar—and you've got a highly nutritious meal. **[Something "acidic" is a MUST!]** The "Feds" say comfrey is dangerous. If that's true, my family and I should all be dead! Plant comfrey once and you will have "free" food forever—food outside the reach of faceless bureaucrats! Maybe that's **"why"** special "interests" had the Feds ban it?

Talk!

Not everyone who reads *Young Again!* is ready for its message. Many people read this book and decide to *"Think about it!"* — and that is as far as they will ever go! Others cut and run or conjure a flimsy excuse why the *Young Again*™ message does not apply to them. It is said that *"Talk is cheap!"* Car dealers use the expression *"tire kicker"* to describe a "talker" instead of a buyer. A cruder version is "money talks and BS walks!" And don't forget *"An empty wagon rattles the most!"* To summarize and make my point, remember this: ***"When all is said and done more is said than done!"*** **Talk solves nothing!**

"Moody" Water!

A Japanese scientist with IBM in the 1960's demonstrated that water could be "programmed" to create radical mood swings of anger, joy, laughter, depression etc. Water is a "living" substance that can be "programmed!" This idea captures the essence of BFRV.™ [See Wall Street Journal 3/10/06]

What Is A "Precursor"?

A precursor is a molecular substance that precedes the formation of something else—as in making your "own" hormones. A racemized™ precursor is the accelerated version of the same—providing greater value and better body response. Body response is the *name of the game*—and the *Young Again Protocol*™ is how you make it happen!

Pesticide Free?

"Think" about this! It was a *huge* canola oil display . The sign said,"Pesticide Free." What they didn't mention was that canola oil is a "systemic" **poison!** If insects won't eat it *"Why should you?"* "Pesticide Free!" Right! Give me a break!

27

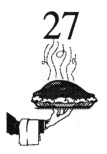

Liver & Onions

"As goes the liver, so goes the terrain!"
John Thomas

The liver is **"THE"** most used, abused and important organ in the human body—and in animals, too! It is the body's **primary** waste removal organ that, in conjunction with the bowel, processes fully 90% of all body-generated waste. Obviously, a healthy liver is essential to good health—and it is **CENTRAL** to the aging-reversal process.

The liver is a phenomenal chemical factory, and it is responsible for **thousands** of biochemical reactions. The liver is the second largest organ in the body—and the **ONLY** organ that can **"regenerate itself by its own volition"** with only 25% of its functional cells intact. The liver's regenerative ability is an indication of its importance!

The liver's **"functional"** cells are called **"hepatocytes"** (*hepat*-liver; *cyte*-cell)—and they are classified as "parenchyma" cells. They are the "functional" cells that perform the "magic!"

The liver metabolizes food, drugs, pesticides, wastes and alcohol. These substances are transported to the liver via the portal vein—and they impose heavy stress on the liver. How efficient incoming substances are processed depends on the "terrain" in general, stomach and intestinal digestive capability and the health and vitality of the vital organs and glands. The liver is absolutely **"CENTRAL"** to good health!

All food—even good food—exerts stress on the liver. Eat junk, and violate the simple rules of the Young Again Protocol™ and your liver will fail—and so will you!

Nails & Pellets • Scarred Liver
When the liver becomes overly toxic, the hepatocytes die. The spaces left behind fill with **amyloid tissue** which eventually "morphs" into scar tissue. "Scar" tissue is comprised of **"stroma"** cells that normally cover the **"outside"** of the liver. Stroma cells CANNOT "double" for the parenchyma cells. Loss of stroma cells means loss of liver function!

As the liver "filters" wastes from the blood, debris and bile salts can "solidify" into "pellets" and "nails." Liver **"pellets"** are supposed to flow into the gall bladder in **semi-soft** form— and eventually into the gut, bowel and toilet. Pellets that "settle" in the gall bladder and "calcify" into **STONES** are called *gallstones!* Waste that "settle," in the **"biliary"** ducts of the liver itself and "calcify" become rock-hard "nails" and can sometimes be heard "clinking" in the toilet bowel during and after the *Young Again! (Tissue and Liver) Protocol*™.

Cirrhosis of the liver is a "condition" of **EXCESS** masking as a deficiency dis-ease—which it is **NOT!** Cirrhosis of the liver causes it to "yellow" and "harden" and become "fibrous" due to amyloid plaque and scar tissue formation. [You do **NOT** have to drink or be an alcoholic to suffer or succumb to cirrhosis! It is a "terrain" issue and can occur at any age!]

Cirrhosis comes with aging! Sooner or later everyone becomes "cirrhotic"—a condition that is reversable if the liver is given the opportunity to "restore" itself!

Blood & Filter Issues

The liver is **heavily** vascularized with blood vessels. It receives a DOUBLE supply of blood. *Oxygenated* blood from the heart is supplied via the hepatic artery and nutrient laden, partially *deoxygenated* blood feeds from the intestines via the hepatic portal vein. When *amyloid* plaque collects in the portal vein, blood pressure rises. This is called *portal hypertension.*

The Kupffer's cells lining the blood vessels of the liver are of **"IMMENSE"** importance to health and vitality. Kupffer's cells are **BOTH hepatocytes** and **phagocytes** (*phag*-to eat, *cyte*-cell.) Phagocytes are specialized cells that remove microbes, foreign matter and worn out red and white blood cells from circulation. Kupffer's cells are **"parenchyma" cells.**

Liver-filtered waste from the blood and lymphatic systems is deposited into the gallbladder in the form of "bile." Bile emulsifies dietary fats. Poor bile flow is **"THE"** issue when it comes to any kind of digestive or bowel disorder. Proper digestion is very dependent upon adequate bile flow. [So-called Acid Reflux Dis-ease is **"nothing"** more than a messed-up liver and a sluggish bowel.]

Fats provide **needed** "cholesterol" for the production of corticosteroid hormones made by the adrenal gland and for creation of sex hormones like estrogen, testosterone, progesterone and DHEA. Insufficient intake of fats and oils spells trouble—especially for women!

Cellulite—as seen on women's butts and thighs—is "abnormal" fat and it is confirmation of an **"acid"** terrain! Cellulite is "aging-in-progress!" Women wanting to rid their bodies of this awful "stuff" should follow the *Young Again*

Protocol(s).™ Those who stay with the program and use the Biogenic™ Body Roller will see the cellulite "disappear!" [Cellulite is **NOT** an "exercise" issue! It is toxic, waste fatty tissue!]

[The liver consumes massive amounts of energy which is provided by the mitochondria. This area of the body is sometimes called the "solar plexes" because of the heat associated with liver function.]

Acidification of the blood, lymph, joints and soft tissues of the body ALWAYS involves a sick liver. The doctor CANNOT test for this because an acid terrain is "SUBclinical"—and precedes diagnosis of a dis-ease condition by 5-50 years! Please read this statement again!

Hepatitis (*hepat*-liver; *itis*-inflamation of) is a liver, "condition"—**NOT** a dis-ease. So is mononucleosis, Epstein-Barr, Lyme, Malaria, Nile Fever and Chronic Fatigue. Practitioners blame nature's garbage crew—the viruses—for damage inflicted upon the liver—but they are wrong! [Terrain and liver issues are **not** difficult to reverse if the individual is willing follow the *Young Again (Tissue and Liver) Protocol.*™]

Impose mental and physical stress on an already toxic body "terrain"—along with insufficient sleep—and the liver will succumb and illness will follow!

*[Thanks to Dr. Guenther Enderlein, we know the **exact** progression of microbial "**metamorphosis**" that occurs along the path called degenerative dis-ease. Restoration of the "terrain" so dis-ease cannot manifest itself is a very "proactive" and "defensive" approach! See Chapters 13 and 14!]*

Personalities

As people age, their personalities change. One personality type—the **choleric**—reflects the condition of a person's liver. The *choleric* has a **bitter** personality that is vile and difficult. The word "choleric" comes from *chole* which means "bile" in Greek. *Chole* refers to the liver's digestive juice and waste product "bile." A "bilious" person has a foul personality. Alcoholics and some older folks are notorious for being *bilious*. [The Greeks believed there were four basic personality types: choleric, melancholy, sanguine and phlegmatic.]

Western medicine's **disastrous** history was the result of the theories of Greek physician and medical writer Claudius Galen (circa A.D. 130-200). He was personal physician to Roman Emperor, Marcus Aurelius. Galen enlarged the personality "idea." He spoke of four personality types based on **"humors."** A humor is a **body fluid** that was believed to influence people's personality. "Bleeding" sick patients at the time of the American colonieswas a version of humor "letting!" Galen's **"MODEL"** was faulty and so is medical science's "model" today! Just because we know how to successfully replace worn out body parts, fails to answer **"WHY"** they wore out! Galen's ideas are still in vogue, but under different "personality" names like type-A, type-B, etc. Children in the "fifties" remember the "good humor" ice cream man who plied the streets daily.]

"Humoral" immunity is taught in current medical science curriculums—and refers to "circulating" antibodies and antigens in the blood and lymphatic fluids.

Bile • Digeston • Hiatal Hernia

Poor bile flow and leaky-gut limits our ability to digest food. Leaky gut **"floods"** the blood stream with an endless procession of over-sized food molecules each time we eat. Insufficient production of hydrogen chloride by cells in the stomach wall **"LIMITS"** protein digestion and absorption—and allows parasites and their eggs to take up residence in the gut and blood stream. Incompletely digested proteins "putrefy" in the gut, causing heart burn, mucous congestion and acid reflux type issues. "Excess" stomach acid is the "TV" version of indigestion when exactly the **"OPPOSITE"** is the case.

Indigestion—like so many other problems—is a *terrain* issue. Increased bileflow—and High Enema Therapy™—are the ultimate keys! Thoroughly chewing food helps. Avoiding liquids—especially "cold" liquids—helps considerably. High Enema Therapy™ relieves "hiatal" hernia complaints by relieving abdominal "pressure" on a **"deteriorating"** diaphragm—a common complaint associated with **"acid reflux."** [As the body turns "acid," the connective tissues break down—and the diaphragm is nothing but connective tissue "wall" separating the pleural cavity (lungs) from the peritoneal cavity (belly). Solving the digestion "riddle" is rather easy if your "model" is realistic—and you learn to think outside the box!]

Stomach Acid & Vitamin B-12

Stomach acid has a pH as low as 0.80. It is so "acidic" that a drop of it on the skin will eat a hole in it. **Healthy** mucous membranes "protect" the stomach wall from powerful acids secreted by cells within the stomch wall. Stomach "peptic" ulcers are the product of H. pylori bacteria that "survived" due to low stomach acid production and "bored" into and set up house in the stomach wall—causing bleeding and pain! Duodenal ulcers occur in the wall of the small intestine immediately below the stomach. [The "duodenum" is followed by the jejunum and the ileum.]

Vitamin B-12 **"assimilation"** is a "stomach" issue and is dependent on the secretion of **"intrinsic factor"**—which is also "secreted" from cells in the stomach wall. Dietary B-12 must be "encapsulated" by intrinsic factor for "safe transport" to the blood steam or B-12 is **"lost!"** Sublingual B-12 tablets and B-12 oral supplements fail to solve the "absorption" problem for the reasons given above.

Vitamin B-12 is a **HUGE** female issue because women deplete their stores of this vital substance 20-30 years ahead of men, due to the loss of menstrual blood. The "odd" thing about Vitamin B-12 is that it is **NOT** specific for anything—and yet B-12 affects virtually everything—especially in women "30" years and older. [Racemized™ Cobo-12™ transdermal creme remedies the absorption issue by using a proprietary "transport" for absorption by the blood capillary beds beneath the skin. Cobo-12™ is useful for anemia issues, too!]

Healthy livers produce about **1 quart** of bile a day. "Bile" is a yellowish-brown and olive-green "juice" of the liver. Bile contains mineral ions, **chole**-ster-**ol** and bilirubin from worn-out red blood corpuscles. "Excess" bilirubin in the blood is responsible for "jaundice" in babies and sickly adults. People with liver "conditions" often have a jaundiced appearance.

[Gall stones are confirmation of liver problems and are ***"10" TIMES*** *more prevalent in* **women** *than in men because women grow "acidie" earlier and faster than men. Gallstones are* **LIVER pellets** *that "settled" in the gallbladder and "calcified." Gallstones range in size from lentils to golf balls.]*

[Partially digested food called "chyme" enters the intestinal duodenum, it mixes with pancreatic secretions and bile from the liver which are **HIGHLY** *alkaline and designed to elevate chyme pH so carbohydrate bonds can be broken and sugars digested.]*

Micelles & Heme Iron
Bile works like **dish soap**—and so does Yucca Blend.™ They break up and emulsify large fat globules into pin-head sized droplets called *micelles*. Micelles have more surface area, making it easier for the body to process and absorb fats. Micelle formation is central to the absorption of the fat soluble vitamins like A,D,E and K. [Fat-free diets and foods are not a good idea—especially for women!]

Poor absorption and assimilation of dietary fats spells trouble because 40% of energy production should come from the burning of "fat!"

The gallbladder "stores" bile secreted from the liver. Eating "triggers" the release of bile into the gut. Insufficient bile release robs the body of nourishment and energy from assimilation of fats and oils and "oxidation" of them by the liver.

Bile contains "heme" iron from worn out red blood corpuscles. Heme iron is **NOT** something you "eat!" It is something your body **"MAKES"**—and it makes a lot more heme iron when **Cobo-12**™ transdermal creme, racemized,™ predigested organic **liver** and **algae** are taken on a daily basis. [Women respond very well to this approach.]

Ideally, **heme** iron should be **"reabsorbed"** in the gut, but it is often "lost." Heme iron is not the same as dietary iron. A shortage of heme iron will reflect a corresponding shortfall in mitochondrial oxidation of glucose into "ATP"—our energy molecule—and diminished blood oxygen levels. Elevated **"blood sugar"** levels are closely "linked" to low heme iron levels, hormone issues and leaky gut. That is why Type ll diabetes (aka *adult onset/sugar diabetes*) is so prevalent during pregnancy and in females over "35" years of age. [Gluco Factor X™ helps.]

*[Iron supplements are bad news! Iron is an "oxidizer" and participates in the production of free radicals by providing the perfect "substrate" for pathogenic bacteria overgrowth. Pregnant women should **NOT** take so called "iron pills!"]*

Acne, boils, constipation, appendicitis, psoriasis and "learning" issues—in children and teens—are symptomatic of liver problems—and an acid terrain.

Lecithin is the fat "emulsifier" in bile responsible for keeping cholesterol in **"solution."** When cholesterol, mineral salts and drugs settle **"out of"** solution—arteries **"clog"** and gallstones develop and grow in size. If gallstones **BLOCK** the duct(s) connecting the gallbladder to the small intestine, "gangrene" will develop. A gangrenous gallbladder must be removed immediately to prevent septic shock and death from blood poisoning (toxemia).

Loss of the gallbladder usually results in diabetes within 20 years unless action is taken to "prevent" it.

Modern medicine has made quick work of gallbladder removal. However, people need to understand the **CAUSES** behind gallstone formation and **NOT** rely on "magic bullet" technology and invasive surgery to save them from death's pall. Gallbladder issues cause 8,000 **deaths** and 50,000 **surgeries** and 1 BILLION **dollars** in medical costs in the USA every year.

Gallstones are a confirmation that the aging process is accelerating—no matter what your calendar age!

People and animals can live without a gallbladder or an appendix, spleen, tonsils, testicles and ovaries—but health and vitality suffer. It is better to keep these "parts" because they are **NOT** "vestigial" organs! The health minded individual should try and **AVOID** organ loss and make the effort to **"offset"** metabolic slow down where these organs are removed or have **"atrophied"** and are no longer "functional."

Without a gallbladder, the liver "drips" bile directly into the intestine—denying the digestive system a "volume" release at mealtime. Insufficient and untimely bile secretion means **marginal** health and **DICTATES** use of the racemized™ digestive enzymes like DiSorb Aid ll,™ R/BHCl™ and Yucca Blend.™

Liver & Cancer
People with cancer should temporarily abstain from eating meat, cheese and fish to provide their body "rest." Heavy, high-stress proteins **"DRAIN"** the system unless **heavy** digestive supplementation is used. "Healthy" eggs and nutritious **SUPER FOODS** work well. The more energy that can be directed to healing—rather than processing of food—the better and quicker healing occurs. [There is a "healer" in Los Angeles with a wonderful track record for reversing cancer. His patients eat **"RAW"** organic beef 3 times a day. Don't over cook beef!]

Dr. Max Gerson used fresh, organic calf liver "juice" to treat cancer patients. It is **LOADED** with biologically active nutrients and enzymes—but horrible to ingest. In the USA, fresh liver is **NOT** an option due to the sick condition of the animals. The same goes for "dessicated" liver. A better alternative is **predigested, racemized™ organic liver capsules!** They allow everyone—and especially vegetarians and vegans—to add some balance to their lives. [See page 383.] Fresh, organic "beet" and "carrot" juices—are **VERY** therapeutic to the liver. [One "raw" egg blended in juice is a great source of good protein. "Raw" milk and products like "kefir" are healing. Kombucha tea and **un**pasteurized saurkraut are superb!

Location Of The Liver • Pot Bellies
The liver is located directly **under** the anterior, right rib cage, **above** the ascending colon, **below** the right lung, **next** to the stomach and **opposite** the spleen. [See page 46!]

A distended abdomen—as in a "pot belly"—is a classic **SIGN** of a **compromised** liver and **acid** terrain, and goes hand-in-hand with colitis, irritable bowel, leaky gut, diverticulitis, prostate issues, gout, arthritis, heart problems—and cancer! [Dis-ease and illness is spelled "liver!"]

*[Intestinal parasites reach the liver via the portal vein and by "traversing" the common bile duct. It is not uncommon to find E. coli "colon" bacteria in the **liver** and **prostate!**]*

Liver Breath
Foods like raw onion and garlic cause "liver breath." These foods are potent detoxifiers—and so are fresh vegetable juices and many Super Foods.™ People with **"stressed"** livers are the ones who suffer with psoriasis, dandruff, ringworm, impetigo, athlete's foot, dry skin, poor nails, cancer, periodontal gum issues, constipation, diverticulitis, colitis, Crohn's and celiac "conditions," acne, irritable bowel, leaky gut, parasites, Alzheimers, and more. Fully, "98%" of the population have "marginal" livers. The need to **de**acidify the terrain and restore liver function is an **"ONGOING"** project. The "terrain" controls! ***By age 45, your author was "aging"—but he "got***

it all back" and more after developing the Young Again Protocol™—and following it!

Mineral Baths & The Liver

Throughout history, mineral springs, hot pools and mud holes have attracted health-minded people. Epsom salt in a "hot" bath is a good "remedy" if water and reacemized™ minerals are drunk **"beforehand!"** Racemized™ clay and charcoal are very useful for absorbing intestinal toxins and rendering them harmless. [See Hot & Cold Therapy on page 399.] The liver is the **"KEY"** to becoming *Young Again!*

PREVIEW: *Our next chapter deals with energy flow, limitless vitality, and the body's toll road system.*

Health & sickness are matters of choice!

High Fructose Corn Syrup

High fructose corn syrup is **MUCH** harder on the body than is sugar because it is a "freak" molecule—and one of the **MAJOR** driving forces behind obesity and diabetes! **Avoid it!**

Prostate Issues

Sooner or later men develop "prostate" trouble. Most men choose **NOT** to deal with their prostate and hide from it until they are in "trouble!" Others swallow the "bait" and go for the cut, burn and poison approach. "Smart" men realize that once upon a time, they did **NOT** have the problem and that "something" has changed! The smart men choose to deal with the prostate **BEFORE** serious trouble erups. [The *Young Again! (Tissue and Liver) Protocol*™, High Enema Therapy™ and R/Prostate™ l & ll solve the dilemma. The point here is if you do like everyone else, you will end up just like "them!"

Racemized™ SUPER FOODS

Here is the list of basic and advanced racemized™ SUPER FOODS used in the *Young Again Protocol(s)*.™ Use them to nourish your body and restore your "terrain."

BASIC Super Foods:
Racemized™ L_sP_cC
Racemized™ Liver
Racemized™ Algae
VitaLight™ Tablets
Harmonic™ Pollen

Harmonic™ Royal Jelly
ADVANCED Super Foods:
H/E™ Powder
TRP Powder™
5 Elements™
High Performance™

SPECIAL Super Foods: Skin & Body Toner™; R/J Factors l & ll™ and Biogenic™ hGH. [See page 149 and Chapters 36-37.]

Heavy Metal Poisoning

Aluminum is a **heavy** metal and is extremely toxic to the body. It—along with mercury, cadmium and lead—accumulate in brain tissue, short-circuiting neuron function and eventually becoming **contributors** to "Alzheimers."

Aluminum alloys contain fluoride, and the "paste" part of common tooth paste comes from the aluminum industry. Put fluoride and aluminum together and you have a very potent recipe! Cities use aluminum to "treat" water. In the presence of the halogen gas "fluorine," aluminum becomes aggressive *and* biologically active. In the body, sodium fluoride—a fluoride "salt"—**dis**associates releasing fluorine gas. [See Chapter 16.]

Aluminum cookware "leaches" into food. The "pits" in cookware are proof! Non-stick resin coatings on aluminum cookware kept at *reasonable* cooking temperatures are **not** an issue—unless the coating deteriorates—exposing the aluminum surface. Stainless steel and cast iron have their share of metal leaching issues. Use descretion and don't over cook.

Some of the **least** suspected **MAJOR** sources of aluminum ions are common baking powder and dill pickles. Look at the ingredient list on a can of baking powder and you will find "alum" listed. **AVOID** all commercially baked goods that use baking powder as the leavening agent. [Non aluminum baking powder is available from health food stores.]

Alum is an "approved" food additive and is listed on the FDA's "GRAS" list ("generally recognized as safe"). Obviously, government watchdog agencies don't have the public's interest in mind or they would not approve alum and thousands of other additives and colorings for dietary consumption. In the body, aluminum reacts with acid wastes and attacks the *nervous system*—accelerating onset of degenerative dis-eases like MS, Peripheral Neuropathy, Cerebral Palsy and Alzheimers.

The human body **needs** "all" of the elements listed on the periodic table of elements. The **deciding factors** are **FORM** and **SOURCE**. Molecular "form" determines toxicity! Ideally, metal ions **should derive** from home-grown and so-called organic foods. [A dependable source is racemized™ sea mineral ions that have "traversed" the **carbon cycle** as discussed in Chapter 28. Colloidal mineral products—and products from "ancient sea bed and plant deposits" are loaded with heavy metals and are in the **WRONG MOLECULAR FORM.**

*[SOC™ and racemized™ algae are chelating substances that shuttle heavy metals across the blood/brain barrier and out of body. VZ II™ "digests" **amyloid** and **scar tissues**—freeing "bound" heavy metals ions for elimination. L_sP_cC™ and PAC's function as "buffers." High Enema Therapy™ speeds the process. Vegetable juice "pigments" help greatly!]*

"Racemization"™

"Racemized™ formulas are exoteric combinations of circular, overlapping energy fields unified to deliver maximum viability and biological activity in the dynamic environment of a living system."

Racemized™ products **"work"** because they are extremely biologically active esoteric **"energy"** formulations that provide maximum benefit and effect in the body's "terrain."

The word **viability** best describes the "effect" racemization™ has on FOOD nutrient molecules. Viability refers to biological *usefulness* and *activity* rather than potency. Racemization™ **"enhances"** food nutrient energy profiles by expanding the esoteric aspects of their "footprints."

Racemized™ products carry a dual rating: "biological activity" and "energy footprint." These indicate *potential* available energy and **expected** biological response. Ratings are **NOT** a measure of carbohydrates, fats, proteins or calories; they are a measure of *life force activity* in living systems.

The racemization™ scale is 0-10. All right-spin substances receive a **static** reference score of "0" keyed to their energy profiles. The reference score is then elevated by a factor of "10x." This four-step *proprietary* process **unifies, boosts, stabilizes** and **locks** energy frequency(s) so esoteric aspects of their energy profiles can be stabilized and utilized.

[Energy is never lost; it merely changes form! The benefits of racemized™ formulations are Fourth Dimentional in nature, and their esoteric aspects are not contained in "physical" form; therefore, they are not contained in physical shipment format. "Transfer" of energy is the issue here!]

Racemization™ does **not** involve the use of magnetics, homeopathy or other processes. Racemization™ has **NO** historical analog. It is **NOT** a physical process!

Racemized™ products carry a 10/10 reference score, giving them far more *viability* in the body than the same formulation in a non-racemized™ energy state. Racemized™ products offer good **value** and **results** to the user despite their cost. Racemized™ products have **NO** equal in the marketplace and are **ONLY** made available directly to the end user and **NEVER** through distribution channels. People who follow the *Young Again Protocol(s)™* know the value of these concepts.

*[The **"hallmark"** of the Young Again Protocol(s)™ is personal "mentoring" made available to everyone **without** fee regardless of individual status. People "like" being treated as human beings, and John Thomas makes himself available to anyone desiring help from "The guy who wrote the book!"]*

"Everything In Excess Is Opposed By Nature."
Hippocrates

28

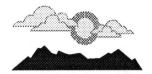

Soil To Sea

"Man does not die; he kills himself."
Seneca

People love the seaside because the "ionized" air and water makes them feel good! It buzzes with electricity! "Ionized" air and water invigorates them! Walking barefoot in the sand siphons away toxic energy from the reflex points in the feet. **"Charged"** mineral ions gives the sea's air, water and sand "healing" qualities! [Charged ions are (+) or (-) electrons.]

The sea is nature's storage battery of right-spin **ENERGY!** It is a phenomenon of tremendous importance. Understanding the source of the sea's energy is central to good health and the aging reversal process.

Mineral **ions** in solution are called **electrolytes**. Ions are atoms that have gained or lost electrons—signified by the + or - sign and a number in raised position next to the atomic element symbol such as Na^{-1}. The + or - indicates the atom is long or short on electrons and that the atom is looking for a way to complete the "valence" of its outer electrical shell so it can "stabilize." Ionic stability occurs when competing atoms "share" electrons. For example, sodium + chlorine = sodium chloride. Table salt is "stable." [**"Oxidized"** (+) and **"reduced"** (-) are chemistry terms describing the electrical **"charge"** of atoms in regard to extra or missing electrons.]

Ionic **"compounds"** are composed of two or more atoms that "bond" by **"SHARING"** electrons. Usually one is an acid "gas"—like chlorine—and the other is an alkaline earth mineral—like sodium. Ionic compounds are crystalline "salts." "Salts" has an "s" because thousands of such compounds are salts. Salts are "chemically" **STABLE** until "hydrolyzed" in water or body fluids—causing them to **"dis**associate" and take on a **"charged"** condition. [Mineral ions that have not gone through the carbon cycle—like table salt or calcium carbonate—have a unhealthy affect on the **"terrain"** of the *bio-electric* body. Racemized™ sea mineral ions have all the desirable characteristics needed for a healthy "terrain"]

Some mineral ions "conduct" electricity in "solution." Others do not! Electrolytes that are capable of conducting electrical current are always **"metal"** ions like sodium, calcium, potassium and magnesium that **"SHARE"** electrons with other elements in order to "stabilize." [The only exception is nitrogen gas in its "metallic" form.] Sodium, for example, is highly unstable in elemental form—and must be stored in oil to avoid exposure to air and moisture to avoid **VIOLENT** reactions in an attempt to "bond." [Racemized™ sea minerals are broad-spectrum electrolytes that **"conduct"** electricity. They are so active that they can STOP an electrolytic heart attack if given at the time of or immediately after the event. They work similarly for heat stroke or heat exhaustion.]

Death by "electrocution" is dependent upon mineral electrolyte conductors, a power source and a ground!
Blood and lymphatic fluids carry electrolytes. The nervous system cannot function without them. Electrolytes **"conduct"** electrical energy and **"transfer"** electrical signals from one end of the body to the other via the nerve fibers. [Insufficient fluid electrolytes or a sodium-dominated "terrain" environment produce pathological dis-ease.]

The sodium "ion" is the most common electrolyte— but that not mean sodium should serve as the body's "primary" electrolyte.
We need sodium in **VERY** small amounts. Too much sodium upsets the sodium : potassium ratio—setting the stage for cancer. Given **"no choice,"** the body will use sodium ions in lieu of a balance of many electrolytes. [Electrolytes derived from sea water "balance" the electrical terrain of the body. Unfortunately, they are lacking in the food supply. Plants cannot absorb mineral electrolytes from soil if they do **NOT** exist or if "terrain" conditions in the soil make them "unavailable" or prevent biological "transmutation." See Chapter 18.]

The best way to insure sufficient electrolytic balance is to use racemized™ sea minerals in each glass of drinking water. Body electrolytes MUST be supplied all day every day to avoid premature aging.

Toll Road
It is helpful to think of the nervous system as a toll road where a price must be paid **BEFORE** each nerve signal is allowed to cross a synapse on its way to its destination— perhaps a finger or leg. Think of synapses as **"toll booths"** along the nerve axon. Schwann's cells keep the gate open by producing hormones that polish the receptors at the synapses. Mineral ions supply the energy that **BOOSTS** nerve impulses so the **signal** can **"jump the gap"** and continue to its destination. [See axon diagram on page 248.]
The body conducts its affairs using "electrical" currency. A unit of electrical *currency* is called a mineral *ion.* As

nerve impulses jump the synapses, mineral ions **"give up"** electrons that supply the energy to fuel the process. The body needs a **constant** supply of biologically active mineral ions. Minerals **not** in ionic form—like colloidal minerals and so-called "mined" ancient earth deposits—do **NOT** suffice. [The word "colloid" refers to a state of "suspension" and particle size. "Ionic" refers to a state of electrical "conductivity!" Disrupted electrical signals produce **"spastic"** motions, making it difficult to move smoothly and function normally. Nerve disorders are classic examples of sporadic, *uncontrolled* electrical impulses. Shingles and Peripheral Neuropathy involve deterioration of the neurolemma (myelin sheath), a vitamin B-12 shortfall, and diminished Schwann's cell activity at the synapses. [SOC,™ Cobo-12™ creme and FG creme (women) and MG™ creme (men) help restore nerve function and synapse activity.]

Athletes & Sports Drinks

Athletes associate performance, strength and vitality with "electrolytes!" They know their bodies will **NOT** perform or hold up to heavy physical stress without enough electrolytes. They drink **"sports drinks"** to get by—and in the end shoot themselves in the foot because of the imbalances and "excess" they create in their bodies. [Smart athletes make their own sports drinks using **racemized**™ sea water ions and water— and they make and drink Kombucha Tea, too! See pages 106,133, 133, 162, 340 and Chapter 38.]

[Non-athletes also need balanced electrolytes—but unlike athletes who burn out in a few short years, non-athletes burn out over many years in slow motion—a day at a time!]

*[All mineral ions are **NOT** equal. Those that have gone through the carbon cycle—like racemized™ sea minerals ions— provide indisputable results! Synchronized earth-mineral deposits dug out of the ground and hydrolyzed into a liquid—and minerals in colloidal form, are poor choices because their **signature** is unfriendly—and they are **LOADED** with heavy metals like lead and cadmium in the wrong molecular forms.]*

*[Children need mineral electrolytes for their brains to "function"—and for their bodies to grow. Teach them to make their own sports drink and avoid sugar and bio-junk! My children **voluntarily** lugged their ionized BFRV™ water to school each day in their special BFRV™ bottles. They loved it and did better in the classroom and in sports. They called it "power water!" All their friends bummed water from them so they could benefit, too! Instead of being "weird," they turned a simple idea into an advantage—socially speaking!]*

As for drinking water, BFRV™ water has a "conception point" ORP potential. [See page 306!] The water's high-energy *footprint* comes from the **restructuring** of the water molecule and erasing of the **memory** of the contaminants the water contained "before" it was transformed into BFRV™ water. BFRV™ water resonates a "healthy" frequency—and when racemized™ sea minerals are added it truly is "power water" because of its electrical affects on the terrain.

[*"Wanna be" water competitors can't get past Third Dimension mentality that says "water is water"—so they ride your author's coattails and the "terrain" concepts of the Young Again Protocols.™ They just don't get it!*]

Electrical "current" is the movement of energy along a conductor—like a copper wire. In blood and lymph, ionic mineral ions ARE the wire!

$10,000 For A Bag Of Salt

Ions in solution cause electricity to "flow!" No flow means no conductors (electrolytes) are in "solution!"

Dr. Carry Reams was once paid $10,000 for **solving** a electroplating problem at a chrome "plating" shop involving electrolytes in "solution" and "electrolysis!" No one—including the manufacturer of the equipment—could get electricity to "flow" and electrolysis to occur. Reams poured a few pounds of common table salt into the solution and bingo, the plating process went to completion! Sodium chloride solved the electrolysis problem because sodium is an *electrolyte.*

The human body requires a "balanced" and "constant" supply of electrolytic mineral ions for optimum health. Substitution of table salt—with its **"unbalanced"** mineral ion load of sodium—creates "terrain" conditions that "mask" fundamental health issues and set the stage for dis-ease and the doctor's diagnosis. [The poor patient never sees it coming!]

Excess sodium accelerates aging and makes things "seem" fine—until cellular potassium levels are depleted! Excess sodium is a poison and a preservative!

Sugar

Sucrose (table sugar) is a "crystal"—but sucrose **CANNOT conduct electrical current when dissolved in water.** Sucrose is **NOT** a conductor because it contains **NO** electrolytes. Sugar is a "concentrated" left-spin energy substance in crystalline form that lowers the body's vibratory frequency and dims the aura by **depleting** the terrain of **"electrolytes!"** [Sugar consumption causes hair to turn "gray" by withdrawing electrolytes from the hair itself!]

Sucrose *sabotages* energy flow, causing the *bio-electric* body to eventually "collapse!" It does it by **"bonding"** with trace mineral electrolytes whose job it is to "conduct" electrical impulses at the nerve synapses along the nerve fibers. When mineral ions "bond" with sugar, their energy potential is **NEUTRALIZED!** When the supply of trace mineral electrolytes is low enough, a health crisis occurs—and aging accelerates! *If you choose to eat food laced with table sugar, you will lose your vitality and grow old.*

[People live their lives on the edge of starvation; their diets are totally inadequate and loaded with enough sodium ions for them to "exist" between subsistence and dis-ease.]

[Earlier, we discussed Kombucha tea. It is important that the reader understand that the Kombucha organism has the ability to convert the most powerful left-spin substance—white sugar—into an equally powerful right-spin energy substance that is loaded with enzymes and healthful "organic acids." The organism uses biological alchemy—as discussed in Chapter 16—to flip-flop the energy footprint of the "solution." The sugar is "gone"—and healthy energy remains!]

The Second Law of Thermodynatics states "energy is never lost; it merely changes form!" Believe it!

"Experts" tell us sugar is sugar. **They** tell us there is NO difference between sucrose, maltose, invert, dextrose and lactose—except in their molecular structures. **They** tell us that mannitol, sorbitol and "aspartame" are harmless! **They** tell us *"The body does not care because in the end, sugar is sugar!"* **They** tell us the "sugar blues" haunting millions of people are "imagined!" The experts are **wrong!**

The body differentiates between sugars as it does with oils based on their energy footprints.

Some sugars accelerate aging by neutralizing the body's supply of mineral ions. Table sugar and artificial sweetners **destroy** food energy by stealing electrons from food molecules through "ionization." [Translation: food molecules are altered through gain or loss of mineral electrons.] **Purified** sugars like table sugar, fructose, high fructose corn syrup and inverted sugar are a biological "disaster" and **MUST** be avoided!

Artificial sugars—like aspartame which is better known by the red, white, and blue **"swirl"** and the latest **"xxxx from sugar"** artificial sweetener have **radiomimetic** qualities that "alter" cellular DNA. Food additives and coloring agents do the same thing! These poisons "zap" body energy and are no different than eating irradiated, microwaved food. All of them bring on gray hair, aged skin, diminished glandular activity and hormone imbalances by **stealing** mineral ions and **"locking up"** body receptors—while **DEVASTATING** the "terrain!" Their effects are characteristic of "zeno" estrogen analogous molecules found in drugs and in the environment.

Foods processed with large amounts of sugar and salt do **not** spoil because their enzymes have been scrambled and deactivated. Bugs do **NOT** eat white sugar and sodium chlo-

ride-laden food. They are **NOT** stupid—but humans are "dumb!"
If you MUST choose between table sugar and arti-ficial sweeteners—choose sugar! VitaLight™ tablets and racemized mineral ions buffer the effects of sugar by "loading" your system with active trace mineral ions.

Major & Minor Minerals

The body needs both **major** minerals and **minor** (trace) minerals to function. Science has known about the major minerals like calcium, potassium, sulphur, and phosphorous for a very long time. Trace minerals—like manganese, boron, iodine, molybdenum, and 60 or so others—have only recently been recognized to be of any importance in human nutrition. [Science is reluctant to acknowledge man's mineral dependence, yet it **"rubber stamps"** the use of soy, canola, aspartame and genetically altered "stuff!"]

We **KNOW** minerals are crucial to maintaining good health and longevity. What is **NOT** widely known is that the "form" of the mineral is as important as the mineral itself. Molecular "form" determines a mineral's **effect** on health.

Elemental mineral compounds are of no use to the body. Calcium carbonate is an elemental compound used to supplement *so-called* calcium "deficiency"—but instead it creates a condition of **"EXCESS!"** Supposedly, lack of calcium is responsible for osteoporosis—but calcium "deficiency" has **"NOTHING"** to do with it—and everything to do with why women are dropping like flies with heart attack. [See pages 38, 58, 85, 91-4, 152, 157-8, 170, 274, 300, 338 and 373.]

Elemental mineral compounds do NOT belong in the body. They foul our nest and create secondary health problems because the body cannot use them.

The "**-ate**" at the tail-end of the word "carbon**ate**" tells says the compound is in "salt" form—meaning a crystal! Taking calcium carbonate to get more "calcium" is the equivalent of a postpartum woman drinking milk so she can produce more breast milk for her baby—or taking chondroitin sulfate and glucosamine sulfate to make "cartilage," which they do not!

Synthetically "chelated" minerals cause problems. "Chelated" means elemental mineral are "bonded" to amino acid "transports" to get them into the blood. **This is NOT desirable!** Tricking or forcing the body to accept that which it otherwise would **NOT** accept creates conditions of **"excess"** which leads to dis-ease and aging! Elemental mineral compounds have **NOT** gone through the carbon chain. Do **NOT** use them.

Biologically active mineral ions should derive from vegetable juices, "unprocessed" food, healthy animal tissues, racemized™ sea mineral ions, and SUPER foods like racemized™ algae, predigested, racemized™ liver capsules, Harmonic™ pollen and Royal Jelly.

Enzymes • Minerals • Nitrogen

Enzymes are nitrogen-containing protein "molecules" that function as **ENGINEERS** in charge of the "toll gates" that control the flow of "energy!" Enzymes are mineral ion **dependent**—and they create energy "hot spots" that "throw the switch" so blood and lymph fluids can transport energy and waste. [Biologically active "soil" and healthy plants function on the same basis using the bacteria as the "mediators!"]

Nitrogen plays a **KEY** role in the life process. All body tissues are made of amino acid "proteins" containing "nitrogen" in their molecular stucture. Nitrogen is **NOT** a "metallic" mineral ion in the "physical" sense of a metal. Nitrogen is a "gas" that occurs in several "states." In its "metallic" gaseous state, nitrogen conducts electricity [Think of "lightening" in the sky!] and functions just like a metal ion "electrolyte!"

Nitrogen—atomic symbol "N"—is an important factor in building healthy connective tissue and in the health and longevity story. Life **cannot** exist without nitrogen. The atmosphere is composed of 78% nitrogen. Plants and animals require nitrogen to grow. The experts use **synthesized** nitrogen "salts" to FORCE crop production on the premise that *"Food is food!"* But nature does not produce high-vitality food in an unbalanced environment. Nature responds with "left-spin" energy food that is high in **"funny proteins."**

Funny Proteins

"Funny proteins" are "unavailable" proteins—that is, proteins that confuse the body—and soy is a "classic" example. Food protein is measured by its **nitrogen** content. When you hear nutritionists and farmers talk about food and crop **protein** percentages, their "yardstick" is calibrated in **"%"** of nitrogen" content. In other words, they are using a "proxy!"

Nitrogen is a gas. Unbuffered, it is an **acid** gas with a pH of "1-2!" When proteins are fully digested and broken down into their constituent parts, nitrogen gas is released. [Think of a rotting carcass that is off-gassing foul-smelling nitrogen gas!]

Imagine the **"acidic"** effect on the "terrain" that occurs when nitrogen containing dietary proteins fail to "digest" for lack of sufficient stomach acid or when body tissue dies and breaks down—as when someone is very sick or dying and they are consuming their own "muscle mass." [Body odor and the smell of death have much in common!]

When the vegetarian body consumes its own tissues, it becomes a meat eater! Think about that!

"Funny" proteins contain nitrogen in the **wrong** form. When eaten, their nitrogens creates a condition of **"EXCESS"** that requires large amounts of calcium to be **"withdrawn"** from the bones to buffer the acidic effects.

Environmental deterioration from high-powered, synthetic salt fertilizers and poisonous sprays used in agriculture is one reason more and more **"funny protein"** is entering the food chain—and as **"freak"** protein levels rise, so does the occurrence of degenerative dis-ease.

Look at a bag of dog or cat food. It lists total protein and crude (unavailable) protein. If you subtract one from the other, you get available protein. Not so many years ago, the amount of unavailable protein was under 1/2%. Today, it is as high as 2%—and more! The rise reflects the amount of "funny" protein in the food supply. [Undigested proteins "rot" in the gut if **insufficient** stomach acid is secreted. Poor protein assimilation translates as a weak, emaciated, low muscle-mass body. Use R/BHCl to remedy this problem.]

As the level of funny protein doubles—for example from 1/2% to 1%—the amount of calcium needed to stabilize blood pH increases by 200 times! And where does the body get the calcium? From the bones, ladies! And it's called osteoporosis when the condition finally becomes diagnosable about 20+ years AFTER the process began.

Your author has stated **repeatedly** that there is **NO** such thing as a "deficiency" condition or dis-ease. So-called deficiencies result from conditions of **EXCESS!** For example, osteoporosis **ONLY** occurs in a highly **"acid"** body terrain. Medical science shouts **"deficiency"** of calcium—when the problem is acidic **"excess!"** [The body stores excess acidic waste in the fatty tissues beneath the skin.]

Millions of cells die each day—and if the break-down products are not promptly removed, **nitrogen-based** acid wastes **"FLOOD"** the system and force the body to withdraw mineral from the bones to "buffer" the acids. Aging is really nothing more than progressive **"acidification"** of the terrain.

*[The best way to reverse **acidification** is by following the Young Again (Tissue and Liver) Protocol(s).™ Drinking small amounts of fresh beet and carrot juice along with Kombucha Tea and unpasteurized sauerkraut help greatly. High Enema Therapy™ is an absolute "must!"]*

Nitrogen & Plants

Nitrogen is the unit of **electrical currency** that opens the plant's "toll gates" so energy and mineral ions can travel to enzyme-created "hot spots" in the plant's tissues.

Chemical agriculture has learned how to trick and force plants into "uptaking" unwanted minerals and poisons into their tissues. [This is the same idea of using "chelated" elemental mineral compounds in supplement form.] "Forcing" crops to grow on hard-core chemicals in soil water "solution" is based on the **assumption** that God, Nature, plants and the body are stupid—but the *experts* are smart! Chelation of minerals smacks of the same mentality that says "*Genetically engineered and hydroponically raised food is no different than food grown on healthy soils.*" These bogus practices supposedly render "moot" the need for healthy soil—and the same can be said for microwaved vs. conventionally cooked food!

Nature designed things so the elements would have to "pass through" the carbon cycle before gaining legitimacy and a ticket into plant, animal and human tissue.

The Carbon Cycle

The "carbon cycle" explains how earth minerals are *ionized* and *assimilated* into food molecules—and how mineral ions become part of sea water. The carbon cycle *transforms* biologically inactive earth minerals into active, right-spin *energy* fields that people can use to maintain or regain their health. Here is the formula.

CARBON CYCLE = rain + soil + sun + microbe + plant + animal = biologically "enlivened" mineral ions.

Bacteria in the soil are the **bankers** for earth mineral ions. Ions are "made available" when elemental earth mineral compounds react with weak organic acids—like carbonic acid— **secreted** from plant roots. [Atmospheric carbon + hydrogen = carbonic acid!] Bacteria "retain" and "modify" mineral ions— and live on their electrical energy until the plant withdraws the mineral "ions" from its "account." **Enzymes** are the **tellers** overseeing the exchange of mineral ion "currency."

Plants use solar energy to make proteins, fats, carbohydrates, vitamins and enzymes that contain biologically active mineral ions supplied by the microbes.

Animals eat plants and deposit their waste on the soil for the microbes to consume. Plants grow, die and leave their residues on the soil for bacteria, yeast, and fungi to consume. In time, nutrient ions find their way to the sea where they become a **"solution"** of biologically active ionic minerals. Mineral ions give sea water its characteristic salty flavor and "energy"—and they are responsible for the "energy" associated with the seaside. [Racemized™ sea mineral ions provide the body with electrical "currency" for maintenance of health and vitality. Their beneficial affect on body physiology is **"confirmation"** of their electrical **"valence!"**]

Vitamins

Vitamins **cannot** perform their job unless needed mineral ions are available in **BOTH** balanced and active molecular form. Vitamins are NOT well understood—but we do know they are mineral "dependent." Science has had to *shadow box* with vitamins, learning of their importance through so-called **deficiency** conditions.

The word **vitamin** derives from "vital"—meaning *necessary*, and "amine"—which is the chemical name for a nitrogen bearing "—R group" molecule. [See Chapter 33!]

The word *amino*—as in **amino acid**—also derives from the word, *amine*. Aminos "join" and form molecules called proteins—and proteins contain **nitrogen!** Also common to protein structures is "carbon" and "sulphur!" [SOC™ supplies racemized™ carbon and sulfur for building **sulfhydryl** bonds that are critical to healthy tissues.]

SOC™ capsules and SOC™ lotion boost blood and nerve activity in congested and traumatized tissues. VZ™ DIGESTS amyloid plaque and scar tissue. L$_s$P$_c$C™ stimulates the body to lay down additional "new" collagen.

Amino acids, fats and carbohydrates are organic molecules resulting from **"anabolic"** activity in living things. [See pages 21 and 198!] Organic molecules contain oxygen, nitrogen, sulfur and carbon. The presence of **carbon** in a molecule qualifies it as "organic!" **Carbon**aceous matter (leaves, grass, wood, etc.) contains carbon. **Carbo**hydrates contain carbon. Life is impossible without carbon. A vitamin is a nitrogen containing substance containing a **carbon** amine "—R" group.

[Earlier, we talked about a family of toxic chemical molecules found in "chlorinated" municipal drinking water called "chloramines." The chemicals cities use to treat public drinking water produces "chloramines!" Chlorine gas molecules in "solution" bond to carbon-containing organic substances in water-forming "chloramines." Organic means anything that is carbon based. Toxic chemicals and chloramines in bathing water "penetrate" the skin and damage the "liver!" They DEVASTATE the gut wall, causing a leaky-gut condition in people of ALL ages—including children.]

Man-made vitamins stress the liver and are toxic—and do **NOT** build healthy tissue. Real, live food and vegetable juices are the best vitamin source! Your author prefers **food-based** vitamin supplements. In biochemistry, vitamins are referred to as **cofactors** or **coenzymes.** Vitamins and mineral ions need each other to work. Please **ENGRAVE** the following statement into your consciousness—and never forget it!

Man DOES NOT live on vitamins, minerals and enzymes—but from the energy released by the chemical reactions they fuel! Believe it!

The Carbon Connection

In his timeless book *The Carbon Cycle*, my friend, Leonard Ridzon defined carbon as *"The governing element that determines the vitality of food crops [and life on Earth]."*

Carbon is extremely important to the aging process. It is **THE** common denominator in high-vitality food and healthy soils. Carbon is the barometer of the soil's aura and magnetic field. It is the basis of all life.

Carbon can combine in **millions** of combinations because of its unique molecular form. *Bogus* science uses carbon to create organic poisons—like pesticides and herbicides.

Highly magnetic soil is called, **"para**magnetic" (*para*-beyond). Paramagnetic soil grows right-spin, high-energy food with a "healthy" energy signature.

Devitalized soil has **NO** "paramagnetism"—and food grown on it does **NOT** sustain human beings, barnyard animals or plants. Sick soil is **LOW** in carbon and microbial activity. Sick food translates *"sick people!"*

The fastest and best way to convert sick dirt into vibrant soil is through *biodynamic principles* as described in *Biodynamic Farm, Biodynamics I & II and Introduction to Biodynamics.*

Avail yourself of biodynamic principles and turn polluted soil into a nice garden the first year with the product "BioGrow." [See pages 147 and 305.]

The ideal food is fresh, home-grown fruits and vegetables that are packed with life-giving nutrients and right-spin energy. Next comes store- bought "organic" food. [Racemized™ supplements boost both.]

[Your author wants to stay YOUNG—and biologically active mineral ions are the electrical currency he uses to "trigger" biochemical processes, stabilize the heart, boost energy and endurance and prevent Rouleau in the blood!"]

Tend to the "basics" and you won't grow old and die prematurely. Tend to the basics and you will **NOT** need doctors **OR** the **"sick care"** system. Implement the information in this book and you, too, will become *Young Again!*

PREVIEW: *Our next chapter is about the immune system and cancer and how to avoid dis-ease.*

Beatings!

"The beatings shall continue until the morale improves!" This approach does **NOT** get good results—at work, in your personal life or in matters of health. Stop the blame game and make meaningful changes in your life and your "moral" will improve!

Hard Wired!

The reflex points in the feet are **hard wired** to the "vital" organs—and so are the nerves flowing from the colon wall. High Enema Therapy™ stimulates nerve-flow and increases bile-flow from the liver. Acupuncture and reflexology work on the same principal. Does the reader "see" the connection?

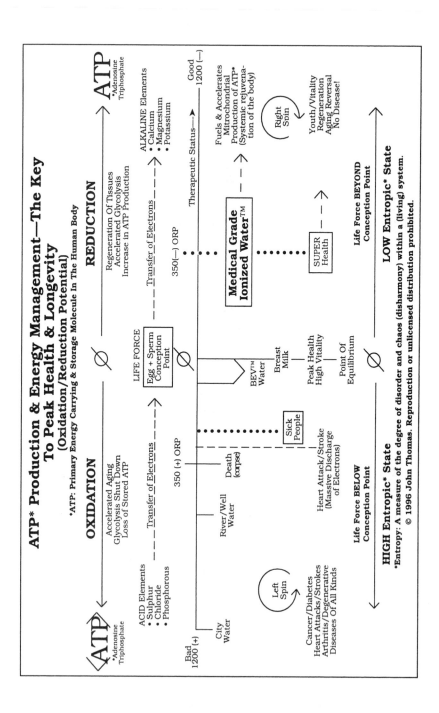

Cancer Tumors vs. Cancer Masses
They are NOT the same!

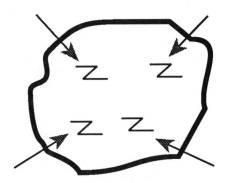

Cancer Tumors
Import & Condense Energy
Tumors calcify; appear on
X-rays, CAT Scans, & MRI's;
can be felt with hand; do not
have an "occult" phase.

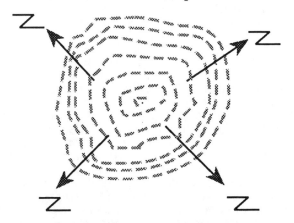

Cancer Masses Export And Disperse Energy
True masses do **not** calcify or
appear on X-rays, CAT Scans or MRI's;
they are soft to touch; and they
are invisible during occult phase.

High Blood Pressure

Hypertension is **NOT** a good thing—and neither is the hard core
drugs used to control it. The Young Again™ answer to these
problems is called NTV.™ It's effective and there are no side
effects like "drugs!" [See pages 315 and 316.]

The Rouleau Effect

The battle for health and longevity is a "terrain" issue that is **won** or **lost** at the "cellular level" where the very fine blood capillary beds "interface" the cells.

Blood corpuscles "tumble" through the very fine blood capillaries one at a time! A corpuscle is a *denucleated* blood cell, that is, a blood cell **without** a nucleus. [A cell and nucleus looks like a chicken's egg without a yoke. An egg is a single cell.]

As cells and tissue spaces overload with **amyloid acid wastes,** the body's energy *footprint* shifts to the left—and blood assumes a "sticky" appearance. Sticky blood is the **EFFECT** of a condition called *Rouleau.* When Rouleau occurs, free movement of blood corpuscles servicing the cells "stalls"—causing the tissue "stress" due to insufficient oxygen, carbon dioxide, waste and nutrient movement. Eventually the condition manifests as a "not-so-nice" dis-ease.

Racemized™ sea minerals break up the *Rouleau Effect* in blood. A short squirt of these ions in every glass of water you drink—regardless of the type of water it is—does the job! The "ionic" effect is an energy response that **translates** as good health and high vitality. [See pages 136 and 294 for a better understanding of these issues.]

SLOWDOWN in the *bilateral movement* of oxygen, nutrients, carbon dioxide and waste in the tissues leads to **aging!** Aging is another word for "self-inflicted" fouling of our own nest—and the fouler we become, the faster we age!

"Stagnation" of **intra**cellular fluids **"within"** the tissue spaces causes the cells to die. Conditions like cancer, arthritis, fibromyalgia and hundreds of other so-called "dis-eases" have their roots in stagnant **AMYLOID** fluid and unbalanced **intra**cellular (inside the cell) fluids, which are an invitation for sodium to invade the cells as potasium is withdrawn to meet they body's needs. [The body does **NOT** "store" potassium. Removal of cellular potassium is shuts-down the cell!]

[SOC™ "triggers" increased **blood flow** and **nerve activity** in scarred and traumatized tissue. VZ™ "eats" amyloid plaque and scar tissue. In time, aches and pains **go away** and the body becomes more "limber" and free moving. SOC™ provides the raw materials the body needs to build **sulfonyl bearing** connective tissue proteins that replace damaged and "digested" amyloid and scar tissues.]

If you wish to regain your health—or hold onto what you have—it's **VERY** important to provide your body with a **constant** flow of racemized™ sea mineral ions. These inexpensive ions provide the benefits of free-flowing blood without the dangers associated with pharmaceutical "blood thinners." They also assist in getting sound sleep—and leg cramps and charleyhorses go *"bye" "bye"* when a liberal dose of these ions are taken immediately before going to bed. Elimination of the **Rouleau Effect** has profound implications for health and longevity. In the end, good health is a matter of **choice!** Rouleau is a **TERRAIN** issue! Don't forget it.

29

Body Fluid Dynamics

*"When science falters, it is because no one
is asking the right questions."*
Charles Walters

Blood is **central** to all body metabolism. Blood carries oxygen and nutrients to the cells by way of the arteries and capillary beds "imbeded" in the tissue spaces. Blood hemoglobin transports oxygen into the tissue spaces and carbon dioxide (CO_2)from **"cellular"** respiration **OUT** of the tissues spaces and **OUT** of the body by "external" respiration in the lungs. [Low "hemoglobin" and blood-iron levels equate to low energy and **EXCESS** accumulation of highly acidic CO_2.]

"Tissue" waste is **NOT** removed by the blood—but by the lymphatic system which deposits the waste into the blood. The waste is filtered from the blood by the liver and deposited as "bile" in the gall bladder. The kidneys process about 10% of body waste—while liver-produced bile transports 90% of the body's waste via the bowel. [Poor liver function and low bile flow cause the body to turn **"ACID"** and age very rapidly!]

Blood is *systemic* because it **"interfaces"** all body systems. It is an excellent "test" medium and a "clinical" barometer of present or pending dis-ease. Blood is the primary fluid "tissue" for determining "state" of health. Urine and cerebral/spinal fluid tell their own stories. [Lymphatic fluids are **"ignored"** and considered "moot" by the medical system.]

The blood system's fraternal twin—**the lymphatic system**—complements the blood circulatory system and **"interfaces"** with all body tissues, organs and systems. [Think of the lymphatic system as the "other half" of the body's plasma protein communication network—the **MOST** important half.]

The lymphatic system does **NOT** have a "heart" to pump its fluids. Lymph fluid is straw-to-clear in color—not red—and unlike blood, no one will buy lymph fluid from you. And, if there is an emergency, no one will ask you to donate lymph fluid.

It is impossible to reverse the SIGNS and symptoms of aging and dis-ease if the lymphatic system is ignored.

"Lymph" circulation occurs when we walk, run, swim or exercise—and when we breath deeply or do load-bearing work.

We do more of these activities when we are young and healthy—and **"avoid"** them as we grow "older!" [We must perform load-bearing physical work if we expect to stay young. [Women are trained to "avoid" hard work. These days—2006—men are "choosing" to do the same. Both sexes are paying the price!]

The lymphatic system is a network of capillaries and vessels similar to the blood system, but with some notable differences. Lymph capillaries begin as blind alleys while blood capillaries "transition" from **oxygen**ated arterial blood capillaries to **de**oxygenated venus blood capillaries that are "continuous." The lymphatic system has "nodes;" the blood system has none. Lymph vessels are "valved" for one way movement of fluids; the blood system has no valves. Lymphatic capillary walls are more "permeable" than blood capillary walls.

The lymphatic system is a plasma protein **"communication"** system responsible for returning acidic, waste-laden, tissue fluids to the blood for filtering by the liver. Tissue fluid entering lymph capillaries cannot escape until deposited into "returning" blood at the subclavian vein just "prior" to the where returning **de**oxygenated blood enters the heart.

It is **IMPORTANT** to recognize that lymph "nodes" are energy storage sites where **TOXIC** energy is "held" for safekeeping until the liver can deal with it. That is why lymph nodes in the armpits, under and outside the breasts or in the groin swell and become hard. They are holding "condensed" energy. [The tonsils are lymph nodes that swell and become inflamed during illness.]

*[The "rebounder" and Biogenic™ Lymph Roller are used to circulate lymphatic fluids. The **best** way to improve lymph **drainage** and cerebral spinal fluid **circulation** is with the L/CSF™ machine. People who are physically limited or who hate to exercise can benefit greatly from using the L/CSF.™ See Pages 107, 160, 381 and 385.]*

The 10% Leak

The blood circulatory system has 10% "leakage" built into the system! Blood is pumped into the arteries under **pressure** from the heart muscle—but only 90% of blood "volume" exiting the heart returns as "blood!" The 10% leakage is through the blood capillary walls **INTO** the tissue spaces as **"plasma"** proteins. These fluid proteins "service" the cells with oxygen and nutrients and become the "medium" for removal of intercellular (inside the cell) fluid waste.

The lymphatic system performs critical functions the cardiovascular system is NOT designed to perform.

Tissue fluid picked up by the lymph capillaries is called "lymph" fluid. Tissue fluid **not** picked up by the lymph system is called **"AMYLOID"** fluid. About 10-15% of tissue fluid is

"NOT" absorbed by the lymph capillaries. Fluid left behind is **"soluble,"** "stagnant" amyloid fluid. In time, **STAGNANT** amyloid fluid morphs into **"non-soluble"** amyloid "plaque"—and eventually **"scar"** tissue! Amyloid plaque is **STRUCTURAL** "brick and mortar" that **"cannot"** circulate because it is no longer in a fluid "state!" [VZ™ "digests" amyloid plaque, returning it to a "fluid state" so the lymphatic system can transport it to the liver for removal in "bile." Yucca Blend™ acts like dish soap by emulsifying tissue wastes so they will **"FLOW!"**]

Lymphatics & Aging

The lymphatic system is the **MOST IMPORTANT** system in the body because failure to circulate highly acid waste causes the body **OVERLOAD** and "collapse!" A functional lymphatic system and heavy bile flow translate as good health.

Aging and dis-ease are **"confirmation"** of an acid "terrain" and sluggish lymphatic system. "90%" of routine blood-waste removal falls upon the liver. And if the liver fails to do its job, the body's **"ONLY"** option is to **"STORE"** circulating, "soluble" waste in the fatty tissues beneath the skin. [These wastes are in "soluble" form; they are not in structural form like amyloid plaque and scar tissue.] Waste is taken "out" of circulation and stored to get it as far **"away"** from the vital organs as the body can "park" the stuff! [Ideally, these soluble wastes leave the body each day in "bile!"]

Waste "congested" tissues **"PREVENT"** the body from "cleansing" itself while denying needed oxygen and nutrients. Waste accumulation **"RAISES"** tissue "pH," speeds breakdown of connective tissue, and skews the sodium : potassium ratio in **BOTH** circulating and non-circulating "tissue" fluids. [Blood and lymph fluids are "liquid" tissues!]

[The lymphatic organs are the lymph nodes, thymus gland, tonsils, spleen and red bone marrow. Lymphocytes and macrophages are also part of the lymphatic system.]

Cancer BEGINS in the lymphatic system and metastasizes (spreads) by way of the body's plasma protein highway—the lymphatic system.

Fats & The Immune System

lymphocytes and **macro**phages in the blood and lymph fluids protect the body from invading microbes and foreign substances entering the blood stream because of a "leaky" gut!

Lymphocytes include T-cells and B-cells. B-cells originate in the bone marrow, and some become **plasma** cells that secrete **"antibodies."** **Anti**bodies conduct warfare against invading **anti**gens in body fluids. [Nail fungus and skin "conditions" are external **SIGNS** of acid waste overload—and trouble to come. **SIGNS** and **symptoms** always give way to dis-ease.

Edema is confirmation of systemic OVERLOAD and stagnation of amyloid fluid and waste in the tissues.

Exercise & Lymphatics

The "primary" purpose of exercise is to circulate lymphatic fluid. Exercise enhances "lymph flow" through body movement and muscle contraction. Brisk "walking" is one of the very best exercises. Women who "exaggerate" arm movement when walking would be smarter to allow their arms to swing naturally. Naturally swinging arms are **"FAR"** more effective than the ridiculous antics prescribed by the "experts!"

[Let's demonstrate the dynamics of lymph movement and "electrolyte" activity. First, have the person stand erect and extend one arm straight out to the side of the body level with the shoulder. Next, attempt to gently but forcefully pull down on the arm and note the amount of "resistance" generated. Then have the person **run in place** *for about 10 seconds. Now, repeat step one and note the loss of resistance and strength. We are demonstrating lymph displacement and loss of* **"charged"** *mineral ions as discussed in Chapter 28.]*

Lymph • Red Bone Marrow • Fluoride

Red bone marrow is that part of the lymphatic system responsible for red blood cell production. Red bone marrow is located in the "flat" bones of the body [chest, hip and back] and in the "epiphyses" (ends) of the *long* bones. **Between** the *epiphyses* and diaphyses is where the growth plates are located. The growth plates give us our physical height when hormones "elevate" at puberty—which is also the *beginning* of our "middle" years. [The diaphysis is the **"shank"** of the long bones. Do you remember *William The Longshanks*—the enemy king of William Wallace in the movie *Braveheart?*]

Fluoride interferes with production of red blood cells, **"blocks"** enzyme activity, and **"hardens"** bone collagen matrix—causing the entire body to become **"stiff and "brittle!"** Collagen matrix is the basis of strong, flexible bones. Fluoridated toothpaste and drinking water suppress red blood cell production and promotes anemia in females as well as limiting blood's ability to carry oxygen. Anemic people have poor vitality and tire easily. [Fluoride's affect on health and energy is similar to taking chemotherapy for cancer—except fluoride poisoning occurs in **SLOW MOTION** one day at a time!]

The lymphatic system services the colon—which **begins** at the cecum. [See drawing on page 46.] The cecum is the **"juncture"** of the lower small intestine (ileum) and the beginning of the large intestine (colon). The **appendix** "dangles" from the cecum—the **MOST TOXIC SITE** in the body and the site where the "chocolate pudding" is housed! [Chocolate pudding is the "stuff" of **CANCER**—and the reason the colon is the "**cancer alley!**"] The appendix is heavily surrounded with lymph nodes called "**Peyer's patch.**" These lymph nodes isolate and manage toxic-waste "overload" to prevent "**death!**" An "**appendectomy**" removes the appendix to prevent "bursting"—but **FAILS** to deal with the causes. [High Enema Therapy™ avoids ever having to deal with "appendicitis!" Surgical intervention is too little, too late! A word to the wise!]

Appendicitis is confirmation of toxic waste overload that ONLY occurs in a highly acid "terrain!"

A sluggish bowel and lymphatic system is **symptomatic** of poor bile flow. People who experience appendicitis, diverticulitis, colitis or irritable bowel are under "*indictment*" for more serious health problems to come—unless remedial action is taken to restore their "terrain" and change-lifestyle.

Acne & Scars

Acne is also indicative of a leaky gut, a stressed liver, poor bile flow and a sluggish bowel! Scars and skin blemishes go with a congested lymphatic system and acid waste accumulation in the tissues **beneath** the skin. [An acid environment **prevents** the *parenchyma* cells from "restoring" damaged tissue. Parenchyma cells are the active, functional cells of healthy organ tissue!]

[Scars and skin blemishes are repaired using VZ™, L_SP_CC™ and SOC™ capsules "internally" and racemized™ Skin Creme™ and SOC™ Lotion "topically." Deacidification of the "terrain" is addressed with High Enema Therapy™ and the Young Again (Tissue and Liver) Protocol™. Contrary to "myth," skin bacteria do NOT cause acne—but bacteria DO feed on acid waste "oozing" from the membranes beneath the skin.]

An astute surgeon can tell the physical age of his patient by the amount of "scarring" in the tissues.

*[Your author underwent hernia repair in 1981. The surgeon was **amazed** at the good "condition" of my **vital organs,** but was **puzzled** by the "breakdown" in the connective tissues of my "belly" that made the surgery necessary. Twenty-five years "later"—age 61—your author is "physiologically" younger. Gone are the dietary issues that led to hernia and knee surgery! Complete "regeneration" has restored these tissues!]*

[Vegetarian, fruitarian and macrobiotic diets lead to "systemic breakdown" of the connective tissues. A diet VOID of eggs and meat is "INCAPABLE" of sustaining a strong body! Your author is younger and stronger at age "61" than at age "36" because he eats "healthy" meats and eggs!]

Burns • Scars • New Limbs

The body can regenerate itself—limbs, nerve tissue,

bones—and brain! We are talking **total** limb regeneration and restoration of function with no evidence of trauma or scarring. These possibilities were amply demonstrated by Dr. Robert Becker and Dr. Melvin Saunders 20 years ago—and recently by the Japanese who helped a diabetic "grow" a missing foot using Medical Grade Ionized Water™! The Japanese CD is available and is best understood with the help of the "water book." [See Source Pages 39, 108, 184, 220 and 306.]

*[In 1983 your author suffered a severe burn in a welding accident. The skin and underlying tissues of the inside of my right elbow were burned and destroyed by a hunk of red hot 5000° F steel that fell and landed in the crook of my arm. I should have scarred "horribly"—but instead healed without **ANY** scar formation. I did **not** see a doctor and I did **not** scar because I performed High Enema Therapy™ daily and "juiced" to move "bile" and keep from going "acid!" I also made **SURE** that I consumed plenty of high quality "protein!"]*

The miracle of "regeneration" was personally experienced by Mitchell May who made medical history by growing new skin, bone, and nerve tissue after suffering over 40 breaks to his femur (thigh bone).

*[Medical **miracles** are closely parallel the principles of vibrational medicine and the manipulation of subtle energy forces in the bio-electric body.]*

Clogged Arteries & Lymph

Atherosclerosis—"clogging" of the arteries—is a major problem in the USA. Yet **nothing** is mentioned of the **inter**relationship between the liver, bile flow, the lymphatic system, amyloid waste build-up, hormones—and their effects on the heart and blood circulatory system. Before we discuss the **inter**relationship, a little **anatomy** and **physiology** is in order.

*["Waste-laden" lymphatic fluid join the blood just prior to where retruning blood enters the heart. The heart then pumps blood to the lungs where **TWO** things occur: blood is **re**oxygenated ; carbon dioxide waste and waste energy is **RELEASED** into the atmosphere. The blood then returns to the left side of the heart for distribution to the body. As the blood leaves the heart, the left and right **"coronary"** arteries branch off and supply the heart muscle itself. These are the arteries that become "blocked" requiring coronary bypass surgery in critical situations. Bypass surgery is a short term "fix!"]*

Waste and toxic substances in the blood **COMBINE** with *chlorine, fluorine, chloramines* and amyloid waste from the tissues forming atherosclerotic plaques that "clog" the arteries feeding the heart and body. Cardiovascular problems, therefore, are "confirmation" of an acid terrain, a sick liver and the cumulative effects of poor choices in lifestyle.

Somebody "terrains" age so rapidly that people simply "drop dead" from a massive heart attack. **Angina pectoris** chest pain results from poor blood flow in the chest, low ATP production—and a magnesium "electrolyte" shortfall. **"Ischemia"** (*ischein*-to hold back. *hemia*-pertaining to blood) is specific to an "oxygen starved" heart muscle. When heart attack occurs, heart muscle tissue dies or becomes non functional. This is called *myocardial infarction.* If a blood clot is involved, it's called *coronary thrombosis.* A clot is a *thrombus.* A stroke involves a "clot" in the brain.

[*Medical experts "wrongly" blame and cut out dietary Vitamin-K to stop blood clots. Vitamin-K is known as "clot factor." Without Vitamin-K, blood will not clot and you will bleed to death—like a hemophiliac! Instead of using aspirin and ending up in the Alzheimers ward—or so-called "blood thinners"— use Racemized™ Sea Minerals and NTV™ and VZ.™ Never use Nattokinase if Vitamin-K2 has been removed! Blood clots are confirmation of a terrain that is "out of control!" Clot factor does NOT cause blood clots—but "EXCESS" waste accumulation and poor bile flow sure does!*]

People & Plants

Human beings and plants have **MUCH** in common except for issues of **mobility** and fluid **movement.** Humans [and animals] rely on physical activity to move lymphatic fluid—and we have a heart to pump blood. Plants have no heart and depend on capillary action, osmosis, enzymes and mineral ion energy to **overcome** gravity for moving energy, water and nutrients into their tissues and back to their roots. Humans depend on the mitochondria in the cells to produce the ATP energy molecule to fuel metabolism. Plants rely on mineral ions, photosynthesis and solar energy to fuel their metabolic processes. Humans rely on red blood corpuscles and hemoglobin to supply oxygen. Plants rely on chlorophyll and chloroplasts. Human body fluids are called "blood" and "lymph." Plant fluids are called chlorophyll and sap. Humans have total control over their environment. Plants are dependent on available sunlight, soil, water and food.]

Movement and activity are critical to good health and longevity. Failure to "move" accelerates aging.

The lymphatic system **"CONTROLS"** the "terrain"— and dis-ease develops in lymphatic system **"before"** it appears in blood. Instead of **"limping"** into old age, **"lymph"** your way back to your anabolic "peak" where you become *Young Again!*

PREVIEW: *Our next chapter is the "cancer" chapter! Learn HOW to avoid becoming a cancer statistic.*

Ring! Ring! Goes The Bell!

And so it does—sometimes 150+ times a day. Will it be "conversation" **or** "communication?" Do we have a "chicken" or do we have a "duck?" To solve the riddle, see Chapter 36!

Protein Digestion

Protein "digestion" occurs in a highly "acid" stomach. Racemized™ R/BHCl™ is extremely helpful for protein utilization, good health and longevity; DiSorb II™ works in the "gut!". Proper digestion kills "parasites," too! [See pages 69, 156, 180, 234 and 318.]

Stroke & Heart Attack

To minimize "stroke" and heart muscle damage, a smart doctor will give the patient 50 drops of racemized™ sea minerals in a glass of WARM water **immediately** following the "event!" To minimize brain damage, a smart doctor will place the victim in a tub of tepid water and lower the temperature to 86°F for 12 hours before slowly raising the temperature to 98.6°F. [SOC™ capsules, NVT,™ VZ,™ L_sP_cC™ and TCM™ help, too!]

A Dual Perspective!

Deacidification of the body requires a **dual** perspective to be effective. For example, we grow old in the **invisible** realm of the Fourth Dimension **BEFORE** we see and experience aging in the world of the **visible** Third Dimension—where we live out our lives. Why we become acidic and what to do about it is the thesis of the "terrain" management concept. High Enema Therapy™ accelerates the release of acid wastes on the physical level—while Enhanced Homeovitic™ remedies clear the tissues in the **"invisible"** realm. When we **"ERASE"** toxic energy signatures in the Fourth Dimension, we deal with **"underlying"** health issues and promote healing in the Third Dimension! Good health and rejuvenation demands a dual perspective! Aging is the manifestation of opposing energy forces at "odds" with each other. The "terrain" controls!

Howdy Doody Facial Lines

You did **not** have those "Howdie Doody" lines from the corners of your mouth to the sides of your chin when you were **"younger"**—so **WHY** do you have them now? The answer is that your **"terrain"** is acidic and out of balance—and you are **FULL** of parasites! So what's it going to be, dear reader? Deal with the problem now or lose control of your life later? The solution to these problems is the *Young Again Protocol(s).*™ [See pages 163, 203, 234, 262 and 318.]

A Typical Day!

1. **Wake-up** at same time each day and immediately drink a two glasses of water with a short squirt of racemized™ sea minerals plus lemon if desired. If using VZ,™ L$_s$P$_c$C,™ Pu,™ SOC™ caps, R/C™ and CWD™ (for weight)—take them now.

2. Do a one-bag enema"—time needed: 3-5 minues (important)!

3. Use L/CSF™ machine for 5-10 minutes (stay near toilet).

4. Stretch and do calisthenics followed by lymphatic "rolldown." (If low back problems, take "hot" tub or shower "before" doing stretching or exercises; no cold water after!) Then "hang" by feet for 5 minutes using an inversion table.

5. Drink a glass of Kombucha tea; 1 cup of organic coffee is fine!

6. Do pull-ups (both over and under hand); get on an impact-free aerobic exerciser to raise heart beat and HOLD it there for 10 minutes in *cold, fresh air* with a minimum of clothing. Use some type of "low" impact equipment.

7. Maybe drink another glass of water on way to the shower.

8. Take a hot shower/bath followed by a **ice cold** shower. Shave, make-up and dress, etc.

9. **First food:** Take 1/2 cup of fresh, raw "beet" and carrot juice plus other juice(s) you like—plus one **"raw"** egg. [Whip mix with a hand-held blender. Take food supplements and Super Foods™ (page 292) you are using. Eat "physical" food that is good for you—like eggs, meat, oatmeal or multi grain cereal (with prunes). No junk! Proteins are extremely important.

10. Each time you urinate throughout the day, drink a cup of water with the racemized sea minerals in it.

11. **Lunch:** Eat something that is good for you—no junk—and avoid "heavy" food! Super Foods™ are an ideal "quick" lunch, along with some fruit. Take CWD™ and/or Gluco Factor-X™ before food to control blood sugar/lose weight. Take a walk, read, enjoy music, meditate, pray or "whatever!" *P.S.* Avoid other people's problems! [Early/mid afternoon—take more PU™ to keep from going into adrenal "overdrive!"]

12. "Hold" bladder throughout day to improve bowel activity. Use Colon Prep™ and Yucca Blend each evening before bed.

13. Do some load-bearing activity [Move boxes; Lift things; do garden work, yoga or Pilates; walk to the store and "carry" your groceries home; pump some iron.] **Hang** and **stretch** twice daily, preferably by the feet. [If hanging by the arms go easy!]

14. **Evening Meal:** Take CWD™ before meal for "weight!" Eat a healthy meal. Take supplements and digestive supports.

15. Do a one-bag "enema" 30-60 minutes **before** bed!

16. Retire at same time each evening. Sleep in a well-ventilated cold room. Pray and give thanks for being alive.

17. **Bedtime:** Take VZ™, L$_s$P$_c$C™, PU™, SOC™, R/C,™ Skin & Body Toner™ and racemized™ hGH with shot of racemized™ sea minerals in water. Use FG/MG/BT/HST creme(s)

18. *"Get a life!"* and people will notice! Share a free copy of this book; offer **NO** advice; let them do some homework!

19. Never forget, poor health is a matter of **"CHOICE!"**

20. Try and develop daily discipline. The "return" is huge!

Parasites!

Parasitic infestation is at **"epidemic"** levels—but it is a "silent" epidemic! People can't see parasites, so they don't think about them. "Parasites" are something that happens to "the other guy"—but they are everybody's problem! Common symptoms of parasites are: foul gas, bloating, body odor, bowel disorders, joint and muscle ache, allergies, skin conditions, nervousness and Howdie Doodie lines.

"Intestinal" parasites are a problem. But it's the **"microscopic"** parasites that "leak" into the blood through a **"leaky"** gut wall—and set up shop in the heart, brain, lungs, pancreas, spleen, liver, ovaries, testicles and thyroid—and anywhere they find a happy home. [Intestinal parasites are easy to kill. The microscopic "critters" require ParaPurge I & II™ and Yucca Blend.™]

EVERYONE has parasites and some people are overrun by them. **The question is:** *"Why do you have them?"* and *"What can be done about these unwelcome guests?"*

The **number one** parasite issue is "terrain" management. Once you get your terrain in order, managing the parasites is easy. Parasites **"love"** a toxic environment! They need a "friendly" environment with food, warmth and safety—like all other life forms. Provide the environment—and parasites will be there!

Hand-to-mouth "tramsmission" is responsible for 99% of all parasite and pathogenic infections. Sanitation is the best offense—meaning short nails and clean hands **immediately** before eating. [Supplemental use of racemized™ R/BHCl™ and DiSorb Aid II™ are **CRUCIAL** to "protein" digestion. All life forms are **"proteins"**—and protein digestion occurs in a highly "acidic" stomach!]

Deacidification of the "terrain" creates an environment hostile to parasitic infestation. Sanitation and digestive support manages the balance of the problem here. [Kill parasites, dismantle them and dispose of the debris via High Enema Therapy™ and the *Young Again (Tissue and Liver) Protocol.*™]

Did You "Go" THREE Times Today?

Laxatives **"FORCE"** bowel activity—but there is a **BIG** difference between **artificial** bowel activity and **"bile-induced"** activity! The flow of **"bile"** from the liver and gallbladder transports *acid wastes* which causes the bowels to "move!" Without **HEAVY** bile flow, the body grows acid and old. **Deacidification** of the "terrain" is the issue here! After the "terrain" is cleared of "excess" and bile-flow issues are addressed, then comes body restoration and aging "reversal!"
P. S. Three bowel movements a day is "desirable!"

30

Cancer & Salt

*"Well organized ignorance, unfor-
tunately, often passes for wisdom."*
anon.

Salt—"sodium chloride"—is a paradox. It is part of life,
yet it is involved in death. A little salt will hurt you a little bit.
More than a little will ***eventually*** kill you.

History can be written according to salt. In ancient
China, two big tablespoons of salt was a socially acceptable
mode of suicide. Salt has served as money, an item of barter
and a cathartic (laxative). For over 100 years, medicine's focus
has centered on salt's *"supposed"* relationship to *high blood
pressure.* We will focus on salt's **EFFECTS** on the "terrain."

Mankind has chosen to upset Nature's balance. We use
salt to ***hype*** food and hasten old age in so doing. Healthy food
does **NOT** need salt because it has plenty of mineral ions in it
that give it ***flavor!*** Unhealthy food requires salt to create the
"illusion" of taste—and to keep it from ***spoiling!*** Look at any
can or package of processed food and you will find that it is
loaded with sodium or sugar—as preserving agents!

"Canned" foods became fashionable in 1859 when H. J.
Heinz Company produced the first of its Heinz 57 varieties. Salt
was used to create a "brine" environment hostile to "clostridium"
bacteria. Clostridium is a ***facultative*** anaerobe that can live
with or without oxygen. Clostridium **endo**toxins cause systemic "shock!" The deadly "condition" is called ***botulism!***

Sailors of old suffered miserably from *salt*-preserved
beef and pork—so did civilian populations. When meat is
preserved with salt, it loses its energy force and nutritive
qualities. Excess sodium chloride (table salt) in the diet upsets
the potassium : sodium ratio—creating cellular and terrain
imbalance that eventually **transfers** your money to the medical cartel or to the mortician—or both!

"Healthy" food is naturally high in potassium and low

in sodium, while bio-junk and processed foods are exactly the opposite. [Synthesized "salt" fertilizers create conditions of **excess** in the soil—just as table salt creates conditions of **excess** in the body. Arthritis is a condition of "excess!"]

A little flour, salt and water mixed together makes wonderful play dough for children—and when it dries, it turns as hard as concrete!

Natural Preservatives

Dr. Carey Reams *taught* that quality produce will dehydrate before it will rot. He proved his point by entering a watermelon he had grown in the local county fair for three years in a row! Your author at this moment (February 2006) has two home-grown potatoes that have been in the refrigerator for over 2 years! Quality food is high in natural sugars and earth mineral ions—and has a right-spin energy "signature."

Acres USA once carried a story about a salesman who carted around three cabbages in his car for nine months without spoilage. On the weekends, he would roll them under a shade tree until Monday morning when he would peel away a leaf and hit the road again. When the salesman was challenged, the nine-month-old cabbages were cut and eaten raw!

Vegetables and fruits high in natural sucrose and earth mineral ions "keep"—and sustain life, too!

Homemade ice cream made with too much white **sugar** will **NOT** "set-up" regardless of how much salt is applied to the ice to "raise" the freeze point. Oranges high in natural sugars wither and shrink rather than rot. Home-grown greens stay crisp and tasty in the refrigerator for over a month with no spoilage! Healthy crops—like healthy people—can withstand more stress and not succumb to dis-ease as easily as people who eat bio-junk diets.

Trace minerals and humic acids sprayed on plant foliage raises sucrose and mineral ion levels in plant juices—and protects crops from frost damage. In humans, blood electrolyte and glucose levels are important "markers" of health and the ability to handle "stress!"

[In the old days, a bushel of fresh green beans weighed 32 lbs. Today, a bushel of beans weighs only 24 lbs. The difference is the lack of earth mineral ions and lower concentration of sugar energy in crop tissues. The more concentrated the energy footprint of a crop, the more food will weigh. Crops grown with salt fertilizers and poisons produce sick, weak populations of human beings.]

SALT: Paul Bragg vs. The Athletes

Here is a true story about how salt affects health and vitality. In the early 1960's, Dr. Paul C. Bragg, a famous health crusader—and one of my mentors—challenged a group of college athletes to a 30-mile hike across Death Valley. The temperature in August was 130° Fahrenheit.

The *experts* advised the athletes to take **"salt tablets!"** The athletes were given all the "cold" water and food they wanted. Bragg drank *only* warm distilled water, [In those days, BFRV™ water was not available!] took no salt, and fasted—taking no food. Bragg was the only one to finish the hike. The athletes—every last one of them—were carried off for medical care. They suffered from heat exhaustion and heat stroke. Bragg finished the hike in 10 1/2 hours, camped overnight, and repeated the return hike the following day. He was in his mid *sixties!* He was **YOUNG** and active. **He avoided all salt!**

Rommel's German-Afrikan Corps used no salt in their diets, yet they fought tremendous desert battles. When they were finally captured, they were in peak condition and unaffected by intense desert heat. [The Americans used salt tablets and salted their food and ate "heavy" food.]

Native peoples consume little salt. When *civilized* man introduces salt into their diet, their health deteriorates. Salt is **always** a factor in the development of **sub**clinical illness that eventually leads to **SIGNS** and diagnosis of "dis-ease."

Cells • Sodium • Mitochondria

High sodium levels in the tissues impose stress on the system. High sodium intake upsets the sodium : potassium ratio—speeding the LOSS of potassium from the cells. Because the body is totally **dependent** on daily dietary intake of potassium to meet its needs, the body will *steal* potassium from the cells and *replace* it with sodium when faced with a potassium shortfall. Potassium and sodium ions have a positive (+) valence "charge"—and both are electrolytes. But sodium spins left while potassium spins right. Potassium is the *predominant* ion *inside* cell membranes. Sodium is the predominant ion **outside** of cell membranes in the **"amyloid"** fluid.

Edema (fluid retention) is a SIGN of excess sodium and excess amyloid waste in the tissues.

[Once inside the cell, sodium short-circuits cellular machinery, sedates the mitochondria and eventually kills the cell. Dead cells release waste "acids" that must be removed from the terrain. Weak cells produce little ATP and put a drag on the system—"squandering" vital energy that should be used for growth and repair. The mitochondria "cannot" function or replicate in a high sodium environment! ATP production is hard to restore once cellular balance is lost.]

Energy • Free Radicals

Throughout this book, much space has been devoted to

discussing and describing "energy"—using terms like: *left-spin, right-spin, negative, positive, aerobic,* and *anaerobic*—in an effort to help the reader understand the **nature** of energy and its **relationship** to aging and dis-ease.

The term **"free radical"** is a term that comes to mind in regard to energy and cancer. A free radical is a molecule that contains an *odd* number of electrons, which makes free radicals highly **REACTIVE** and extremely **UNSTABLE!**

Free radicals are part of **everyone's** life. Poor choices in lifestyle, diet and water are compounded by environmental free radicals bombarding the bio-electric body from every direction. For example, healthy reactions occur continuously and look like this: $O^2 + O^2 + H^2 <\longrightarrow> H_2O_2 + O_2$. The double arrow indicates the reaction can **reverse!** In a stressed body, **reverse** chain reactions cause electron "theft" to go out of control. The product of such reactions is accelerated aging!

Free-radical production greatly influences aging and the formation of cancer in the body's "terrain." Please understand, these **"wild"** reactions drive the production of **"non-differentiated"** tissue and systemic excess. Cancer tissue—by definition—is **NON-DIFFERENTIATED TISSUE!**

Timely hormonal *influence* causes non-differentiated tissue to **"differentiate"** and form organs and glands to become cartilage instead of muscle, bones instead of brain, etc. Cancer is **"OUTLAW"** tissue "without identity." Tissue *insurrection* best describes a cancer situation. Free radical reactions cause a steady loss of control over the "terrain."

Uncontrolled free radical oxidation of healthy tissue produces EXCESS in the system, eventually manifesting as so-called deficiency dis-ease.

Cancer uses cellular ATP to proliferate. In compliance with the Second Law of Thermodynamics, energy is **NEVER** lost, it merely changes form. When excess toxic energy **EXCEEDS** the body's ability to cope, tumor or mass "formation" begins. We will discuss their individual characteristics shortly.

*[Uncontrolled free-radical oxidation can be prevented through **deacidification** of the terrain and the use of various racemized™ products and protocols outlined thus far. Consumption of Medical Grade Ionized Water™ is perhaps the ultimate tool for terrain control. "Health" is a "cumulative" state of being—as are all "states" of dis-ease!]*

Health and dis-ease are "cumulative" reflection of the choices we make.

Cancer's Energy Footprint

Cancer is a manifestation of a **negative** energy condition. Cancer **tumors** surround themselves in a zone of **SODIUM.** They **concentrate** energy by acting as anaerobic "black

holes"—stealing away and concentrating the host's "life force."
[Tumors are **NOT** the "enemy." Rather, they is a statement that all is not well. Tumor formation is a self-defensive
measure by the body to **preserve** itself through the **condensation** and **isolation** of deadly, toxic energy. We are talking about
toxic energy that the body is unable to neutralize or dispose of
through healthy bile flow produced by the liver.]

*Tumors are warning SIGNS and should NOT be
ignored, even when they are "benign!"*
In the early stage, a cancer tumors goes unnoticed. As
it concentrates more energy, it becomes more "dense." It can
now be seen by X-ray, CAT scan and MRI. It can be *felt* with the
fingers if it is not too deep in the body. Cancer tumors are **NOT**
the same as cancer masses. Tumors are energy *importers.*
They "form" in order to take toxic energy **OUT** of circulation.

Tumors are **"nationalistic!"** They stay within their
territory and import needed energy by **hijacking** it from other
parts of the body. Tumors multiply as the body terrain weakens—but tumors do **NOT** **"spread"**—unless they are "messed
with!" Removal of a cancerous tumor is **NOT NECESSARILY** a
good idea. Surgical intervention often makes matters worse—
and the trauma of surgery definitely "weakens" the patient!
[The word "tumor" is **NOT** a synonym for the word "death!"]

Sometimes the body chooses to **dissolve** a tumor. In
most cases, however, it chooses to **calcify** the tumor by
depositing calcium into the sick tissue to petrify it in an effort
to "synchronize" the toxic energy on a **permanent** basis. [The
tumor is an effort by the body to preserve itself!]

Serious healing requires *focused* effort and *total* repro-
gramming of the way people **think** and **perceive** their "situation." **Perception is reality!** There is no room for negative
thinking because "time" is **FINITE** when you have "cancer!"
"Thought" is a creative force! **The mind is 90% of the battle.**

A positive thinking, happy and loving person can
outlast the worst of cancers—but only "if" they choose to
exercise correct choices on the **"physical" level.** Death of the
physical body is a "physical" issue! [God performs miracles for
people who make correct "choices!" Choice is the issue!]

When a **malignant** tumor (or mass) is discovered, it is
time to get serious! Radiation and chemotherapy are **NEVER**
wise choices. Why pay someone to "torture" and "cheat" you of
what time you have left? [If the patient is disciplined and willing
to take responsibility for their life—*live or die*—and is will
follow the *Young Again Protocol*™—they can **face down** death!]

People with cancer must take a laid-back, happy-go-
lucky attitude and outlook—and live one day at a time! There
is **NO** room for doubt, fear, worry, hate, blame or anger—only
love! ➥ The desire to live must be **greater** than the **fear** of death.

[Two highly recommend the books, *Your Body Believes Every Word You Say* and *Holographic Universe.* [See Source Page.]
The ONLY thing cancer tumors and cancer masses have in common is that they both are virus havens and both like left-spin, anaerobic, high sodium environments.

Cancer Masses

A "mass" is **not** a "tumor," and these terms should **NOT** be used interchangeably. A mass is **NOT** dense like a tumor. It cannot be felt because it has no definitive boundaries. A mass is "soft" tissue—never hard—and difficult to detect!

As a mass takes "form," it grows and establishes **outposts** quietly. Masses exist in the "twilight zone" **between** life and death. They rarely appear on X-rays, CAT scans, ultra sound, or MRI's until the late stages—and it is difficult to tell where sick and healthy tissue begin and end. Masses are **invisible** because they have "low density" and are usually hidden behind other tissue structures.

Masses are **"offensive"** in nature! Think of them in terms of outposts for colonial expansionism in a third-world country—in this case **"your" body!** Masses "colonize" during a **seven year`** period referred to in medical circles as the "occult" period. [Occult means hidden!] Long before a cancer *mass* announces itself to the host—it is **"there"** growing and spreading! Masses use the lymphatic highway to **spread** while **sabotaging** the host's immune system. During this time, the host notices nothing—and usually feels "good!" By the time a mass announces itself, the individual is in **DEEP** trouble!

Cloaking Period & Sodium

During the occult period, cancer masses are concealed, invisible and non-detectable by the host. In other words, a mass employs a **"cloaking"** technique so as to go "undetected!" The years preceding the end of the occult period are often some of the very best years in terms of **"OUTWARD"** appearance of good health. On the inside, however, confirmation of the person's lifestyle, thought patterns and choices are coming home to roost—and aging is in full swing.

Masses often cause the body to gain weight with little or no increase in body measurements because water is heavier than fat on a volume basis. Therefore, weight gain without increased inches is reason to question *"What is "going on?"*

A person who is waste-and-sodium "toxic" generally suffers from edema (water retention of the tissues) partly due the sodium and **MOSTLY** due to the accumulation of "amyloid" waste which attract and hold water in the soft tissues.

Edema is a **SIGN!** Edema is abnormal! Chronic edema is the equivalent to a quiet proclamation of **WAR**—and must not be ignored. **Edema is a "red flag!"** Look for puffy, water-filled skin that "dents" easily when pressed and does not spring back quickly. Be alert to swelling in the legs, ankles, feet and hands. Look for an increase in clothes size.

Edema goes part and parcel with congestive heart failure—a condition affecting the elderly.

People in the early stages of cancer "mass" formation often experience substantial weight gain for **no** particular reason—usually **WITHOUT** noticeable change in dietary habits. Near the end of the occult period, they get the *"I just don't feel up to par!"* syndrome. Then—out of nowhere—the person becomes **skin** and **bones** as their body **evaporates!**

When "mass type" cancers remove their cloaks, the occult period is over and the final struggle begins.

➥ Edema is cancer's cloaking device! People do **NOT** recognize edema for what it is! They think everything is okay— *"Just a little old age!"* During the cloaking period, the cancerous body literally **"cannibalizes"** itself—by digesting its own protein-rich muscle mass. [Eventually everyone's body becomes a "meat-eating" cannibal!]

*[Free-radical oxidation accelerates **simultaneous** to the "**cannibal effect"**—as the body digests its own tissues—a process called **auto digestion.** Here, the body "lives on" stored energy. The body is now in a catabolic, high-acid "state." Once the body exhausts its energy reserves—BANG—the game is over! Because of the invisible nature of cancer masses, unsuspecting patients fall for "exploratory" surgery by "mad" experts in white smocks! Exploratory surgery "**sabotages"** remaining energy reserves—further weakening the patient.]*

*[The word "cancer" **devastates** the psyche of the sick person. Conventional cancer therapy **steals** what is left of the patient's life, body weight and energy! When **intra**cellular sodium levels and **inter**cellular amyloid waste levels reach the "tipping point," cancer turns **"off"** its cloaking device—and announces itself!]*

A positive "confirmation" of CANCER is NOT a blessing! LUCKY is the person who is sent home to "die" because then they are free to do what needs to be done!

It's Your Life

➥ There are **NO** tests to determine sodium toxicity at the cellular level—but there are **SIGNS!** There are **NO** tests for *amyloid* invasion of the tissues or to determine the extent of acidification of your "terrain"—but there are **SIGNS!**

Learn to pay attention to the SIGNS! When you see adults and children gaining weight—*take notice!* Be **alert** to gyrating blood sugar levels manifesting as mood swings and depression. Pay **attention** if your menstrual cycle is "off"—or you don't feel "right!" Acne, boils, balding, "subclinical" illness, low energy, bladder infection, prostate issues, bowel problems and hair—all tell a story!

If you are in trouble, seek help. But be forewarned! If you are diagnosed with cancer, you will be bullied into conventional cut, burn and poison therapy.

People feel **"relieved"** when the "enemy" [Cancer!] has been identified. They want to **"believe"** their physician. **FORGET IT!** Identifying the enemy means you are focusing on what you **don't** want. Ignore medical "fairy tales" they are a **"trap!"** Realize, the "health-care/sick-care" system is a complete **"fraud!"** Ignore the "wonderful" and "promising" new treatments and drugs tendered under the pretense that they will "cure" you. Better to take responsibility for yourself, get away from these people—and **GET A LIFE!** You do **NOT** cure disease, rather you change the "terrain!"

Forget about dying. You could have died any day of your life—but you did not die. If you want the **MIRACLE**, you have to do your part. *"Stop the games!"* The **body** does the healing. **Your job** is to provide a healthy terrain "environment" where healing can occur. Follow through is **"CRITICAL!"**

High Enema Therapy™, juicing and tissue deacidification are mandatory terrain protocols.

Use of Super Foods—**mandatory!** Juicing—**mandatory!** Restoration of liver function—**mandatory!** Electrolyte management—**mandatory!** Lymphatic drainage—**mandatory!** Yes, hormone issues need to be **addressed!** Yes, biological-friendly water is **crucial.** You get the idea!

Walking is very beneficial. Positive thinking and visualization are crucial. Use of the L/CSF™ machine has no substitute. Laughter and fun are basic prerequisites. Worry and fear are **not** allowed. **GUARD** your thoughts or you will become a self-fulfilling prophesy. Remember the power of prayer—for yourself and for others. Meditation and deep breathing are powerful tools. Time spent "barefoot" in the garden growing food and flowers and enjoying Nature is as close to heaven as you get on planet Earth! Take time to **focus on** and **help others**. The more you give, the more you receive. Get plenty of rest at night and naps during the day. Get rid of "stress"! Sleep on a Biogenic™ Medical Grade Mattress Pad. Be happy and thankful you are "alive!"

Rules Of Personal Responsibility

There are three rules of personal responsibility.

Rule 1. Keep your mouth shut and stay away from doctors! They will *confuse* you; cause you to *doubt* your instincts—and make you fearful! They are **not** your friends!

Rule 2. Keep your mouth shut and avoid well-meaning

family and friends who will pressure you to "go conventional!"
Rule 3. Keep your mouth shut! And if the "pressure"
from medical "bullies" becomes intolerable, don't hesitate to
pull the "God" card! Tell them you are going home to pray about
it and you will let them know when God gives you your answer!
Repeat it as necessary until they "get it!"

*[It is **not** easy to drive sodium from the tissues when
cancer is involved. Organic potassium should come from fresh
vegetable juices (cabbage, celery, beet, carrot, etc.) **Sip** and
chew your juices. **Do NOT gorge!** Juices are like jet fuel! Use
moderation and be certain to take some Yucca Herbal Blend™,
DiSorb Aid II™ and R/BHCI™ for digestive support.]*

Fresh vegetalbe juice is a **VERY** powerful detoxifier—
and can flood the body with wastes to the point that the liver
becomes **exhausted** and the kidneys **overload.** High Enema
Therapy™ **EASES** the waste burden on these organs. High
Enema Therapy™ and plenty of sleep are 50% of the prerequisites for healing. Better to **stay home** and recover instead of
chasing a guru master in the mountains of India or Peru.

Liver is good food—if you can stand it! Better to use
racemized™ **predigested** organic beef liver capsules. Cancer
therapy should **always** include liver. Domestic liver is bad
news—avoid it! If a vegetarian or vegan or heavy meat eater, you
"MUST" change your dietary habits—and address the things
in your lifestyle that led to the "diagnosis!" [Kombucha tea is a
good tonic. Lymphatic drainage using the L/CSF™ machine
and body roller are very helpfull! Raw saurkraut is a "superb"
food! Keeping "regular" hours! Get "8-10" hours sleep nightly.

Expect To Feel Crummy
"EXPECT" to feel crummy as you **de**acidify! You are
paying for your sins! Do **NOT** forget the power of prayer and
positive thinking. Try to find strength within yourself to finish
what you have begun. Prayer is a direct phone line to God—*ring
it often!* Find a "strong" person to help you through the
transition back to the world of the healthy. Do your part!

*[Once potassium begins exchanging places with the
sodium ions "inside" the cells, the mitochondria will come alive
and replicate themselves. The more of them that come alive—the
more **ENERGY** there will be available for your body to rebuild
itself. At first, you will feel worse. In time, you will feel better.
Think, two steps forward, one step backwards!]*

Talk To & Reassure Your Body
Deacidification can be tough. It's a kind of **"mind
game."** The body will shout, *"I feel crummy!"*—but you must
ignore the complaint and **reassure** the body that things are
under control and that you **"want"** the body to "heal itself!"

Talk out loud and tell your body *what you expect* and *what you desire.* Never "freak" at the first **SIGN** or symptom of a metabolic slump! Guard your energy reserves at all cost! Good days are followed by bad days. In time, you will enjoy more good and fewer bad days. If you **"panic or cut and run,"** you will **NEVER** be healed and you can kiss your life "good-bye!"

God does miracles, but they are usually dependent upon you doing your part!

Chemotherapy • Not Approved

Chemotherapy is defined as the prevention or treatment of infectious disease by *chemicals* which act to promote "anti**sepsis**" in the body while avoiding serious side effects in the patient. If we dissect the word *antisepsis,* we get *anti*-against' *sepsis*-a general fever-producing condition caused by bacteria or their toxic by-products. In light of this dictionary definition, do you think that *chemotherapy* as used on cancer patients meets this description? Did you know that you must *"Sign a little form!" before* you get your *magic-bullet* cancer therapy? [See Chapter 6.]

Cancer drugs and radiation/chemotherapy are "magic bullets!" They are NOT safe—but they are "Approved!" under the PRETENSE that they work. They don't!

Drugs of "death" are administered to unsuspecting people by egotistical, well-meaning "mad men" in white smocks. Medicine and the pharmaceutical companies **side-step** the "liability" problem by having people *sign away their rights* **beforehand**—so patients cannot bring suit later! Those "forms" are unilateral [one-sided] contracts giving you **"NOTICE!"**

When people sign *"standard"* forms, they are giving the legal and medical systems *jurisdiction* over them. The name of the game in our legal system is *jurisdiction!* Either medicine and the courts have jurisdiction or the person does—but **NOT** both at the same time.

["Standard" forms are no different than entering a courtroom where the judge has committed constructive treason, perjury of oath and contempt for the constitution by **placing** *a "yellow fringe" on a Title 4 U.S.C. 1 flag of "peace" of the united [note small "u"] States of America or displaying the flag inferior to a ball, eagle or spear on the pole, or placing it on the right as you face the judges bench, or placing it inferior to any other flag, or substituting a flag of "different" dimensions. Judges "knowingly" do these things to "create" a foreign "state" in order to deny citizens their constitutional rights.* **JURISDICTION** *is everything! [from the Constitution: No STATE shall create another "state" within a STATE or from a combination of "states"...]*

When the medical system has jurisdiction, the patient does not. When the patient grants jurisdiction over their body, medical "science" is free to maneuver with impunity. Parents must give "permission" for children in non-emergency procedures to grant "jurisdiction!" Believe it!

For the cancer patient, the options "within" the medical system are nil. Sign the form or be refused treatment because **jurisdiction** was not granted—a limited liability, unilateral contract where ONE side shares the benefits and the patient assumes ALL the risk! The medical system needs *jurisdiction* because they are using **EXPERIMENTAL** drugs in the treatment of cancer and destruction of YOUR body—with the blessings of "so-called" watch-dog agencies, of course!

[Everyone MUST understand something known in legal AND medical circles as the "Rule of Probable Cause." It states: "...experimental drugs may be used IF the side effect of the drug is NO worse than the end effect of the untreated disease."]

"For Experimental Use Only"

Regardless of the specie of cancer drug, it will be stamped with the tell-tale sign of a **"magic bullet"** medicine— "For Experimental Use Only." Once a drug is "approved," they don't bother to tell you that it is still "experimental!" How do you like that? How does it make you feel to know that the **MAXIMUM** risk to the poor patient is **no worse** than if treatment were not rendered at all. What an alternative, *"Sign on the dotted line and let us milk you of your life and savings —or go home and die!"*

"For Experimental Use Only" is a fact that should be sufficient **SHOCK THERAPY** to motivate every thinking person to immediately begin the aging reversal process. No matter how you figure it, *"You are on your own!"* So go home and get a life! "Magic bullets" don't work! Self-treatment is less risky and the odds of recovery far greater—*with a fraction of the suffering!*

Health and life are worth more than all the money you can throw at the medical system in the **futile** effort to buy back your life! **Good health isn't for sale!** But it requires commitment, discipline, responsibility and choice. **AVOID** the horror of cancer and degenerative dis-ease by implementing what you have learned throughout the pages of this book!

Cancer & Root Canals

The *terrain* is **"THE"** issue when it comes to teeth and gums! As people age, teeth and gums spawn **MAJOR** health problems! The mouth **"mirrors"** the "terrain" and the rest of the body. Dental "issues" are the earliest of warning signals!

ROOT CANAL QUESTIONS: Why did the tooth die? Is it safe to have a dead body part in the body? What effect will a decaying, dead body part impose on the immune system? Will the spread of decay into adjoining bone tissue cause further loss of other "healthy" teeth? [Don't expect a candid answer!] Root canals are bad news!! They are **"stop-gap"** measures that lead to "cancer!" Unfortunately, dentures, bridges and implants have shortcomings, too! Now that **CERAMIC** bridges and caps are available, bridges are the best option to real teeth.

According to Dr. Issels, a German doctor, "Only 20% of the population has root canals, yet 90% of cancer victims have root canals in their mouth!" [The COMMON DENOMINATOR behind dental issues is an "acid" terrain. Major dental problems generally appear after age 25 when body acidity levels accelerates.]

As "dead" root-canalled teeth *decay*, they flood the body with **highly toxic poisons,** causing an antigen/antibody response within the immune system and a **rise** in "CRP" (C-reactive protein)! CRP is a "marker" of **sub**clinical non-febrile "infection" within the body's terrain! The scale is 0-.50. If your "CRP" numbers are elevated for "no obvious" reason and you have root-canalled teeth, find a holistic dentist and get those dead teeth **OUT** of your mouth! Please call and learn how to **"prepare"** your body. What you do **BEFORE** major dental work is vitally important!

The "terrain" CONTROLS!. Dental procedures are an after the fact "fix!" Take care of your teeth and gums!

Control the TERRAIN and you control the aging process. Terrain control is how you become *Young Again!*

PREVIEW: *Our next chapter deals with the world of Time and Space and its relationship to the Fourth Dimension, ageless living and the vast UNKNOWN!*

The Basics!

Drink plenty of quality water with sea mineral ions; make fresh juice with one raw egg; eat healthy; do enemas; avoid sugar; get plenty of sleep and exercise; avoid salt; keep your life simple!

It's Your Life!

Some things are worse than "death"—and becoming a victim of *conventional* cancer treatment is one of them. **Never** rejoice because *insurance* is paying the bills. **Do** be concerned about what "they" are doing to you. **Do** be independent; keep your dignity! **Do** keep control of your life. **Do** stay away from doctors. **Do** these things and you will not leave your loved ones with the ugly memory of the **"torture"** that preceded your death! And **just maybe** God will **NOTICE** that you are doing your part and grant you your "wish!" And if it is *"time to go,"* perhaps you will be able to leave worthy family members or a worthy friend an inheritance! Naked we come—and naked we leave!

CHOOSE to live and die on your own terms!

31

Time & Space

"Time and Space are the shadows by which man defines his existence."
Sepio

TIME is duration. **SPACE** is extension. We do not think of Time and Space as entities, but we do consider the bodies and events that occupy them as entities. If we acknowledge the existence of material bodies because they occupy space, then what is an event? An event is a group of circumstances that occupy **TIME** . Therefore, material objects are also events, and both are entities.

Mankind attempts to define those intangibles we call "time and space" using words and concepts. We have **NO** physical sense organs for **TIME** and **SPACE**. We interpret them through "intuition." Intuition, then, must be a sixth sense—a projection of the physical body—something we invoke to comprehend **TIME** and **SPACE**.

Philosophy tells us that **TIME** and **SPACE** consist of relations between entities—that there is co-existence and succession of entities or events. Metaphysics (*meta*: beyond) tells us that **TIME** and **SPACE** are indistinguishable as long as neither is excluded. Yet, we are aware of the *passage* of Time.

Plato stated *"Time and space is the "substance" which contains identity and diversity in one."* If we think of **SPACE** as something that is created, then something must create it. What? *Meta*physics answers *"Time."* Okay. If there is creation, then motion must also exist. If there is motion, then there must be a mover or source of motion. Metaphysics tells us **TIME** is the source of motion. If so, then **Time is** *ENERGY*.

Is **TIME** "energy," or is energy created in the passing of time? If energy is created, the results are perpetual motion which is not a straight line, but a curved line that returns to itself—like a circle. Therefore, **SPACE** becomes Time's "trail." But a trail does not move, so **SPACE** cannot move either, since it was **TIME** that generated **"energy"** in its expansion—

creating **SPACE! TIME** and **SPACE** can be demonstrated to be static, indistinguishable or non-existent. Let me illustrate.

Suppose we are in an airplane that is traveling at the same speed as the Earth's rotation or approximately 1,080 miles per hour, and we are heading West following the sun at its own speed. We begin our three-hour trip in New York City at exactly twelve o'clock noon, and, when we arrive at Los Angeles, it is still exactly twelve o'clock noon.

What has taken place here? **TIME** became a motion of **SPACE**—and **SPACE** the relaxation of **TIME**. We moved from one point to another point on the surface of the earth, but Time did not change. We are in a quandary—caught between **TIME** and **SPACE**—a kind of cosmic cul-de-sac. The mathematician working on our dilemma would have difficulty making his calculations respond to our problem—so he would give the *unknown* condition a name: "fourth variable," and reestablish his equilibrium by imposing the ingredient **"TIME"**—so his calculations could continue as if **TIME** were a fixed point.

When we ponder the situation, we must conclude that **TIME** is **"not"** a fixed point to which we can anchor our lives, but a mirage on a phantom's shroud. Once we admit that **TIME** is not a fixed point, we **lose** our center and our reference point—yet, intuition tells us there should be such a center.

To compensate, man divides **TIME** into three parts: *present, past,* and *future.* However, this does not solve the problem, because present is but the transition from past into future—a transition that lacks both dimensionality, and duration. The present is the future before we think of it, and the moment we think of it, it is the past. Under these circumstances, self examination of our thought processes and sensory experiences becomes impossible. Is "present" but the "living fringe" of memory tinted by expectation? And if it is, what of our dilemma between the poles of eternity—past and future?

These extremes—past and future—have delivered us into the ***enigma*** we call the Fourth Dimension—the "unknowable." Because man *seems* capable of comprehending only three dimensions related to his physical world—that of length, width, and height—the idea of the existence of another dimension that is totally invisible only compounds his dilemma. **Yet, the existence of the Fourth Dimension cannot be denied. Intuition is real. It is more than an intangible tool by which we interpret Time and Space. It is an extension of our mind.**

Perhaps the Fourth Dimension is not unknowable, but simply misunderstood. If so, there is no reason for man to have to die and emerge from his terrestrial envelope before he can come to know this ***Unknowable*** Dimension.

Knowledge of the existence of this *other* dimension is quite different from understanding it. Consider Jesus, who passed through the wall in the Temple. He was a Third Dimensional being with a physical body, yet He passed through that wall! Since both He and the wall were solid matter, shall we chalk up this event to Deity? Did He violate some Natural Law? Or did He invoke knowledge of the Fourth Dimension? When we enter the arena of the Fourth Dimension, necessity demands that we visualize a **hyper-space** that is measured with *meta*geometry (*meta*-beyond). Our three-dimensional world of length, width, and height becomes but a section of **hyper SPACE.** Let us examine this in more detail.

The *length* of a procession of events is not contained in three-dimensional space. Extension in **TIME** is a projection into unknown space—or the Fourth Dimension. Because **TIME** and **SPACE** are interchangeable at specific points, **TIME** becomes a dimension of **SPACE**—therefore, **TIME** "is" **SPACE** in motion—becoming the future or the past. Therefore, **SPACE** is time projected—"horizontal" **TIME** that persists; **TIME** that moves. And since **SPACE** can only be measured by **TIME** and **TIME** is defined by the *speed of light,* we must conclude that there is **"no"** difference between **TIME** and **SPACE** *except* that **"consciousness" is defined in "TIME!"**

Therefore, we are forced to acknowledge that **"present"** is eternal—that **TIME** per se does **not** exist; that it is "relative" to the person with the *notion* of **"TIME!" Events do not ebb and flow' it is we who pass them by!** The more we attempt to understand, the deeper we sink into the vast unknown.

The creature we call man "exists" in two different worlds: visible and invisible. The invisible world is the realm of negative and positive "energy" forces that ultimately determine our perception of reality in the visible world in which we find our existence. The visible world and the physical body, in turn, act as our compass and bridge into the sphere of the unknown —where the *electric* body exists and functions.

People who **become OLD** say *"Time seems to fly, and the older I get the faster it flies!"* Their day seems to disappear before it has hardly begun. Is this a figment of their imagination or is it reality? And if it is reality, by what measure do we scale this phenomenon?

We cannot measure the phenomenon of **"TIME"** of **"SPACE"** in Third Dimension terms for it does not exist— leaving us, once again, wrestling in the shadows of the *un-known* of the Fourth Dimension world where we are totally dependent on **"intuition"**—*our SIXTH sense!*

We must invoke *intuition* to measure the passing of **TIME** because it passes at the **sub-atomic** level of our existence—where the invisible "electric" body resides. Therefore, **"TIME"** does move faster for those who are "catabolic" and who have passed their "anabolic" peak! Their "terrain" is aging at an *accelerated* rate. Terrain management is the key here!

TIME passes slowly when we are young—when we are climbing on the anabolic side of the pyramid where we experience "slow" **TIME**. After we pass our anabolic peak, we experience "fast" **TIME**—as we *slide* down the catabolic side of the aging pyramid [See page 198.]

We have "arrived" at the answer we have been seeking. It is the *Young Again* "thesis"—summarized as follows: **The "terrain" CONTROLS aging and the passing of TIME!**

Slowing the aging process slows the passing of Time and transcends the physical world. The physical body is "defined" in **TIME** and **SPACE**, but the *electric* body is an extension of *self* and a fixture of the **unknown** Fourth Dimension where mind and emotion are "windows" of the soul. The *electric* body is spirit!

Buying Time! By "stopping" our *bio-electric* clock, we buy **"TIME"**—providing us the opportunity to **exchange** an old body for a **young** body. The process is the "equivalent" of recycling the sand in an hour glass. This recycling process does **NOT** mean that we "relive" our earlier experiences. Rather, it means that we recycle **TIME** itself. This is what is meant when your author speaks of becoming *YOUNG AGAIN!*

PREVIEW: *Our next chapter deals with rejuvenation of the bio-electric body through rest, fasting, and avoidance of self-imposed physiologic stress.*

| **Hair, Skin & Thyroid** |

Hair is as an "extension" of skin! Balding and thinning are **SIGNS** of "dormantcy" of the hair follicles—and confirmation of "rising" **ACID** waste levels in the tissues **beneath** the skin. "Thyroid" is a "factor" in the hair story—as is "terrain" management. Direct intervention is accomplished with HST™ creme and by following the *Young Again Protocol(s)*.™

*"The purpose of life is not to be happy. It is to be **useful**, to be **honorable**, to be **compassionate**, to have it make some **difference** that you have lived and lived well."*
Ralph Waldo Emerson

Bran Muffin Recipe: 1/4 C honey, 1/3 C blackstrap molasses, 1 tbsp. non aluminum baking powder, 1 egg, 2 C **"unbleached" white** flour, 1/2—1 C water, 1 C bran, 2 tbsp. olive oil, 1/4 C sesame seed, 1 C raisins, 1/4 C wheat germ, 1/2 C chopped walnuts, perhaps a little pumpkin pie spice. Recipe makes six muffins. Bake @ 400° until medium brown. Mix ingredients lightly. Do not knead. Enjoy! [Whole wheat flour is too heavy!]

Taoism & Taoist™ Super Foods

Ancient Chinese Taoists (pronounced *Dowists*) saw man as a "reflection" of the universe. They perceived that **cyclic** change governs all living things. They laid down principles and correlations describing Nature's effect on man—and man's response to Nature. These principles are called **Yin** and **Yang**.

Taoist Masters believed that Five Elements describe the natural cycle of life—and that man follows Nature's *cyclical* patterns through the "universe within."

Taoist herbals were formulated to help man adapt to Nature. Taoist Masters strove for **balance** and **harmony** while promoting *self-cultivation*, enhancement of thought and **Yin** clearing and **Jing** building by manipulation of Five Elements. Toist discoveries are now confirmed by advanced physics.

The **Wood Element** represents the liver and gallbladder which control emotional harmony—and the smooth flow of Chi (energy) necessary for a strong nervous system and the clearing of toxins from the body. The **Fire Element** is represented by the heart and small intestine—and addresses blood, lymph, and cerebral-spinal fluid systems, plus physical and mental health and growth. The **Earth Element** represents the stomach and spleen addressing *extraction* and *separation* of good and bad "chi." The **Metal Element** represents the lung and colon—and is said to dominate respiration and maintain defensive Chi (the immune system). The **Water Element** represents the kidney and bladder systems. Taoists believed that *Jing* (the very *essence* of life) is **"within"** body "humors" as expressed by the hormonal and reproductive systems responsible for maintaining youthfulness and glandular function.

Taoist philosophy teaches that the body has the power to **"regenerate"** if physical and mental **STRESS** are "managed!" Taoists believe that the body is designed to function on the basis of "whole" food—and that **"accountability"** underwrites good health as *reflected* from the "universe within." Taoists discovered **"truth"** and **"enlightenment"** through **balanced** lifestyle and *expression* of the person "within"— which leads to **"understanding!"**

Taoism captures the essence of man's "physical" dilemma on planet Earth. Taoism is **NOT** a religious concept, but it does seek to explain man's sojourn on Earth. Consumption of Taoist™ SUPER foods; doing High Enema Therapy™—and use of fresh, "live" vegetable juices are simple ways to enjoy Taoist Principles. See Page 292.]

Taoist™ SUPER foods derive from "3500"
year old formulations.

Especially For You!

Young Again! was written to help people **understand** the forces in their lives that **CHEAT** them of health and happiness and **CONTROL** them and **LURE** them to an early grave. The author has endeavored to use examples that are meaningful. Every effort has been made to help the reader develop a foundation in conventional science plus in the **para**sciences. The reader is reminded that knowledge must be **"applied,"** and that the return of health and rejuvenation requires much **time, focus and patience!** Sometimes rejuvenation isn't fun, but the rewards are worth the effort. Each day brings new opportunities to make "healthy" choices. Each step in the right direction brings improved health and slows physical degeneration. Each day is the **first** day of the **rest of your life!***Young Again!* is a testimony, an offer and a template all in one. It is the product of the author's personal life experiences, observations, philosophy and lifestyle. It was **NOT** written to satisfy pretentious **"experts!"** The author is **NOT** an "expert!" Experts claim to have answers, but they can't demonstrate proof in their own lives. They suffer from dis-ease despite their knowledge. Their *magic bullets* do **NOT** save them. They **"talk"** a good story, but they can't walk it because their model is "defective!" Medical science will **NOT** be fond of this book. They will quote chapter and verse from "their" literature in *defense* of themselves. They will scorn and belittle—and even accuse the author of oversimplification. They will demand "scientific proof!" Their demands will be *ignored!* This book was written for people who seek results rather than *endless* debate. It was written for people hungry for **TRUTH** and who will implement *Young Again Protocol(s)*™ *and principles in their lives.* Old age is **not** fun; it is **not** a joyous process. People age through **ignorance**. Ignorance is a lousy excuse. **You can do better!**

Brush Your "Teeth," NOT Your Gums!

Dental hygienists advise about "proper" brushing—but they **"NEVER"** say *"Do not brush your gums; brushing causes the gums to recede!"* And receding gums cause bone anchoring the teeth to "withdraw"—and the teeth to loosen! Gum grafts are **useless** because the ligaments anchoring the teeth are part of gum tissue, **NOT** tissue from the roof of your mouth!

Autoimmune

An autoimmune condition "means" the immune system **"attacks"** the host—which is "you!" Behind **all** autoimmune conditions and so-called "dis-eases" is a "leaky gut!" And behind **both** is a messed up weak liver and an acid "terrain!" The solution is called the *Young Again! Protocol*™ It was developed to "address" issues of health and longevity.

32

Rest & Fasting

"Dine with little, sup with less; do better still: sleep supperless."
Benjamin Franklin

We dig our grave with our teeth! Powerful words—and true! Do we eat too much? Do we eat too often? Is the problem what we eat? Or is it all of the above? The deleterious effects derived from eating the **WRONG** things have already been discussed. Now let's look at *degenerative* problems that spring from other dietary habits.

Food a'Plenty
In America, food is plentiful and inexpensive—and we have become accustomed to treating our dietary **"habits"** with *total indifference!* As children, we are encouraged to eat as much as we want, to gorge ourselves where less would do, to snack between meals—and at bed time. We are taught that food is food and to eat whatever we like. We **"think"** hunger means it's *"Time to eat!"* We seek a "full" belly—or at least the feeling of one. We carry our beliefs and habits into adulthood—and eventually to the grave.

[Bio-junk diets have become the norm—and they are killing us. But it is our **FAILURE** to develop *discipline* as to *what, when* and *how much* to eat that **"COMPOUNDS"** the discipline issue many times over.]

Food-Induced Stress
When we are physically tired, mentally fatigued or spiritually depressed, we are advised to get extra sleep because sleep "heals!" But when we sleep on a full belly, we deny ourselves quality sleep and actually do ourselves damage.

The vital organs are called **"VITAL"** because they are! They need rest and they don't get it when we sleep on a full belly. Over eating also stresses the vital organs because digestion is **NOT** a voluntary activity. We eat and the vital organs "react!" If we eat too much or too often, they go into **OVERDRIVE** and become "hyper" stimulated which leads to organ "burn out!"

[The digestive tables shown on page 88 indicate that the body requires a certain amount of "time" to digest food.]

Digestion is influenced by stress, exercise, fatigue, quantity of food eaten, hydration levels, time of day, how often food is eaten, enzyme and saliva production, chewing of food, liver function and bile "flow," and the condition of the body terrain as a whole.

Avoid exercise for one hour after eating a meal because the body needs time to get the digestion process going before the blood supply is diverted from the abdominal area. Food imposes stress on the body—and the energy "drain" following a meal is a confirmation of this fact. The "heavier" the meal, the bigger the "effect!" If food is loaded with "additives," high in carbohydrates or laced with sugar, the "drag" on the system can be very noticable. Snacking imposes "stress" on body organs —partly due to the junk nature of snack foods—and partly due to the digestive burden imposed. [The vital organs need "rest!" Without dietary rest, the vital organs burn out!]

Pot Belly/Distended Belly

A *distended* belly hanging over a man's belt line or filling a woman's pelvic area tells a story. People refer to abdominal excess as "fat," when the condition really reflects much more! Distension (stretching) of the connective tissues that anchor the visceral organs in place is part of the "belly" story—as is a constipated, sluggish colon and poor bile flow!

In older people and women over 40 years of age, spinal compression and forward extension of the abdominal "visceral" organs is due to settling of the spinal column from osteoporosis, as illustrated in the skeletal depiction of the dowager's hump on page 100. [The visceral organs include the liver, large and small intestines, spleen, pancreas, ovaries, uterus, prostate and bladder!]

The small intestine ("gut") and the large intestine ("colon") are held in place by connective tissue called **mesentery** —which means "apron!" As the body ages and turns "acid," the mesentery loses integrity and allows the intestines to **"sag!"** [Engorged bowels and gravity contribute to "belly sag"—as does a distended bladder after a hysterectomy.]

Understanding the causes of "belly sag" provides some clues and answers as to what to do about it—meaning **de**acidification of the "terrain!" At the **TOP** of the list is High Enema Therapy™ for dealing with engorged bowel. Next comes the *Young Again (Tissue & Liver) Protocol*™ to increase bile "flow" issues and **de**acidification of the "terrain!" [The more acid the terrain, the faster the connective tissues break down!]

[Loss of physical height is part of the distended belly story because of the relationship of height to osteoporosis in the

spinal column. If you are **SHORTER** *than you once were, your body is very "acid" and your are well into the osteoporosis dilemma that stalks every woman.]*

Hanging by your "feet" using an "inversion" table is an **EXTREMELY** effective procedure for stretching the spinal column and taking pressure off aged "discs" so blood can access these tissues. [Think of an inversion table as a floating "slant board!" They are inexpensive and available.]

Hanging by your hands from a chin-up or trapeze bar drains lymph nodes and vessels in the breast and arm pit areas. [Start slowly if you are female or older because the shoulders are a weak area and easily strained. Hang for "15" seconds at first and **SLOWLY** increase your time.]

"S-t-r-e-t-c-h-i-n-g" the ligaments, tendons and muscles increases blood and lymph flow so the connective tissues can "regenerate." In other words, get oxygen and nutrients in, fluids and waste out. Yoga and Pilates are very effective activities! [VZ™ is used to digest amyloid plaque and scar tissue; SOC™ and Limber Life™ boost blood and nerve flow, eases pain and inflammation and restores limberness; L_sP_cC™ causes the body to manufacture "collagen" for regeneration.]

Gluttony

"Gluttony" is an *old* word. As a child, your author was taught that gluttony was a sin against the Sixth Commandment. Whether it is a sin or not is **NOT** my concern—but premature aging and death resulting from gluttony should be everyone's concern. [These days gluttony is spelled "obesity!"]

When we eat beyond *minimum* satiety [See Chapter 9.], we **overload** the system with excess and free radicals and we **"squander"** vital energy! Drinking liquids with meals and failure to completely chew food makes matters worse!

Gluttony **IS** "driven" by genuine hunger due to dietary starvation. In other words, the body's nourishment needs are going unfulfilled! The way avoid the need to snack and "pig out" is to eat **"nourishing"** food with plenty of healthy "fats" and proteins to meets the body's energy needs. Good food automatically "limits" overeating. Poor dietary choices and the inability to digest food is why 75% of the population is "obese." [Racemized™ DiSorb Aid II,™ R/HCI™ and Yucca Blend™ boost digestion and ease the burden food imposes.]

Sleep

An overly full belly interferes with quality sleep—and lack of quality sleep interferes with all **"EVERY"** aspect of good health and longevity. [Deep sleep is when the body grows and repairs damaged tissue. Without it, we grow old!]

[Plants have a cycle too. They manufacture food during

the day—and they grow and repair at night. Visit your garden in the wee hours of the morning to "hear" corn growing. It crackles and pops! [During the day the Earth exhales. At night it inhales. The "dew point" is when plant and microbial activity are at their PEAK! Everything has rhythm and purpose!]

Lactate • Detoxification • Glycolysis

The body feels refreshed after a "good" sleep because its wastes have been processed and "isolated." *Neutralization* of lactic acid occurs during the sleep cycle. Anyone who has experienced muscle soreness and fatigue from over exertion has experienced the effects of lactate formation in the muscles. "Lactate" formation occurs during "glycolysis"—because of **insufficient** oxygen levels in the cells and, therefore, **incomplete** burning of glucose sugars. Lactate is a **"transitional"** waste product that is converted into the ATP "energy" molecule during the "sleep cycle!" The **"-ate"** in lact**ate** tells us it is the salt of lactic acid. Salts are *bound* energy. [To prevent lactate formation and fatigue, drink plenty of water with racemized™ sea minerals every 30 minutes during heavy work or exercise along with SOC™ capsules and Kombucha Tea. Lactate is a byproduct of **an**aerobic fermentation and the incomplete conversion of glucose to the ATP energy molecule.]

Kombucha Tea uses "aerobic" fermentation to produce a product that fuels glycolysis and prevents lactate formation in athletes who drink it during a game to have more energy and endurance and less muscle soreness.

Cellular oxygen deficiency prevents full conversion of glucose sugars into the ATP energy molecule. The energy "conversion" from glucose to "ATP" occurs **"inside"** the cells, **"inside"** the mitochondria and **"inside"** the Electron Transport Chain of the Krebs Cycle. Lack of oxygen sabotages energy production and healing. Potassium loss from the cells and sodium invasion of the cells greatly **"COMPOUNDS"** loss of energy production.

Get Enough Sleep

You can't put "sleep" in a pill! Fatigue and sleep go together, and sleeping on a full stomach causes **anaerobic** fermentation—and foul gas! **An**aerobic conditions produce **"putrefaction"** of undigested food—and the formation and release of very toxic molecules like indoles, skatoles and phenols—in the gut and bowel. Get "at least" eight hours or **MORE** of good sleep every night—even if you can "get by" on less. **Failing** to get enough rest is no different than **failing** to recharge your golf cart, with one notable difference. **Human beings are not golf carts!** Just because you can "whip" your body and keep it going is **NOT** justification for doing so. Mental "hype" is Fourth Dimension power imposed upon the Third Dimension body! Using "hype" is a "dangerous" skill that comes with a very high price tag called "aging!"

Food Discipline

Avoidance of overeating requires *discipline!* Spacing meals requires *discipline!* Adding *rhythm* and *routine* to daily life requires *discipline!* Health and longevity are the products of *discipline!* The body responds to **"DISCIPLINE!"**

[Your author went from 3-4 meals a day to someone who juices and takes some SUPER FOODS in the am and only eats one regular meal in the evening. He is rarely hungry—and looks and feels better than at anytime in his 61 years!]

Allow 4 hours **between** meals—including so-called "snacks!" Eat wholesome food and the need to snack will end. Children are *growing* and require highly nourishing food if they are to avoid the urge or need to snack. Obesity in children says they are "starving" to death on full bellies! Healthy water and racemized™ sea minerals fulfill another need of both adults and children. Bowel activity should be 3-5 times per day—and water intake very much affects bowel activity. [Children with sluggish bowels should take Yucca Blend™ and do a simple "one bag" enema morning and night. Soft drinks are "OUT"—and artificial sweeteners are "dangerous!" Their long-term effects are WORSE than "alcohol!" Believe it!]

Do NOT encourage children to develop bad habits that will later "morph" into unhealthy lifestyles and lives of misery. Healthy children don't need the "doctor!"

Nourishment and *deacidification* strengthen willpower! The more active the bowels, the more "bile" that is exiting the body. Willpower is the **PRODUCT** of a healthy "terrain!" Smoking, drinking, drugs, gluttony, obesity, etc.—in children and adults—have their roots in **mal**nourishment and and loss of control over the body "terrain."

[Hungry people snack and eat their way into old age and hasten their appointed destiny with the grave—*decades* ahead of schedule. They are *early birds* in the truest sense!]

Rhythmicity

One secret of health and longevity is daily rhythm. *Rhythmicity* is the ebb and flow of energy in our daily life. Up each morning at the same time, meals taken within 1/2 hour of the appointed times, plenty of water, exercise, bed at the same time, a full 8 hours of sleep. Practice rhythmicity, and the lessons in this book will become "patterned habit."

Health and vitality flow on the wires of rhythmicity. The lifestyle of Dr. Paul Bragg and his daughter, Patricia Bragg speaks for itself—as you will see in the following story.

The Miracle of Fasting

This is a true story, told exactly as it happened. Your author hopes you will enjoy it.

It was May 1, 1993. The place: Santa Barbara, California. Your author was attending a dinner party following a publishing seminar when a cute lady approached him and said *"Did you get one of my apple cider books?"*

I answered in the negative. And as she proceeded to hand a book to me, I got a square look at her face and said *"Who are you?"*

"I'm Patricia Bragg!" she answered.

At that moment, I knew that the path upon which Bob McLeod—who you met in Chapter 1—had started me on 22 years before had reached its destination. I was standing before the daughter of the Great Wizard, Paul Bragg!

"Please come sit down," I said. *"We must talk!"*

I began, *"Your father saved my life. I cannot tell you how thrilled I am to meet you! You look exactly like your picture in your father's book on fasting."*

So we talked and laughed. The following day, I was able to sneak away long enough to visit the Bragg Worldwide Headquarters in Santa Barbara, where I stood in awe of a 20-foot-high painting of the wonderful Wizard, Paul Bragg.

"How did your father die?" I asked. *"I have heard several rumors and I am anxious to know the truth."*

"He died in a surfboard accident in Hawaii. He drowned. They could not revive him!"

"Please tell me, what was his age?"

"My father was 97 years YOUNG!—and if he had not died when he did, I have no doubt he would have lived to be 125 years young!" she snapped.

"What is your age, Patricia?" I asked with a lump in my throat.

"I am like my father. I AM AGELESS!"

And so she was. Sweet! Cute! And very much a senior citizen by the calendar, but you would never, ever guess! Patricia looked to be in her late forties, but had the energy of a teenager—and the figure to go with it, too!

Paul and Patricia are PROOF positive that each of us can experience agelessness. Your author is forever thankful for having met this wonderful human being—the daughter of the Great Wizard himself. Like her father, she has helped millions of people. I am proud to continue in their footsteps.

Many readers will be too young to remember Paul Bragg. If the reader elects to read his wonderful book *The Miracle of Fasting*, be sure you are *wide awake!* Bragg speaks

simple TRUTHS—and in simple terms, too! He was a man among men who will be read and remembered for the **TRUTH** he spoke and for the lifestyle he promoted.

Thanks to Paul Bragg and Patricia Bragg—to whom this book is dedicated—your author was **inspired** to create a realistic "model" so everyone who desires to experience "agelessness" can become *Young Again!*

PREVIEW: *Our next chapter deals with the world's MOST toxic element, and it's in YOUR body and drinking water. You will also learn what you can do about it.*

Purpose!

We have to live with the consequences of the choices we make in every area of our lives! Yesterday is "gone"—but tomorrow is available—so why not get started "today?"

Stones & Nails

"Stones" in the gallbladder and "nails" in the liver are "calcified" waste material removed from the blood by the liver. These anomalies take many years to form and are major impediments to restoration of health because they block the flow of "bile" from the liver and gall bladder. Gall stones are liver "pellets" that settled in the gallbladder and calicified. They range in size from B-B's to golf balls. "Nails" take their characteristic shape from the biliary ducts within the liver itself and only appear in very sick people. Nails "clink" against the toilet bowl when doing High Enema Therapy.™

Failure of the liver to remove blood borne wastes, forces the body to store this "soluble" material in the **fatty tissues** beneath the skin—out of circulation and under lock-and-key. [Release and disposal of stored wastes is why the *Young Again Tissue and Liver Protocol*™ was developed] "Soluble" acid waste in the joints and connective tissues is called "amyloid" fluid— and if allowed to **stagnate** it will "morph" into **STRUCTURAL** waste along with pain, stiffness, deterioration—and a doctor's diagnosis. Acne, wrinkles, psoriasis and graying hair are also symptoms of acid waste overload of the body's "terrain!"

[*Detailed instructions come with the Tissue and Liver Protocol.™ Adults follow the program over a two-month period. A "normal" life is followed during the process. Epsom salts are toxic and are not used. OX™ controls cleansing "reactions!" R/ C™ restores the integrity of the "gut" wall and enhances immunity to protect the body from highly toxic waste "released" into circulation during the process. Systemic overload is avoided by doing High Enema Therapy™—as needed!*]

Meat Eating vs. Vegetarianism

Turn to page 367 for a discussion of a volatile health issue. As for your author, *"I've been there! I've done both!"*

Ear Problems!

From ancient times to the present, people have had trouble with their ears—things like: ear wax, infections, water in the ear, pain, poor hearing, tinitis (ringing) and so on. Over 600,000 **adenoid**ectomies and **tonsil**ectomies [Think, ear and tonsil surgery!] are performed each year as a result of ear infections. 50% of all children's surgeries and 25% of children "admissions" are due to ear-related complications. [If outer ear wax is the issue, put one drop of Taoist™ Ear Oil in each ear before bed. Upon rising, use a baby syringe to flush out wax. For adults, the Bio-Magnetic™ Dental Irrigator doubles as a ear cleaning tool by simply turning-down the down the pressure. Use hydrogen peroxide to fill the outer ear canal to "boil" and dislodge wax and "infection!" If the problem is **INSIDE** the ear and you have pain, ringing, fever and pressure—take Yucca Blend,™ MX,™ OX™ & R/C™—and perform High Enema Therapy™ [adults] and simple enemas [children] until things ease. Use MX™ for congestion and void medications where possible. MX™ causes mucous to break up and "flow"— denying bacteria, yeast, fungus and viruses a "medium" in which to breed. MX™ is microdosed DNA at "nano scale"—and it works extremely well on congested sinuses, lungs, bronchioles and ears in waste-filled bodies. Clear Head™ is used to irrigate the sinus cavities and destroy microbial overgrowth.]

Israel "Warns" Against Soy

The State of Israel issued a **health warning** [August 2005] to its people to **avoid** consumption of soy products. The Israeli government said the list of disorders associated with soy are: digestive problems; thyroid dysfunction; ADD and ADHD disorders; dementia; reproductive disorders; and cancer. Perhaps the most **"telling"** thing here is all the "flim-flam" and **hype** given soy in the uSA. Your author "broke" the soy story in this book in 1994—and caught "hell" for it, too—especially from upset vegetarians who did **NOT** want to hear that their darling "soy" was bad news! I rest my case!

Acres USA

This publication has had **profound** influence on my life—and on this book! If I could only receive one publication, this is the one. Order a trial subscription, and see what I mean. Call (800) 355-5313. I accept your thanks in advance.

33

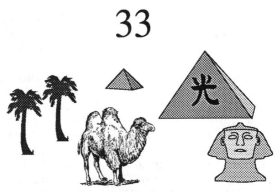

The Camel Or The Palm Tree?

"Truth will come to light; murder cannot be hid."
Shakespeare

"Kibyo" is Japanese for **strange disease.** Kibyo described the series of strange conditions that appeared during the 1950's in the small fishing village of Minamata on the southwest coast of Kyushu, Japan.

The conditions came to be known as "Minamata Disease." In 1957 mercury was discovered to be the toxic **"agent"** behind the strange **symptomatic** conditions and **SIGNS.**

Cats went crazy. Crows fell from the sky. People experienced dizziness and tunnel vision; their nervous systems failed; numbness was experienced in their extremities; and their legs burned! ALL life forms in the area suffered from the high mercury levels in the air, water and soil. The mercury came from an industrial plant up the coast from Minamata.

Mercury & Aging

Mercury is the **MOST** toxic "element" known to man! It's also the only elemental metal that occurs naturally in the "liquid" state. Sometimes it is referred to as *quicksilver* due to its elusive nature. A broken thermometer allows mercury to splatter and run. It **evaporates** like water!

Mercury is a **BIG** part of the "aging" story because of its toxic nature and ubiquitous presence in the environment—and in peoples "dental" fillings! It has been used in industry for hundreds of years. The fur industry used mercury to process animal furs in the "1700's." Mercury poisoning was first diagnosed in 1865—but mercury continued to be used by the fur industry into the "1950's!" The expression "mad as a hatter" refers to the tremors and insanity that plagued hat and garment workers. Ignorance and making a living "snared" workers because mercury came with the territory in many industries. Doctors who **DARED** to create a fuss quickly found themselves **without** a "license!" [Can the reader say the word "control"...for the good of the "public?" of course!] In those days, a hat worker's widow was given a "gold watch" and a wreath on the casket. No longer!

Mercury is a **BIG** part of life in "2006!" But these days, medical "science" assigns new names to mysterious dis-eases— usually with the word **"syndrome"** attached. The English equivalent of "kibyo" is "syndrome!" Today, everyone is a victim of mercury poisoning because there is no escaping it! The only practical answer is to keep it from building up in body tissues and to remove existing residues—a process that takes **"YEARS"** to do! [Mercury, sodium and carbon monoxide are easily absorbed, but **VERY DIFFICULT** to remove from the body.]

It took 8 years for your author's body to release and dispose of "tissue-bound" mercury! SOC™ shuttles mercury and heavy metals out of the tissues.

About Mercury

Mercury crosses the placental barrier and deforms the unborn. It lodges in the vital organs and short circuits their activity. It causes disintegration of the central and peripheral nervous systems and damages the kidney's nephrons (blood filters). [People who die of **heart attack** have **MASSIVE** mercury levels [from their "teeth"] in the heart muscle!]

Acute mercury poisoning causes vomiting, bloody diarrhea, tremors in the extremities, eyelids and tongue. **Moderate** mercury poisoning has a "ghost type" profile with symptoms like fatigue, insomnia, headaches, anxiety and loss of appetite. Erythrism (redness or blushing) is also a characteristic symptom, as is nighttime leg pain.

Dietary sources of mercury include tuna fish, shell fish, the air we breathe, and the water we drink. Mercury is a component of military munitions and fire works explosives— hence, it's in the air! Other sources are house paint, insecticides, fungicides, "pressed" and plywood building materals, wall sizing, and thousands of products people use everyday.

[Growing a garden is one way around mercury. The bacteria in healthy soils denature toxic substances; they are the "mediators" between Earth and sky. See Chapter 18.]

The Young Again! Tissue and Liver Protocol™ "shuttles" heavy metals OUT of the body through increased "bile flow" and systemic buffers!

The most **"OVERLOOKED"** source of mercury poisoning is **amalgam** dental fillings. These so-called "silver" fillings are a death sentence—and there is absolutely **NO EXCUSE** for any dentist to **EVER** use mercury amalgam in the mouths of innocent children and ignorant adults.

As far as your author is concerned, dentists who

*put mercury into innocent people's teeth should be in-
dicted for "murder!" And that is precisely the reason the
American Dental Association will NEVER admit the truth
about mercury and fluoride!*

The next most common source of mercury in the United
States comes from tap water. Mercury—in the form of mercuric
acid salt—is widely used to treat public water supplies in an
effort to control the spread of dis-ease. During the fall of 1993,
hundreds of innocent people became sick and some DIED from
drinking tap water contaminated with pathogenic bacteria and
laced with "mercury!" The cities were Milwaukee, Washington,
D.C. and Chicago. The worthless **authorities** blamed bacteria— but the real problem was "mercury!"

Here is the problem. Cities treat water with **"mercuric
acid"** to kill bacteria. This is done "without" public knowledge
and is **vehemently denied** by authorities. Mercuric acid is
used during the "warm months" when demand outruns water
processing capability. Cities don't have time to treat water
before distribution, so they use **mercuric acid** to control the
spread of "in-line" pathogens!

Cities use the dirty sand filters over and over—seldom
changing them! Instead, they use mercuric acid to kill the
bacteria and viruses that breed in the filters and send the water
to the gullible public to drink! In the Fall when the hot season
is over, cities stop using mercuric acid. If cities "miscalculate,"
the result is sick and dead people from an explosion of
pathogenic bacteria. [Safer treatment methods are available—
but yellow fringed flag "corporate" government isn't interested.]

Without mercury, public water supplies are a potential
source of *pathogenic* dis-ease. With mercury, people "drink"
their way to *systemic* dis-ease and old age without ever
realizing the problem. Mercury keeps the hospital lines full of
sick people demanding a *magic bullet!* Sick people are good
business. All toxic chemical agents in public water supplies are
"time bombs" waiting to manifest as dis-ease in the bodies of
people who are ignorant enough to drink it.

*[Do **NOT** drink "raw" tap water! Either make your own
biologically friendly water with a BFRV™ home unit or, buy
expensive bottled water, or fill your own bottles at the store and
haul it home. Raw tap water is at the **"ROOT"**of "leaky gut"
which is behind all "auto immune" conditions and dis-eases.]*

**Municipal water is "potable"—but it is not good for
your health! Drink biologically friendly water instead!**

Deregulated Death • Bombs And Munitions
The U.S. Department of Agriculture has established a
"ZERO" tolerance for mercury. Yet, the FDA established a
"safe" level for mercury. The word "safe" **implies** a safety and

watch-dog function—so people will "feel" protected! Regulatory agencies are *supposed to* "protect" the public. But powerful "interests" make sure mercury's use in industry goes unrestricted. Mercury is a $6,000,000,000 (billion) dollar industry!

Mercury occurs in three forms: Elemental vapor (mercury evaporates like water); mercurous/mercuric salt solutions and mercuric acid; ["Mercurochrome" was used on cuts and scratches in the 1930's, 40's and 50's—before it was "removed"]; and a third form called methyl mercury that **"binds"** to "proteins." [Body chemistry **requires** protein enzymes. Mercury blocks vital biochemical reactions and lodges in protein-based collagenous tissues.]

Corporate yellow fringed flag "government" is "OWNED" by certain unseen "interests!"

"Corporate" government—by way of the Atomic Energy Commission—supplies mercury to industry. After WWII, government held **HUGE** stockpiles of mercury—and policy "shifts" ushered this "silver death" element into the marketplace.

[Bombing of the Oklahoma City Federal building probably involved large amounts of mercury to accelerate the explosion. Pictures show that the explosion GAINED velocity as the force went up the face of the building—instead of dissipating as in non-mercury-related explosions.]

Agriculture uses **massive** amounts of mercury in the production of **FOOD!** In 1914, chemists discovered that mercury was an effective fungicide. Over six million pounds of mercury have been used in **FOOD PRODUCTION** in the past 40 years and over 200 million pounds total use since 1900. These numbers do **NOT** account for the disastrous "effects" mercury imposes on people's health when it is put into their **"teeth"** by dentists who should know better! The air we breathe is a **MAJOR** source of "mercury!" [Please see the BFRV™ Air Processor on page 114.]

Mercury is used to treat agricultural "food" seeds and in the paper industry as a slimicide. **AEROBIC** bacteria convert industrial mercury into highly toxic *methyl* mercury. Methyl mercury is difficult to remove from protein-bound body tissues. [The *Young Again (Tissue and Liver) Protocol*™ was developed to get the mercury out of "your" body! Homeovitic™ remedies are then used to "reprogram" tissue vibratory "frequency!"]

Mercury Fillings In Teeth

Dentistry has used *mercury* amalgam "silver" fillings for over 100 years. In the mouth, bacteria convert elemental mercury into *methyl mercury* "which bleeds" into the tissues and is "inhaled" and absorbed in the lungs.

Amalgam fillings are BIG business! Young, dumb, unsuspecting, starry-eyed dental students are **"taught"** that mercury amalgam fillings are "stable" and "non-toxic!" The *ignorant* patient is told the only difference between gold and amalgam is the cost and appearance. Dentistry avoids using the word **"mercury"**—preferring to call these fillings *amalgam* or **"SILVER."** It is **CRIMINAL** to fill teeth with the most toxic element on Earth. Like the "fur" industry, mercury fillings bring on dis-ease and S-L-O-W death. [Dentists who install amalgams **claim ignorance and lack of "scientific proof"**—while their patients lose their health and their lives. Dentists have the **HIGHEST** suicide rate. They reap what they sow!]

Dentistry likes mercury amalgams because they are a fast and profitable "drill and putty" procedure!

Gold also creates problems—but of a different sort. Gold fillings, bridges and crowns are composites of **dozens** of different "metals." Elemental metals are toxic to the body, and their energy "footprints" are measured in milli-volts that interfere with brain signals and body metabolism. These are extreme low voltage electrical signals similar to what spews from cell phones. If you need a crown or bridge, insist on pure **CERAMIC** crowns and bridges! Never metals!

If you have **mercury** in "your mouth"—do **NOT** remove it until you have prepared your system as outlined in this book! Please, call for guidance before you remove them! Mercury amalgam "removal" is **FAR MORE DANGEROUS** than when they were placed into your mouth. Age, poor immune system integrity, weak thyroid and compromised liver function come to the fore when mercury are "removed!"

Removal of mercury amalgams is EXTREMELY dangerous! The patient MUST prepare beforehand and take protective measures afterwards! Too little is too late!

NEVER, EVER go to ordinary dentists for amalgam removal. They are **antagonistic** to the idea and **careless** in their technique. Be very careful to **AVOID** "johnny-come-lately" dentists who are **NOT** certified, biological dentists and **ACTIVE** members of the American Biological Dental Association [Locate them on the web!] Dentists who **also do** amalgam fillings—on any pretense—are total phonies! Avoid them!

The Camel Or The Palm Trees?

Today, more than ever, people are faced with the dilemma of choosing between conventional medicine and holistic therapies. Making the right choice is easy. Let me emphasize "false" alternatives with a childhood story.

When we were children, one of our favorite pranks involved finding an empty Camel cigarette package and showing it to whomever we could get to listen.

"Assume you are in this picture, and it is raining cats and dogs and you must run for cover. Would you get under the palm

trees or would you get under the camel?" [On the face of the package is pictured a camel, some palm trees and several pyramids.] Some people answered they would "Take cover under the palm trees!" while others said they would "Take their chances under the camel!" Regardless of the answer, the person was wrong! We kids did what conventional medicine and dentistry does to *ignorant* and *desperate* people. We **only** offered two alternatives—and **BOTH** of them were bad choices! [The correct answer was to go around the corner of the package and take lodging in the hotel!]

In the world of conventional medicine and expert opinions, you are constantly faced with "camel or palm tree" decisions. Do not allow yourself to fall for false alternatives in matters of health—or you will grow old and suffer miserably along the way. Heavy metal poisoning—be it from tap water, food, colloidal minerals or dental fillings—is serious business.

Would you rather drink water that is contaminated with pathogenic microbes, mercury, sodium, chloramines and fluoride, or water that is "safe" according to industry standards?

The answer to this camel or palm tree question is, **"NEITHER!"** The world's second biggest manufacturer of mercury amalgam filling material has agreed to post **ALL** dental offices in California with signs **WARNING** patients about the carcinogenic, mutagenic and teratogenic effects of mercury—especially in children—and the unborn! [Good luck finding those signs!] Scandinavian countries and Germany **BANNED** mercury "amalgam" fillings. The American Dental Association—and its **"lackey"** dentists—are too damned proud and greedy to admit their mistakes, so the beatings shall continue until the poeple's moral improves!]

Putting "mercury" amalgam fillings into innocent people's teeth is a crime against humanity!

Dental Alternatives

Mercury removal requires that special protocols be followed for your safety—and the safety of the dental staff. "Composite" plastic is the replacement material of choice. These fillings require more skill and time than "drill and putty" mercury fillings. If composites are done correctly, they have a long life. Your author's composites are "intact" after 15 years!

Do not accept porcelain fillings. A dentist that tells you that composites don't hold up isn't doing them correctly. Cost is **not** the issue here—but your health is! Call your author for guidance and help **BEFORE** amalgam removal. Do **NOT** remove your amalgams if you are female, older or in poor health. You must become "personally" knowledgeable about the issues involved in mercury removal **BEFORE** you begin!

One final comment. Dental problems—be they decay, periodontal, root canals, implants or "cavitations" [infection pockets in the gum or bone from improperly extracted teeth and root canals]—cause illness and early death. Infection in the mouth destroys the heart muscle—as does mercury! [Do **NOT** underestimate the severity and long term consequences surrounding the "teeth!"]

Your "terrain" controls dental health—but once infected the teeth control your terrain! Don't put yourself in harms way by visiting the typical dental "quack!" Locate a biological dentist. Spread the word to everyone you care about! Dental health goes with being Young Again!

PREVIEW: *In our next chapter, you will learn about tobacco and how it relates to health and vitality. The American Indians knew the answer!*

Teeth

Terrain "acidity" controls tooth decay, gum dis-ease and early "death" of the teeth. Acidity manifests as early as "age 6!"

Sins of omission; and sins of comission. "Candor" avoids both of these human shortcomings!

Red Flags

Show me a lady with a cold body, memory complaints, excess fat, thinning/graying hair, yeast/bladder infections, PMS, fibroid tumors, aching joints, receding gums and low energy, and I'll show you a woman whose "terrain" is out of control. **Show me a man who** is fat, impotent, lost his sex drive, has prostate troubles, low energy and gray or missing hair, and I'll show you a man who is **NOT** in control of his body's terrain. [Pay attention to your body's "signals"—they are called **SIGNS** and symptoms; the same ones that lead to a miserable life!]

Take Time For 12 Things

Work. It is the price of success. **Think.** It is the source of power. **Play.** It is the secret of youth. **Read.** It is the foundation of knowledge. **Worship.** It is washes the dust of earth from our eyes. **Help & Enjoy Friends.** It is a source of happiness. **Love.** It is the one sacrament of life. **Dream.** It hitches the soul to the stars. **Laugh.** It is laughing that lightens life's loads. **Beauty.** It is everywhere in nature. **Health.** It is the true wealth and treasure of life. **Plan.** It is the key to the first 11!

The Romans knew the power of table salt. When they defeated Hannibal's Carthage, they made sure Carthage would NEVER rise again by salting her soil!

Hello there!

Few people comprehend the **"true"** state of their health. And only 1 out of 1,000 are willing to take responsibility for their lives and **STOP** the whining! Some folks **rationalize** their circumstance; others **utter** excuses and post **blame**; others simply give up and await the grim reaper! Be willing to do your part. Prevention is easier and less expensive than restoring someone **after** their "terrain" has **crashed!**

What is done to **AVOID** serious medical problems is **EXACTLY** what is done to **REVERSE** them. Everything is a "terrain" issue! In **"my"** younger years before age 43, health food, vitamins, herbs, juice, yoga and exercise were **enough** to keep the reaper away from my door. But these things alone will **NOT** keep the reaper away from your door after age **"35"** because the rules are **different!** **"Fundamental"** issues control the body's "terrain." Traditional "health" fads don't "cut it" once the terrain is in trouble—or when you are over 35 years of age. High-profile, big-shot practitioner's make lots of noise, but they have the same health problems as their followers. The reaper **waits** at their door, too! Results count, and the *Young Again Protocol*™ definitely produces results for anyone who is **short** on excuses and **long** on responsibility. If you need help, *"Ask for it!"* **And please be willing to do your part.** Aging-reversal requires much patience—and lots of work, too!

Feed a cold; starve a fever!

Things fall apart; the liver cannot hold;
Confusion and anarchy seize the terrain;
The dimmed tide is loosed upon the moment,
As hell decends upon the ignorant soul!

Sore Feet, Back & Joints

When your author was in his teens, he had tripple-A width feet. When the US Army was finished with me , they were B-width. By September 2000, they were C-width and I was in trouble. [Due to a freak injury to the ligaments in his feet, I was limping and in severe pain by Thanksgiving, 2000. **"Plantar facitis"** was the diagnosis; fallen arches was the issue! So I paid a visit to Nick's Boots—a local specialty boot maker who made a pair of boots designed specifically for my feet—triple-A width! **The results were astounding!** These boots realigned the bones in my feet and changed my life, overnight! **"I love them and so will you!"** You haven't lived until you wear a pair of Frank Petrilli's Sweedish boots in either work and dress styles.

[P. S. If you wear tennis shoes, you will pay the price in "misery" in the years to come. Get rid of them or at least insert a "good" pair of orthodic inserts before you totally ruin your feet!]
Call (800) 824-2685 or (509) 483-1246

34

The "Sacred" Three Sisters

"First, the Creator gave us tobacco."
["Kanonsionni-Kayeneren-Kowa"]
The Iroquois

When the white man came to the Americas, he discovered that the main staples of the Indian diet were corn, beans and squash. The Indians called these foods the "sacred three sisters." They understood the importance of these food crops in their diet. They also understood the importance of another FOOD—a food which they held in the **utmost** esteem. That food was **TOBACCO!**

The Indians considered tobacco **sacred** because they had discovered tobacco's **NUTRITIONAL** characteristics. Their discovery was incorporated into their religious beliefs. The Indians told the white man *"The Creator gave us the sacred three sisters. But before the Creator gave us corn, beans and squash, He gave us **TOBACCO!**"*

Tobacco's status in the Indian psyche was based on DIETARY need, but it was respected on a religious level. Smoking was the extension of the dietary status tobacco held in the culture of the natives of the Americas.

When native peoples elevate certain foods and events to religious status, there is a reason. Unfortunately for millions of people, the white man failed to take his cues from Indian dietary habits and religious beliefs. The white man did **NOT** make the connection between diet and health until 498 years later (1990). The connection was made by a lone individual named Tom Mahoney.

Tobacco

Despite its negative social image, tobacco has significance to the aging process—and to health and longevity. Tobacco is **terribly** misunderstood by the American public. They know **NOTHING** of its therapeutic or dietary value because they can't see through the "smoke" the government and pharmaceutic companies have "created" to hide the *truth!*

People are told of the negative aspects of smoking—but they know **nothing** of the real tobacco story. The public's "ignorance" is **NOT** an accident; it is by design!

Prior to the discovery of the Americas, Europeans did **NOT** grow or eat corn, beans or squash. These important foods were absent from European diets; dietary imbalances were the norm; dis-ease—as a result of *excess* acid waste build-up— "plagued" the white man and his "civilization."

The *Sacred Three Sisters* were taken to Europe, and for a time people's nutritional status improved. Corn was easy to grow and became the "dominant" food staple of the poor. By the 1700's, corn gained dietary dominance and resulted in **"excess"** and the occurrence of dis-ease—particularly in Mediterranean Italy, Spain, Greece and Portugal. The condition of **EXCESS** had no name—yet!

Casal's Necklace

In 1735, the Spanish physician Casal described a disease condition by one of its key **"SIGNS!"** He called it *mal de la rosa* or "red sickness." People on farms who ate too much corn suffered the most. Typically, they had a red **"ring"** around their neck which came to be called *"Casal's necklace."* [In the American South, corn's dominance among farmers and the poor caused the phrase "red neck" to come into usage.]

In 1771, an Italian doctor described the **SIGNS** of an unknown dietary condition of *excess* when he wrote of "rough, painful skin." *Pellagra* is the English corruption of Italian and summed up the condition nicely. Until the 1900's, however, no connection was made between corn intake and the condition of *excess* that had come to be called *pellagra.*

*[Like most conditions, pellagra operates behind a "cloak" in the early stages. It includes loss of energy, weight loss and poor appetite. The four 'D's'-**dizziness, depression, dementia** and **delusion**-best describe pellagra's **SIGNS!** Today, there are tens of thousands of people suffering from these **SIGNS,** but you will not hear the term pellagra.]*

In the 1850's, a new "condition" appeared in the uSA— with symptoms and **SIGNS** similar to those of Mediterranean peoples. The "condition" paralleled H. J. Heinz' introduction of his famous Heinz 57 "canned" foods in 1859.

Canned food contains copious amounts of salt to keep down botulism. In addition, heat processing destroys and denatures food enzymes and proteins.

The Civil War wrought massive upheaval in people's dietary habits—especially farm people in the South. Conditions of **EXCESS** became prevalent due to lack of dietary **variety** and **insufficient** availability of food proteins. Economic conditions were blamed, but *pellagra* had its roots in the shift from an **unbalanced** agricultural society to an **unbalanced** industrial one. The poor suffered the most; they ate too much corn and **not enough** greens and proteins. [**Excess** corn creates an acid condition in the body's terrain—just as excess intake of "meat" contributes to an acid condition.]

By the turn of the century, the dis-eases of pellagra and beriberi became widespread. Poor people were eating too much hominy, corn meal, grits, and corn meal mush—especially in the South where this practice continues to this day! Worse, the corn being consumed was "bolted!" Bolted corn does not contain the "germ!" The germ is what causes seeds to "germinate!" It is the seed's **"LIFE FORCE"** and contains all of the important B-vitamins and mineral ions.

Food "processing" companies discovered that **BOLTED, "devitalized"** (degermed) corn meal keeps better. Bolted corn was one of the first "natural" bio-junk foods. "White" bread was second. An ignorant public perceived these new foods to be **"status foods."** [Perception is reality!"]

[Processed food became "value added" food and commanded higher prices and profits. People didn't realize that they had been **"taken!"** *They are* **STILL** *being "taken" every time they spend their hard-earned money on "processed" foods!]*

[Pellagra became **"endemic"** *to certain geographic areas and diets. Thousands of people suffered from pellagra and beriberi. In dogs, pellagra is called* **"black tongue!"** *These dis-eases could have easily been* **prevented** *if the white man had payed attention to the Indian diet—including tobacco! Tobacco contains the "entire" vitamin B-12 complex in natural molecular form. Tobacco is very valuable as a* **FOOD!]**

Back to corn. Non-hybrid, non-bolted corn is good food! But too much of anything creates imbalance and conditions of **EXCESS** that eventually manifest as dis-ease! [The diet should include fresh, green leafy alkaloid vegetables, fresh vegetable juices [beet, carrot, celery], and high-quality proteins. [**VARIETY** avoids conditions of "excess!"]

[The Mexican custom of soaking corn in lime water and the **inclusion** *of fresh, green leafy vegetables, offsets corn's acidity and prevents the incidence of pellagra in Mexican populations. The custom was adopted from the native Indians; so was the combining of corn and beans for dietary balance.]*

How the body responds to food is a function of the liver and the "terrain." The terrain controls!

The B-vitamin Story

The B-vitamins (B's) offset dietary excess and rid the body of conditions like pellagra and beriberi by restoring "balance" to the system. B-vitamins are found in "healthy," fresh, green, leafy vegetables—which also contain Vitamin-C along with bioflavonoids, rutin and hesperidan complexes. "Niacin" has been credited as the "active" pellagra curative agent, which is no more true than the **"misconception"** that Vitamin-C cures scurvey! [Isn't it "strange" how half-turths and mistruths find their way into government school books?]

[*A vitamin is a vital amine. Vitamins are vital because they act as cofactors with bio-active mineral ions to create and sustain life. An amine is the active "—R" group on food molecules, giving them certain biological and chemical qualities.*]

Niacin is "called" Vitamin B-3. "Supposedly" niacin is involved in ALL critical metabolic pathways. These pathways are a very complex series of reactions that keep us alive, healthy and happy. Good health is a reflection of strong activity in these very critical biochemical pathways.

Real Vitamin B-3 contains two very important molecules: NAD (**nicotine**amideadenine dinucleotide) and NADP (**nicotine** adenine dinucleotide phosphate). These substances are required in the Krebs Cycle (aka: Citric Acid Cycle) within the mitochondrial "electron transport chain" where our *energy* molecule "ATP" is created, burned and converted into cellular "lightning" as discussed in Chapter 24. [The reader can gain a fuller understanding of things "medical and science" by study and "coloring" at home!" [See pages 233 and 240.]

All of the **REAL** "B" vitamins are involved in **FUSION** reactions of the gut and liver. The body and the mitochondria need the B's to make energy, build/repair tissue and keep the immune system strong. **Isomeric** Vitamin B-3 (niacin) does **NOT** have the same characteristics as food-derived molecules. [B-vitamins that don't derive from real food are useless!]

B Vitamins • pH • Soft Drinks

The Indians knew about tobacco's life-giving properties. Tobacco is the richest natural source of natural B's in the world! Concentrations of real B-vitamins run as high as 30%! We get the B's when we add **"small"** amounts of green or dried tobacco to stews, beans and salads. [Please note, care must be taken in the choice of tobacco variety. Most importantly, fresh lemon juice or apple cider vinegar **MUST** be used to bring "green" tobacco leaf into the "range" of digestion.]

[*The pH of edible tobacco is Ph 10-11. Lemon juice and vinegar have a pH of 2. Stomach acid (HCL) is pH -1 to +1. For each # up or down the scale, pH changes by a factor of "ten." pH of 10 is 1,000 times more alkaline than pH 7. [pH neutral is 7.0. Anything above "7" is alkaline; below is acid.*]

Terrain "pH" is grossly affected by "soft drinks" which **FORCE** the body to **"withdraw"** bone calcium to **"buffer"** the acidic effects soft drinks cause in the "blood stream." Soft drinks "upset" the **calcium : phosphorous ratio** and grossly alter body **physiology**—"stealing" minerals from the "terrain" and color from the hair as noted in Chapters 28, 29 and 30.

Synthetic vs. Natural B's

Real "B" vitamins are potent, right-spin substances—even in small amounts. "Synthetic" B-vitamins are not good; natural Vitamin E in "soy" oil is a joke; cod liver oil beats synthesized vitamin-A; common Vitamin-C [as used by thousands of people] is next to useless as are the B-vitamins of which 95% are lost down the drain!

The real stories of vitamins "B" and "C"—and how to achieve therapeutic blood levels of BOTH—will be discussed in detail in Chapter 37 coming up shortly.

The body is unable to build healthy tissue with synthetic vitamins—which is why your author stresses the importance of juicing and eating fresh, whole, "live" food and avoiding bio-junk diets. [Raise blood levels of real B-vitamins to "therapeutic" levels, and energy levels and pernicious anemia (chronic shortage of oxygen-carrying hemoglobin and red blood corpuscles) disappears and immune activity takes off!]

When we are sick, white blood cell count should go "up!" **Failure** of the immune system to "respond" to a threatening condition is called "aging!" Without plenty of "B's," the body **CANNOT** defend itself. [Excellent food sources for building blood serum hemoglobin and so-called "iron" levels are racemized,™ predigested liver capsules, Cobo-12™ and racemized™ algae. [Cobo-12™ is a racemized **"transdermal"** vitamin B-12 creme developed especially for women!]

After age 30, vitamin B-12 absorption via the mouth and stomach "collapses!" Cobo-12™ absorbs through the skin into the blood capillary beds for instant effect!

Green tobacco is loaded with complexd, naural B-vitamins. Green tobacco juice also contains nicotine in natural "alkaloid" form. Dried tobacco contains "real" so-called nicotinic acid. Bottled forms of nicotinic acid, niacin, and nicotinamide are "synthesized" and not the same as from "tobacco!"

Niacin is "promoted" as the "heart" vitamin, which is true if derived from a food source and fully "complexed!" The "B's" improve blood circulation and prevent blood clots—which has **"NOTHING"** to do with Vitamin-K as the "experts" would have you believe. The "experts" also tell us the "flush" that accompanies synthetic niacin ingestion is due to its "activity"—but it's not so! The "flush" effect is a mild reaction to **synthetic** niacin molecules and binders. Better to get so-called "niacin" from fresh vegetable juices and healthy food. [Digestion and leaky-gut issues prevent full absorption of the B-vitamins—a problem that has now been overcome as noted in Chapter 37.]

Fresh "greens" are one of the best sources of the B's.

Meat has limited amounts of trytophan which the liver **converts** to so-called "niacin" (60 mg of trytophan = 1 mg of niacin). [Isn't it interesting that government outlawed trytophan under the "pretense" that it was "protecting" the public.]

Predigested, organic liver capsules from healthy, free-range animals off the grasslands of South America and racemized™ algae and Cobo-12™ are loaded with B-vitamins and lots of other "factors" that promote health.

Food **"alkaloids"** can be **poisonous** if overdone! Alkaloids are highly active nitrogen-containing compounds with "marker" physiologic properties. Alkaloids make things happen in the body because they are extremely biologically active!

By definition, "alkaloids" have an alkaline pH. Common alkaline vegetables are spinach and swiss chard—which explains why many people have difficulty digesting them. These "potentially" nutritious vegetables **MUST** be eaten or prepared with **lemon** or **vinegar** to bring them within digestion range.

[Some well-known plant-derived alkaloid drugs are digitalis (foxglove), belladonna (nightshade), and marijuana. When real is "synthesized," drug side-effects multiply! Pharmaceutical drugs are isomers and should be avoided!]

The Niacin Story

Nicotine was named for Jean Nicot—the French ambassador to Portugal who sent tobacco seeds to Paris in 1550. By 1571, crude nicotine had been isolated. In 1828, purified nicotine was isolated. In 1867, *nicotine* was demonstrated to **"cure"** black tongue and pellagra—but this fact was **"hidden!"**

[Nicotine in "PURIFIED" or "SYNTHESIZED" form is extremely poisonous. Natural nicotine is different—and that is the point here. The reader must learn to "differentiate!" The Indians used it judiciously, and the white man should, too!]

Nicotine in dried tobacco is **NOT** toxic, as the public has been led to believe! If it were, people who smoke and chew would react and die on the spot. I would **remind** the reader that the mucous membranes of the respiratory tract are the avenue of choice where fast absorption is desired. Cigarettes are "bad news" because of what is in them —and we are **NOT** talking about the "tobacco!" [Cigars do not share the dangers of cigarettes. You can tell the difference by the smell! Inhale a "cigar" and you will turn **"GREEN"** and get sick from too much liver "stimulation!" Regular cigar smokers seldom get sick; old time cigar smokers like George Burns live very long lives!]

Lung cancer is proliferating in people who have **NEVER** smoked or been subjected to ongoing secondary cigarette "smoke!" Christopher Reeve's widow, Dana [who died in March of 2006] is a good example! The government is "lying!" The **REAL** cause of lung cancer [and many birth defects]is people's

"**DIET!**" Specifically, the total lack of **folic acid**—a component of the B-vitamin complex. [Without healthy, fresh juices and vegetables, people are "toast!" Natural folic acid is inexpensive and available. Take 10 mcg. daily whether you smoke or not!]

People who take "folic acid" and smoke will NEVER get lung cancer—and neither will others who breathe the smoke! The government and the bureaucrats are "liers!"

History of Vitamin P-P

From the turn of the century, nicotinic acid was known by the *disguised* name of "P-P factor"—short for **P**ellagra **P**reventive. "P-P" factor was used until the generation of people then alive had died. **Later**—in the 1930's the words vital and amine merged into the hybrid word "vitamin." P-P factor then became known as "Vitamin P-P."

In 1899, Dr. Joseph Goldberger of the United States Public Health Service launched a study into the effects of P-P factor and its relationship to pellagra. He *dragged his feet* for 16 years before he penned his study regarding the relationship between P-P factor and pellagra—something that had been "**KNOWN**" since 1867! The foot-dragging was **NO** accident. There was a "commercial" **reason** for the delay!

In the *meantime,* pharmaceutical and oil industry interests went to work developing "synthetic" P-P factor. They did **NOT** want people to know they could treat pellagra and beriberi—and spin-off dis-ease conditions that resulted from them—by "**growing**" their "cure" in the form of tobacco. They did **NOT** want people to make the association between P-P factor, nicotine and tobacco.

Pharmaceutical interests figured out a way to manufacture synthetic "P-P" cheaply and easily using pyridine carbon rings from inexpensive charcoal and petroleum. Synthetic P-P factor is **NOT** the same molecule. It is an "isomer!" Real vitamin P-P spins "right" and supports health. The fake one spins "left."

The pharmaceutical companies could NOT "patent" tobacco—but they could patent "synthesized" man-made molecules. They are doing the same thing to women with their damnable, synthetic hormone analogs as contained in female replacement "hormones" and birth control pills.

Keep The People Confused!

"Niacin" is a *bogus* term. It is a coined word—like "canola!" It was "popularized" by the medical establishment and pharmaceutical interests in the 1950's to hide the fact that real "nicotinic acid"—the acid form of nicotine in dried tobacco—is the **active** "factor" in tobacco that causes pellagra and beriberi to go *"Bye, bye!"* when added to the diet.

Certain "corporate" interests wanted control over

America's health. There was a massive effort to VILIFY
tobacco. That effort continues to this very moment.
To create "confusion" and cover their tracks, the "experts" **DIVIDED** the B-12 vitamin **"complex"** into separate "vitamins" known as vitamin B-1 through B-12 and offered the public a "fix" using **synthetic** molecules and formulations. The entire operation was a massive "fix!"

*[After age 30, Vitamin B-12 absorption drops dramatically because **intrinsic factor** secretion from the stomach wall "collapses!" Women lose their B-12 reserves from their "vital" organs 20 years before men, due to loss of blood from the menstrual cycle. Cobalt is central to hemoglobin formation. Anemia issues reflect loss of cobalt. The introduction of Cobo-12™ skin creme answered the need for cobalt. Sublingual B-12 tablets and oral sprays do **NOT** solve the problem because both are **dependent** on intrinsic factor production. B-12 is a **HUGE** issue for women because it affects virtually **everything** about female body physiology—and yet it is **not** specific for any "single" condition. B-12 shots are a synthetic "band aid!"]*

Cobalt & Health

Cobalt 60 is known as "cobalt blue" and is a *naturally occurring radioactive substance* that **must** be present in order for life to exist. It is a crucial element in mitochondrial fusion reactions in man and animal. It is "central" to production of the massive amounts of energy needed to keep us alive each day. Tobacco is loaded with cobalt blue and full of the B-vitamin complex. When we eat whole, natural foods—like fresh green leafy vegetables—and tobacco—we provide the body with natural NAD and NADP, cobalt 60 and all of the B-vitamins needed to assist the mitochondria in the production of the ATP.

Everyone should grow and eat tobacco. It is legal to grow. It can be frozen or dried. The tobacco of which I am speaking is a beautiful plant, standing 6-10 feet tall and 3 feet wide. The bugs will **NOT** eat tobacco—it's too potent!

The Dilemma • Lies & More Lies

The public is **told** that tobacco and nicotine are bad for them. Then they are **told** that niacin and the B's are good for them. We are **NOT** being **told** the whole truth! A long-term campaign was begun in the 20th century to get people to stop using tobacco in all forms. Today, the effort is **"massive"**—and the public is being **WHIPPED** into a frenzy! The occurrence of major dis-ease is being unfairly "blamed" on tobacco to keep people ignorant—and to "fatten" pharmaceutical interests!" Don't believe me? Can the reader say Vioxx™? The **TRUTH** of the matter is that people have been smoking "toxic" tobacco "substitutes" instead of the real thing! [If you want to smoke, buy real cigarettes or get a cigar and go outside.]

We have been lied to at a time when our food supply is deteriorating at a fantastic rate! At the same time that tobacco is being vilified, the U. S. Government is "the" biggest grower of **hybridized** tobacco in the world! The implications are scary, but tobacco isn't to blame!

[The **issue** *here is parallel "corporate" government in the form of the "U"nited States Government—which is* **NOT** *the same as the "united" States of America. The "government" operates under the yellow fringed flag—a war flag! America was "formed" under the Title 4 USC, Section 1 American Flag of Peace. The people are* **NOT** *the same as the "government!"]*

Tobacco—like the "War on Terror!"—is a perfect **"COVER!"** The pharmaceutical companies and "corporate" government are the problem here!

The more something is believed to be true and the greater the number of people who believe it to be so, the greater the odds that it is NOT true!

Old-time farmers from Tennessee fed their horses TOBACCO! Tobacco was the American Indian's gift to the white man. He accepted the Sacred Three Sisters, but he ignored the greatest gift of all. Pellagra's "disappearance" in 1935 had **NOTHING** to do with "enrichment" of the food supply as "claimed." Pellagra disappeared when **dietary variety** and **quality proteins** found their way onto people's dinner plates.

When health is lost, medical science says *"syndrome."* The Japanese say *"Kibyo."* Your author says *"old age!"*

PREVIEW: *For the **first time** in 12 years, five "new" chapters have been added to Young Again! Enjoy what follows!*

When you control the dietary health of a nation, you control the people. And when you control a nation's money supply, you have the perfect monopoly.

The Appendix—Not A Vestigial Organ

The appendix **"dangles"** from the cecum in the most toxic area of the body. [See page 46.] It was put there to draw away **"excess"** toxic energy from the cecum. The appendix is surrounded by clusters of lymph nodes called "Peyer's patch." The cecum is the end of the small intestine **(gut)** and the beginning of the large intestine **(colon)**. It's where parasites "hang out"— and it's the **MOST** toxic spot in the body! The cecum is 6 feet "up" from the anus and the **end of the road** when doing High Enema Therapy.™ The medical folks consider the appendix a **vestigial** organ—but God put it there quite "on purpose!"

Making It Happen In Your Life!

Good health is a one-step-at-a-time process—in reverse! Here are some basic steps to health and vitality. **Drink** biologically-friendly water—and enough of it. **Complete** the *Young Again (Tissue & Liver) protocol.*™ Eat "good" food. **Juice** beets, carrots and celery daily. **Avoid** extremes. **Seek** balance in ALL areas of your life. **Get** into the *Young Again*™ *High Enema Therapy*™ *Protocol.*™ **Add** racemized™ super foods to your diet. **Restore** and balance your hormones and **clear** your receptors.

   Avoid processed foods. **Get** some aerobic exercise daily. **Learn** yoga and Pilates. **Use** racemized™ hormone precursors! **Stay away** from doctors. **Get** control of your mind. **Laugh!** Love! Help others! **Reject** hate, anger, greed, envy, blame, etc. **Avoid** medications, recreational drugs and alcohol. **Follow** your instincts. **Visualize** good health and the life you desire. **Refuse** to buy into negative thinking—but be realistic. **Erase** "vaccine" energy fields from your body. **Remove** mercury fillings from your teeth and get the residues **out** of your tissues. **Develop** a healthy, regular prayer and meditation life. **Use** a rebounder or L/CSF™ machine daily. **Use** a Biogenic™ lymph roller on your body 2x a day. **Use** CWD™ for energy and leveling of blood sugar and burning of fat. **Live** today. **Forget** yesterday. **Leave** tomorrow alone. **Drink** Kombucha tea & use GH$_3$+ and HST™ Creme to grow & darken and hair and improve general health. **Do** load-bearing work. **Simplify** your life in every way possible. **Use** racemized™ sea minerals in your water. **Grow** a garden! **Grow** a garden! **Grow** a garden! **Learn** to use a pendulum and vibration chain. **Use** Taoist™ SUPER foods for superb health. **Eat** only healthy food. Don't buy food in grocery stores. **Never** consume soy or canola oils or soy products. **Give** thanks each day to be alive. **Be** patient with yourself; good health takes time to manifest. **Experience** the *miracle* of rejuvenation by living life 90% correct—don't worry about the 10%. **Do whatever it takes** to have a healthy life. **STAY AWAY** from doctors! Good health is a matter of **CHOICE!**

Buffalo Girls

   "Buffalo girls won't you come-out tonight, come-out tonight, come-out tonight; buffalo girls won't you come-out tonight and dance by the light of the moon!"

   The moon has profound influence on womens hormone cycles—as well as their menstrual cycles—as does "diet," bile flow and the "condition" of the woman's **"liver!"**

Hormones & Stress

"Stress," regardless of the source has dramatic effects on womens hormone levels. Stress is the ultimate hormonal "wild card!" Reduce the "effects" of stress with PU.™ [See page 46.]

35

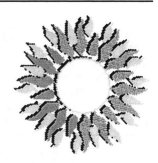

Vorago™ SunRise

"There is value in reading widely and trying to remember seemingly unrelated facts [and] sometimes, the mind will come up with links to memories that will prove useful."
Dr. Linus Pauling

"Something's happening here! What it is ain't exactly clear!"
Unknown

"Let there be light!" In Genesis, the rainbow was given by God to Noah and his progeny as a **"SIGN"** when they emerged from the ark after the great flood. Hidden in the rainbow, however, is another story of importance with meaning for people who wish to experience superb health and longevity.

The rainbow is the **"display"** of the visible light spectrum, ranging from violet-blue at 425 nanometers of lightwave frequency to red at 750 nanometers of lightwave frequency.

Plants ***"capture"*** **and** ***"freeze"*** the colors of the rainbow in their **pigments** as "frozen light.™" Plants comply with the command to *"Be fruitful and multiply!"* —and in the process bring "light" into the soil of Earth for the benefit of all creatures—man, animal, plant and microbe.

Food is **"THE"** most central issue confronting all life on planet Earth! Real food—"healthy" food—is a gift from God for those who choose to partake of it. [Exercise choice!]

Fresh fruits and vegetables are **"stabilized"** energy in the broadest sense and **nourishment** in the dietary sense as measured by their carbohydrate, fat and protein content. But there is a bigger message hidden in the "food" story!

When we eat "healthy" fruits and vegetables, it is their **"pigments"** that produce the beneficial effects we associate with health and longevity. The colors of the rainbow are sunlight "energy" in the form of *lightwave frequency* that is "frozen" and "concentrated" as individual color pigments. What we think of as **nourishment** is actually frozen light™—and the "pigments" contain the **"MAGIC!"**

Sunlight As Food
Fruitarians and vegetarians generally avoid animal

proteins in the belief that they are somehow better off without them. But the *Young Again Model*™ provides a more realistic explanation for the health benefits these folks *temporarily* enjoy. The answer to the "riddle" is hidden in the "pigments" contained in live, fresh food.

Vegetarians, vegans and meat eaters all seem to **think** they have "the" formula for a healthy life. And in a way all of them are correct—but only "partly" correct! "Believing" something is true does **NOT** make it so—and people who nly consume only fruits and vegetables suffer the **exact same consequences** as the meat eaters who refuse to eat fruit and vegetables. Balance is the issue and the "pigments" are the key!

The **odd** part of the "pigment" story is that only a tiny percentage of pigments survive gastrointestinal "passage" functionally intact! But those that do survive the GI tract intact have a **BIG** effect, as told in the following story of "Aunt Bertrena."

Vorago™ Women & Men

At 84 years of age, Aunt Bertrena was very, very active! She was a prolific gardener and a voracious consumer of the wonderful foods she grew on her little "parcel" of land.

When her niece, Catherine, came to visit Bertrena after many years away—Catherine found her *climbing* in fruit trees, picking and eating fruit. Bertrena had **no** signs of arthritis; she was **flexible**; her body was that of a **young** woman: toned, full-breasted, trim, **plenty** of muscle mass, a **full head** of natural color hair; **boundless** energy—and gorgeous at age 84!

Bertrena was a true vorago™ woman. It is estimated that only one in 10,000 women are vorago™ females. These women have a **different** physiology than "normal" women. The **BIG** difference is that vorago™ women do **NOT** age!

At puberty, Bertrena was absolutely beautiful! In her late teens, she "glowed" all the time—like a woman seven months pregnant! Her body was that of a Greek goddess—and she did not lose it as she grew older. Bertrena married young and bore many children.

Your author knows of another vorago™ female who bore 14 children in 20 years—and was absolutely beautiful at age 48 and beyond.

[A less obvious characteristic of vorago™-type women is that they are "loaded" with female hormones—and unlike "normal" women, menses and "ovulation" carry into their 80's and beyond! Some vorago™ women "NEVER" experience a menstrual period in their entire life! These women are extremely fertile—and as you might expect—they usually have a very healthy sex drive to go with it! True vorago™ females consume copious amounts of "healthy" fruits and vegetables!]

[Back to Aunt Bertrena.] From early childhood, until

age 84—when Catherine found Bertrena climbing in her fruit trees—Bertrena ate nothing but fresh fruits and vegetables and home- grown eggs and meats. Bertrena was a creature of the Sun—and the food she consumed was a gift of the Sun. [All food is condensed sunlight energy.]

Bertrena started out as a vorago™ female —and she REMAINED a vorago™ because of the "magical" effects of the "pigments" in the food she grew and consumed.

Hollywood Voragos™

Shades of "true" vorago™ women appear from time to time. Some [Hollywood] examples would be Sophia Loren, Loretta Young and Rachel Welch—all breathlessly beautiful women by any measure! And yet as beautiful as these women are and were, they are **NOT** true voragos.™

The vorago™ story has its roots in the pigments of healthy, live, home-grown food! You cannot buy this kind of food because it is **NOT** for sale. You **MUST** grow your own food or seek it out. [Your author grows his own food on a one-acre parcel of land—and because he does **not** age and has managed to "rewind" his biological clock to age 19, he qualifies as a vorago™ male. The rules apply to both sexes!]

Voragos™ of either sex can be "created" regardless of age. Controlling factors are diet, liver and "terrain!"

Pigments & The Skin Window

So what about 99.9% of the people who will **never** be able to grow their own fruits and vegetables on a grand scale? How can the rest of the world enjoy the benefits of being a vorago™-type woman? The "answer" to the *dilemma* is to be found in SunLight™ Creme—a racemized,™ pigment-based, transdermal skin creme that promotes the vorago™ "effect."

[Each jar of SunLight™ Creme contains 32,000 racemized™ activity units of "frozen sunlight"™ for "uploading" the rainbow through the skin. SunLight™ Creme "bypasses" the GI tract—using the skin as a PROXY! It can be used as a face creme along with SOC™ lotion and racemized™ Skin Creme. SunLight™ creme has "magical" qualities!]

SunLight™ Creme is a SUPERB "breast" creme, and women who use it can remove the big "C" word from their vocabularies and STOP worrying and fretting!

SunLight™ Creme is **NOT** a "hormonal"—but it helps normalize hormonal "swings" with rainbow-based plant pigments that mimic the Vorago™ effect. [SunLight™ creme is part of the *Young Again (Female and Male) Protocol(s)*.™]

Vorago™ females are "insulated" from many aging issues—as they reverse the aging process! Lucky is the woman who never needs to see a doctor!

It's The Food!

It is **assumed** that a woman must experience "menses" or she is not fertile and cannot "conceive"—but this is not so! True Voragos™ **NEVER** have periods—but they are very fertile. [The exact "opposite" of a Vorago™ woman is an anorexic or bulimic female that **STOPS** her menses because she is "starving" herself to dealth. These women cannabalize their body by digesting their muscle mass—becoming "prison-camp" frail. This is also what happen to men and women in the years before they die. In the end, everyone becomes a meat eater, so better to choose and eat carefully to avoid becoming a "cannibal!"

Aunt Bertrena, Today!

Sadly, Bertrena had financial troubles and fell prey to her well-meaning children who made her give up her little parcel of land and move into an "apartment" where meals— *delivered on wheels*—became her way of life. **No more** food "pigments;" **no more** physical work; **no more** nature—and **no more vorago™ Bertrena.** Within six months, Bertrena became a "broken" old woman: arthritic, wrinkled and sad! Her beauty *"Gone with the wind!"*

[Aunt Bertrena's story inspired the creation of SunLight™ Creme. And all of the bits and pieces of information collected over these many years made it possible for your author to write about the possibilities of duplicating the vorago™ effect in regular people. As Linus Pauling said in the opening quote"There is value in reading widely and trying to remember seemingly unrelated facts [and] sometimes, the mind will come up with links to memories that will prove useful."]

If you would like to wake up to a vorago™ sunrise, all the reader has to do is "Make the choice!"

Vorago™ women—and men—can be "created!" They enjoy "health" beyond most people's wildest dreams for as long as they are willing to practice the principles outlined in this book. The **"pigments"** are nature's way of adding an extra "edge" in the pursuit of becoming *Young Again!*

PREVIEW: *In our next chapter, you will learn of a most unique discovery that"reverses" aging and restores the body "terrain" in a way never before attainable!*

"The capacity to blunder slightly is the real marvel of DNA. Without this special attribute, we would still be anaerobic bacteria and there would be no music!
                                                    Lewis Thomas

CATCHEXIA: Wasting away—as in "self cannibalization."

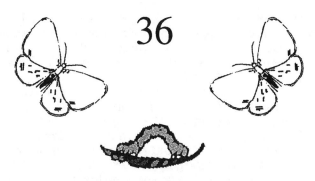

36

SilkWorm Blues

The worms crawl in; the worms crawl out;
The worms play pinochle on my snout!
Unknown

[The above quote is a "clue" as to what this chapter is about. The quote hints at issues that are at the very "core" of the aging process—and what must be done to reverse the process!]

In the body, what goes around does **NOT necessarily** come around—unless you have a little help from a "friend!"
[The reader will soon discover "who" that friend is because your author is going to tell a "wormy" story of profound significance that has "never" been told by anyone before!]

The human heart "pumps" the body's primary "liquid" tissue—blood—throughout the body each time it beats. However, only 90% of the blood leaving the heart returns as "blood"—meaning we have a **10% leak** in the system!

The "leakage" is the **"liquid"** serum/plasma proteins that **"seep"** through blood capillary walls into the tissues spaces—where the **"EXCHANGE"** of oxygen and carbon dioxide, nutrients and waste takes place. [The tissues is where the "real" story of aging is to be discovered—and defined!]

After the **"exchange"** takes place in the tissues, liquid, cellular "acid waste" from the cells is removed by the lymphatic capillaries. This waste is called "lymph fluid!" But the lymphatic system only uptakes 85-90% of "soluble" fluid waste. **"Stagnant"** fluid waste left behind in the tissues is called **"amyloid"** fluid. "Stagnant" tissue fluids are highly **"ACIDIC!"**

*[When oxygen (O_2) is exchanged for carbon dioxide (CO_2), the CO_2 is "supposed" to be removed by the blood for delivery to the "lungs" and disposal by the normal breathing process. But if blood hemoglobin levels are **low** and **insufficient** oxygen is delivered to the tissues, **"excess"** CO_2 accumulates in the amyloid tissue fluids. CO_2 is highly "acidic!"]*

Collection and circulation of waste-laden lymphatic fluids is **TOTALLY** dependent upon **body movement**—as in walking, exercise, work and activity—and without sufficient body movement, acidic tissue wastes do **NOT** "circulate!" Instead, they **"STAGNATE!"**

*[The lymphatic system deposits its payload of fluid waste into the blood just prior to the blood entering the heart. The blood then goes to the lungs for "reoxygenation" before returning to the left side of the heart for distribution to the body. Blood-borne waste is **REMOVED** and concentrated as **"bile"** by the liver. Bile is "stored" in the gallbladder. If the liver is **UNABLE** to remove blood-borne acid waste or if the liver's biliary ducts are "clogged," the body is forced—by default—to "store" excess acid waste in fatty tissues **beneath** the skin.]*

90% of tissue and cellular waste MUST exit the body by way of the liver and bowel or it does NOT leave!

Now that the reader knows where the body stores its "soluble" acid wastes, it should **not** come as a surprise that "skin cancer" generally occurs in skin that is **not** usually exposed to the sun! Sun does **NOT** cause skin cancer! The sun merely serves to "trigger" the acid wastes stored in the tissues "beneath" the skin in a grossly **ACID** body "terrain!" [Read *Sunlight* and *Healing Sun*. See Source Page 400.]

The conventional medical "model" of health, disease and aging is NOT valid! Do NOT rely on it!

Connecting The Dots

We "grow" miserable and we die for what we **FAIL** to do, **NOT** for what we overtly do! In financial, medical and legal matters, that which goes **"unsaid"** is often **MORE** important than what **"is said!"** And so it goes with the "experts!" Reliance upon "experts" causes people to **"assume"** that all pertinent information they need to know has been "given" to them. Consider the following: It's what the doctor or attorney or accountant **failed to** tell you that is the surprise! It's the questions "you" **failed** to ask that ups the ante! What people "think" is important is often **not** the "core" issues. **Failure** to understand the "nature" of the problem and **failure** to "know" what questions to "ask" only makes matters worse!

The "Terrain" Again!

"Aging" is about the "terrain!" Tissue fluid that **fails** to **EXIT** the tissues via the lymphatic system is called **"amyloid fluid!"** Amyloid "fluid" is "soluble," acid waste. In time, amyloid fluid **"morphs"** into amyloid **"plaque!"** Amyloid plaque is **"STRUCTURAL"** waste. It **cannot** "circulate" and **EXIT** the body by normal means because it is **NOT** a "fluid!" It has become **STAGNANT, STRUCTURAL, ACIDIC** waste!

Amyloid "plaque" causes people to grow old, go deaf, develop heart problems, lose eyesight, become arthritic—and learn first-hand the nature of dis-ease!

➡ **NO AMOUNT** of ordinary "cleansing" can remove amyloid plaque—because plaque is "brick and mortar!" It is "structural waste"—**NOT** fluid tissue waste. Amyloid waste is **WHY** health "gurus" age! Its **WHY** high-profile, well-known health **"EXPERTS"** grow old and drop dead! These folks "go-down" just like everyone else because their "model" is **DEFEC-TIVE!** [See page "1" to capture the point being made here!]

➡ Over **"TIME,"** amyloid plaque "morphs" into **"scar tissue!"** Following surgery and physical trauma—amyloid fluid and plaque form "scar tissue" on an accelerated basis. Scar tissue is **"nonfunctional"** tissue! Amyloid plaque and scar tissue are **"ACIDIC"** in nature! ➡ That is why **de**acidification of the "terrain" is the **CENTRAL** point of this book!

Aging is defined as acid waste accumulation in the body's tissues and diminished organ function.

Silk Worm Magic!

The silkworm moth dissolves its cocoon of "silk"—the strongest fiber known to man—with an enzyme made by bacteria in the moth's gut and secreted by the moth so it can emerge from its cacoon and repeat its life cycle.

➡ *[Humans have a life cycle, too—and it's called "birth to death!" Your author is concerned with the **"in-between"** part of man's cycle called "life on planet Earth"—for it is "here" on terra firma that people struggle in ignorance and suffer.]*

Aging reversal is "central" to the Young Again Protocol™—and so is the silk worm's secret!

Intestinal bacteria in the silkworm moth's gut serves as a "proxy" for the laboratory production of the "magical" enzyme. But the enzyme is **"USELESS"** for humans unless properly **"formulated!"** The enzyme has **"NOTHING"** to do with food digestion. Its purpose is to "eat" structural amyloid plaque and scar tissue and return it to "liquid" state so it can **EXIT** the body! The health implications are **VERY** "impressive!" Formulation and racemization of the energy footprint are "key!"

*[The product is called VZ II™—and it is taken **without** food, twice daily, before bed and upon rising. Its **effects** on the **entire** body are cumulative and occur over a "24-month" period. Some folks experience sticky, sludge-like waste that "clings" to the toilet bowl! The "sludge" is the "stuff" of dis-ease and old age! It takes about "2 years" for the body to "digest" and pass the "liquified" amyloid waste from the system.]*

Old Tissue • The Flu • Whiplash

Amyloid plaque and scar tissues are "old" tissues! They

are also sick, unhealthy tissues that "fuel" aging and dis-ease! When people "catch" the flu and become sick, they have crossed the acid-waste "threshold" and their bodies "revolt" because tissue waste provides the **PERFECT** "breeding" ground for pathogenic overgrowth! [The "terrain" crashes when the body exceeds the "tipping point"—**NOT** because of something people "catch!"

*["Angry" tissue is **traumatized** tissue! A "whip lash" results in "angry" tissue. Its angry because it is holding onto the "memory" of the **TRAUMA!** Angry, damaged tissue cannot and does not heal until old blood and old amyloid waste is removed from the trauma site and nerve **memory** is "erased!" The process is called "GUA SHA."]*

Gua Sha is a 3,000 year-old Chinese modality done "at home" with a water buffalo horn and releasing balm. The kit comes with a complete demonstration video.

A Realistic Model

90% of the "physical" body is composed of connective tissue in the form of bones, cartilage, muscle, tendon, ligament, skin and gums. **Acid**ification of these tissues is **"THE"** single **BIGGEST** issue driving the aging process. **D**eacidification is the obvious answer. When **you** have a "realistic model" of how the body actually works—and **you** are willing to do **your** part —**you** are on **your** way to becoming *Young Again!*

PREVIEW: *Our next chapter tells of another secret that has **not** been told before—a secret that is very important to everyone!*

Metabolism

"Blood-sugar management" is a **BIG** problem for millions of people—affecting mood, weight, hypertension, hypoglycemia and diabetes. Sugar "blues" come with poor carbohydrate metabolism and a messed-up liver and terrain. The solution is called Gluco Factor X.™ [See pages 186 and 290]

"Real" Food & Good Health

Food is a "gift" from God—and as Socrates said, *"Let your food be your medicine and your medicine be your food!"* The mandate for those wishing to enjoy good health and a long life is to eat "real" food. You can grow "food" in pots on your patio deck or in your back yard, or you can buy "food" from a friend or neighbor who gardens. *Real food is worth the effort!* Homegrown food is "free" of poisons and is nourishing. Good health means you don't "have" or "need" a doctor—or the services of the "sick-care" system! **Starving to death on a full belly** is what everyone else is doing. You can—and must—do better!

37

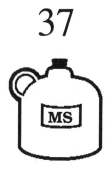

MoonShine

"I feel sorry for all those health food people. Someday, they will be lying in a hospital bed, dying of nothing!"
Redd Foxx

SOMETHING is going to kill all of us! A fall, a disease, an accident—or maybe some "moonshine!" If we could be sure of dying "quick and easy" and know that we will enjoy a good life until we give up the "ghost"—all the fuss made over staying "healthy" would be "laughable!" **But *"We don't know!"***

Lying in a hospital bed or being trapped in some "facility"—*"dying of nothing"*—affords little dignity. Better to choose to *"Go-out with your boots on!"* The problem is that when you are old—or very sick—you can't get your boots on because you are weak and stiff. Weak from a collapsed immune system; stiff from connective tissue breakdown. But life does **not** have to have a miserable ending. God gave man a wonderful body—and if provided the ***means*** and ***opportunity***—the body is very capable of "growing" younger!

Flim-Flam & Moonshine

The word "moonshine" has many connotations. The meaning your author wishes to impart is **something illegitimate**! Not illegal—just *less-than* the real McCoy—like a defective "medical-model" based on bogus "medical facts"—presented to the public in such as way as to ***"appear"*** legitimate by credentialed "experts" who can't even save themselves!

Flim-flam men! Hocus-pocus! Abbra-ca-dabra! Add some cut, burn and poison and "presto"—you are "cured," or so they would have us believe. Pride and arrogance are at the root of it! **Avoiding** "experts" and **ignoring** their "opinions" is the only defense available to us! Exercise it!

"Knowledge"—if valid and applied—takes us off "defense" so we don't need the services of the medical mafia. Better we learn to think outside the box. Better that we have a realistic "model" in our heads to guide us in matters of health and longevity. Better that we follow our "gut" instincts! Moonshine is **not** acceptable!

The "Real" Story of Vitamin-C

The real story of "Vitamin-C" has profound implications in matters of health and longevity. Until now, the only "reported" benefits of Vitamin-C the public is aware of has more in common with "moonshine" than reality. Let's have a look!

Albert Szent-Györgyi [pronounced "saint georgie!"] was the Hungarian biochemist who discovered Vitamin-C. He received the Nobel Prize for his work in 1937. Thirty-two years later, another biochemist named Linus Pauling received the Nobel Prize for his work with, you guessed it—"Vitamin-C."

For the past "37 years," the public has taken Vitamin-C for colds and flu and to boost the immune system—and that is as far as the story went! Grade-school kids are taught that scurvy was a horrible curse to sailors of old and that lemons and fresh vegetables—containing Vitamin-C "cures" scurvy.

The problem here is that Vitamin-C does **NOT** cure scurvy because scurvy is **NOT** a dis-ease! Scurvy is a "condition" of **"excess"**—and excess always manifests as symptoms of deficiency! Stated differently, **REMOVE** the excess and the symptoms of the so-called "dis-ease"—**disappear!**

When people eat "real" food containing natural Vitamin-C, it is the rutin, hesparidan and bioflavonoid complexes—**NOT THE VITAMIN-C**—that provide relief and benefit. These **"other"** factors cause **EXCESS** body acids to "flow" by way of increased "bile" production—and **EXIT** the system so the body can rebalance and restore itself.

The Vitamin-C "molecule" is too large to be absorbed through the gut wall; 95% of it is "lost!"

Linus Pauling knew that **"therapeutic"** blood levels of Vitamin-C **cannot** be achieved by oral dosage. He figured a way around the problem so effectively that he was teaching school at Stanford into his 90's—sharp as a tack—and well preserved, too! [Your author knew Pauling and had many interesting discussions with him in his later years. That's how your author learned of his health and longevity "secret!"]

Pauling said *"The only way to experience the profound* **therapeutic benefits** *of Vitamin-C is to get it directly into the blood "intravenously!"*

Pauling's peers attacked him unmercilessly because they were educated "idiots!" He outlived his critics in grand style and died ...with his boots on!

Now for the first time in history, everyone can obtain **"therapeutic"** blood levels of Vitamin-C without having to resort to an "IV" needle! [The product is called L_sP_cC™! It is taken "orally" 2x a day and provides potentially 100% absorption directly to the blood stream by using a proprietary "transport" technology beyond Linus Pauling's wildest dreams!

The Vitamin-C & Osteoporosis Connection

Vitamin-C has another "aspect" that **never** reached the public's consciousness because the experts *"Just don't get it!"*—and the health folks are "stuck" on colds and immunity!

If **"therapeutic"** blood levels of Vitamin-C can be **achieved** and **maintained,** the body automatically builds massive amounts of new "collagen!" Collagen is the foundational "matrix" for new **SKIN,** new **BONE,** new **CARTILAGE,** new **MUSCLE,** new **TENDONS** and new **GUMS!**

Lay down lots of new collagen and unbelievable things happen throughout the body's "terrain!"

➡ [Collagen is the **"third leg"** of the osteoporosis story. The other legs are tissue acidification and hormones. Deal with all **THREE** factors and aging "reversal" becomes "reality!" **Failure** to address **ALL THREE** of these factors driving osteoporosis and you will grow "old" by default!]

Commonly available "varieties" of over-the-counter Vitamin-C are next to useless because they **CANNOT** achieve therapeutic levels in the blood stream. Health experts have been peddling vitamin-C **"moonshine"** stories to the public for over 37 years! It is time to remedy this situation!

Now everyone can do exactly what Linus Pauling spoke of WITHOUT the need of a needle!

The Rest Of The Vitamin-C Story

Racemized™ L_sP_cC™ is "nanoscaled"—meaning the Vitamin-C "molecule" is reduced in physical size to about 180 nanometers before "encapsulation" in its **"transport"** ("phosphatidylcholine"). The L_sP_cC™ **"transport"** is absorbed wholly intact through the "jejunum" wall (the "middle" portion of the small intestines where fats are "absorbed") creating a new pathway for efficient and meaningful Vitamin-C absorption.

The minus size of the metric system "scale" goes milli, micro, nano, pico. [Each level being 10 times **smaller** than the previous one.] At "180" nanometers, you are "sub-atomic" in .size—and very close to 1,000,000,000 of a meter—making it possible to achieve up to 100% absorption and bioavailability of Vitamin-C to the blood—and **"bypassing"** the absorption problems associated with Vitamin-C in **ALL** other forms.

To grasp the significance of how small a "180" nanometer "molecule" is, please realize that each L_sP_cC™ molecule is about **10,000 times "smaller"** than the diameter of a strand of human hair! Restated, it takes about 10,000 molecules to equal about a strand of human hair. "Tiny!"

Add L_sP_cC™ "jelly" to water or juice and drink

morning and evening—preferably with VZ.™ *[Please see Chapter 36 for the VZ™ story and why it is so very important that these "twin" products be used together!]*

When Vitamin-C is "encapsulated" in phosphatidylcholine, the body **identifies** and **absorbs** the "transport" as a "fat"—not as Vitamin-C. The fat goes to the liver where it is **processed** and the "Vitamin-C is **"released into"** the blood as if given by "IV" needle! The body uses the "transport" material for repairing cellular membranes and rebuilding "brain" tissue! The entire story is an absolute **MIRACLE!**

The same "miracle" has now been duplicated with "real" B-Vitamins. It is called L_sP_cB.™

Alzheimers, Hormones & Vitamin-C

Alzheimers Dis-ease is characterized by brain tissue **"atrophy"** and **"invasion"** by amyloid plaque. "Homemade" hormones provide women protection for brain tissue! But hormone activity drops off starting as early as age "35!"

The incidence of women with Alzheimers compared to men is "3 to 1"—so it's obvious that there is a hormonal connection here. The great part of this story is that women now have a way to "remedy" these issues. Another point to remember is that after age "25," the female anatomy turns "acidic" **10x FASTER** than does the male anatomy. [Use of non-steroidal antiinflammatory-type over-the-counter drugs—like aspirin etc.—is the "fast-track" to the Alzheimers ward! Avoid them!]

An acid "terrain" is filled with soluble and non-soluble amyloid waste that can ONLY exit the body by means of increased "bile flow" from the liver!

A woman's **LIVER** is responsible for **"making"** and **"orchestrating"** her hormones when the ovaries slow or cease their activity—or are lost through surgery. The *Young Again Protocol*™ provides women with the means to prevent and **REVERSE** terrain acidification and "hormone-related" aging issues like "osteoporosis." Osteoporosis **MUST NOT** be ignored! Changing the "terrain" is a **"HUGE"** issue for women—and linked to it is hormonal activity and bile flow. [The entire aging-reversal process just became a whole lot easier with L_sP_cC!™ Achieving therapeutic blood levels of Vitamin-C is the **final missing piece** of the osteoporosis puzzle. [➥ And isn't it interesting that you did **NOT** learn about it from the "experts!"]

When you learn to tell the difference between "moonshine" and the "real" thing, you can forget about *"dying of nothing"* because you have learned to think outside the box and you are free to become *Young Again!*

PREVIEW: *Our next chapter sheds some light on the meaning of the expression "Smoke and mirrors!"*

38

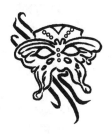

Kabuchi Dance

"In the land of the blind, the one-eyed man is king!"
Desiderius Erasmus

A **"Kabuchi Dance"** is an "illusionary" portrayal using costumes and trickery that is performed without any pretence of a "reality" of the situation. In other words—*a mockery!*

The "health care" system is a kind of Kabuchi Dance—an oxymoron in name and a mockery without question! Healthcare is really "sick care" in an *Alice in Wonderland* game where little is real and everything you are taught to believe in is a **guarantee** that you will end up exactly like everyone else—sick, old, bitter and broken—and just maybe if you are lucky, you will get to die—but only "after" you are dead "broke!"

The best way to avoid the "sick-care" **TRAP** is to change the rules of the game! That is what your author has said a hundred different ways throughout this book. Changing the "rules of the game" is not difficult. All you need is a realistic "model" followed by action and guidance. That's what the *Young Again Protocol*™ provides. Here are a few **examples** of what can be accomplished.

Regeneration

Worn-out bodies can be "rebuilt!" Regeneration occurs during the **sleep cycle**—and to make the process work, you need raw materials and a stimulus. If all of the necessary ingredients are present—and you maintain your course—you will grow younger each day—and watch the miracle unfold.

[At "conception"—when the egg and sperm "join"—a period of tremendous growth occurs within the womb as our bodies are formed from **"antegenic"** *protein.* **Ante**genic protein is "construction" material in the form of Skin & Body Toner™! The stimulus is racemized™ growth hormone "precursor"—so you can make your own hormone! These things "trigger" the regeneration process! Your author did it and become a "young"*

man with bio-electric age of 61/19!]

Life: 24/7/365!

Excess body fat, moodiness, elevated cortisol levels, stress and blood-sugar swings go together. Each of these "factors" feeds the others. But **"STRESS"** is the ultimate wild card affecting the "rate" of aging of the terrain! "Terrain" management is **"THE"** issue when it comes to enjoying a healthy life and staying away from the "sick-care" system. Manage "stress" and the rest is easy. [CWD™ and PU™ manage "stress" by "settling" the effects of adrenal **overload** so people can **GET OUT** of **OVERDRIVE** and return to "normal!"]

Being in constant adrenal "overdrive" day after day is probably the WORSE possible element of modern life that causes people to lose control of their lives!

High Enema Therapy,™ a good diet, exercise, and good drinking water and deep sleep are extremely important "factors" in the aging story. Deacidification of the "terrain" is the health equivalent of *"getting out of jail,"* and it underwrites everything—including "stress" management!

Male & Female Issues

Sooner or later, every **"man"** must deal with his "prostate." Men who **ignore** and **hide** from this issue suffer and die early. Men who follow the *Young Again Protocol*™ and use R/Prostate™ I & II don't have to deal with these issues. Instead, they get to say *"good bye"* to them. "Band-aid" approaches like saw palmeto, zinc and selenium sound nice, but they will **NOT** stop "male" aging and **CANNOT** restore the male "terrain" once it is "over the hill!" [See pages 149 and 162.]

Women who follow a realistic "model" don't have to suffer and age like their female friends. Women who "keep" the puberty window **"OPEN"** and become voragos™ enjoy a very different kind of life—and they live a lot longer, too!

If you live your life like everyone else, you are in a "Kabuchi Dance" by your own choice!

Avoid the "Kabuchi" lifestyle and you will enjoy good health and a long life that says you "are"*Young Again!*

Preview: *Before you read the next chapter, read the title and see if you can guess "where" your author is going to take you. You are going to be surprised!*

Silent Suffering

Growing "older" doesn't have to be a miserable experience! Instead of suffering, why not change your life for the better by implementing the ideas in this book. It's not hard to do!

39

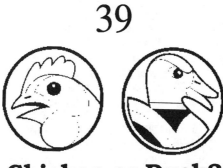

Chicken or Duck?

"And those who were dancing were thought to be insane by those who could not hear the music."
Frederich Nietzsche

Her name is "Patience" and she lives in Singapore. Patience is Chinese and is **both** a friend and a customer. Patience **taught** your author a very important lesson.

Upon receiving fax instructions from Patience, I read them and did what Patience asked me to do. Two days later I received another fax from Patience *"...concerned about a big "mix-up!"* and to please call her. So I called Patience and this is what she said to me.

"In the Chinese culture, we call this 'a chicken or a duck!' Did we have 'conversation' or did we have 'communication?" *[speaking of the fax message.]*

There was *"no question"* that we had "not" **communicated** with each other! In your author's field of work, *"chicken or duck!"* conversations cause **misunderstandings!**

That is **"WHY"** personal "one-on-one" mentoring is provided to everyone at "no cost" **BEFORE** the *Young Again Protocol*™ is begun. It's better to "root-out" issues and "air" histories and "voice" expectations **FIRST!** "Practical" goals and timelines dictate that everybody puts their cards on the table! **No games! No surprises! No unrealistic expectations!**

And remember Patience' lesson, because *"A chicken is* ***not*** *a duck!"*

PREVIEW: *The next chapt*er is a "farewell" from your author with a hidden message enclosed. See if you can figure it out!

| Information Collectors |

"Ever learning, and never able to come to the knowledge of the truth!" Information collectors go nowhere!

"El aur guyazah!" **Hindu saying meaning "1+1=11."**

What is BFRV™?

➥ BFRV™ is a **terrain management** "concept" that is part of the *Young Again! Protocol(s).*™ BFRV™ is also a "trademark" developed by your author to **differenciate** the *Young Again! Model*™ from the very confusing world of "alternative!"

Because BFRV™ is a **"trademark,"** please take notice that anyone "posting" or "using" it except for John Thomas— is doing so **"ILLEGALLY"** and **"WITHOUT"** permission from your author and should **NEVER** be trusted! At "present"—and over the past 13 years—dozens of "bootleggers" have **hijacked** your author's ideas, concepts and trademarks—and some of these characters have "attacked" your author because they have **NOTHING ORIGINAL TO SAY!** It is impossible to police the entire marketplace against infringements, snipping and bootlegging. **Your author offers this book as his answer and defense. What more need to be said?**

Old Body, Young Body?

Women experience *menopause;* men experience *andropause.* BOTH sexes must tend to hormonal issues if they want to "stay" young. Sexual hormones **fuel** the restoration process, and they provide protection from the mental condition known as Alzheimers! B.T.™ thyroid creme helps restore brain function, hair, body temperature, skin and energy. L_sP_cC™ boosts collagen formation and VZ™ "digests" amyloid brain and scar tissue. All aging issues are linked to acidification of the "terrain!" [See pages 72, 164 and 212.]

Deadly "Word" Games

Hydrolyzed vegetable protein is used in hundreds of foods—including health foods—and is a *trade name* for MSG (monosodium glutamate). MSG contains glutamate + aspartame + cytoic acid—known "poisons." **Aspartame** is the *chemical name* for a popular sweetener with the red, white and blue swirl. These soy-derived **"excitotoxins"** destroy nerve/brain cells. Public outrage ended the use of "MSG" in baby food in 1972 because it was causing **"retardation"** by preventing brain development in babies. So "they" changed the name and added a pretty little swirl! Cute! [A baby's brain begins forming in the 7th month and is well developed by age "two"—if adequate nutrition is provided—but it contintues to grow until about age 30 and beyond. Hopefully the reader now understands **"why"** early vaccinations are so dangerous to infants with "undeveloped" brain tissue and undeveloped immune systems. Seems like your author remembers a king named "Herod" who killed children under 2 years old in the effort to kill "The Christ!"]

40

Unforgiven

"Most wonderful; with its own hands it ties
And gags itself—gives itself death and war
For pence doled out by kings from its own store.
Its own are all things between earth and heaven;
But this it knows not; and if one arise
To tell this truth, it kills him unforgiven."

Tomasso Campanella, *The People*

Reversing the aging process is a ***one-step-at-a-time***
process that occurs one-day-at-a-time—***in reverse!***

Ask yourself these questions. *"Am I willing to take*
responsibility for my future and create the miracle of agelessness
in my life? Am I willing to do whatever it takes to keep my youth
and/or gain back the years I have lost? Am I willing to act in my
own best interest today? Right now?

Everything in life comes at a price. Pain! Suffering!
Money! I hope you will join me by picking up your yoke—no
matter how difficult it may be. Never scream *"Uncle!"* Health
and vitality belong to the person who is willing to take personal
responsibility for his or her life.

May you become *Young Again!*

Sincerely,

John Thomas

"Old age is like everything else in life. To make a
success of it, you have to start when you are young!"
John Thomas

Healthy Progress

"What can I do to speed the aging reversal process?" **is the question most often asked.**

Answer: *"Drink biologically friendly water; make fresh vegetable juices; get lots of sleep and do High Enema Therapy.™ Next, restore liver function; deacidify your terrain and remove soluble and structural acid waste from the tissues. Then, clear the liver's biliary ducts and dump those stones and nails; "digest"* **amyloid** *plaque and scar tissue from your terrain; rebuild the collagen matrix comprising your connective tissues; and finally, restore hormanal activity so your body can regenerate.* **The body can't return to a youthful condition when the tissues and organs are sick and old!**

"You" are responsible for **your** condition. How long does it takes to turn things around and look and feel "good?" The answer depends on many factors—and **"you"** are responsible for putting up with **"whatever"** for as long as it takes! That is why guidance and mentoring are provided along the way. Please be willing to do your part. After all, it is **"your"** life!

Pain In The Butt!

Okay! Your author will admit that High Enema Therapy™ is a "pain" in the butt! So what? It's better than losing your health **and** being miserable **and** living out the balance of your life in a "facility!" The best way to minimize heart problems, restore mental faculties and reduce that "belly" is with an enema morning and evening. You will sleep better —and snore less, too! The process only takes about 5 minutes. You decide! [See pages 70, 106,123, 262 and 399.]

Energy Transfer

Energy is never lost; it merely changes form! The benefits of racemized™ formulations are Fourth Dimentional in nature and their esoteric aspects are not contained in "physical" form; therefore, they are not contained in physical shipment format. "Transfer" of energy is the issue here!

Inflammation & Pain

Pain is **confirmation** of "inflammation!" Sometimes fever accompanies pain, but not always—as with a sprained ankle, infected prostate, rotting teeth or touchy bowel. Use Inflame Away I & II™ for effective relief without drugs!

Anal itching often accompanies deACIDification!

L/CSF™

Exercise improves health. The question is why?

People who exercise are healthier than those who do not exercise because you have a heart to **PUMP** and circulate blood—but your lymphatic system "depends" on body movement, work, exercise and activity to circulate. Lymphatic fluids must **"CIRCULATE!"** When the lymphatic system is inefficient, waste plasma proteins do **NOT** get picked up for removal from the tissues—which leads to "aging" of the terrain.

People who **cannot** exercise or who **hate** to exercise can use the L/CSF™ Machine to "effectively" circulate their tissue and lymphatic "fluids" **WITHOUT** the need for harsh exercise or driving yourself to do something you despise!

Use the L/CSF™ Machine to "run" five miles morning and night while lying on your back watching the news. The device is a wonderful invention that "works!" Your author uses the machine morning and evening because he "sits" at a desk all day long talking with people. He wants to stay young and he **must** circulate his body fluids or old wage will "knock!"

Regardless of your "state" of health, if you fail to circulate your body fluids—your days are numbered. You must either use it or lose it! [See diagram of L/CSF™ on page 382.]

Perception

"The difference between an optimist and a pessimist is that an optimist thinks things are going to get better; a pessimist knows things are going to get a hell of a lot worse!"   Bosnian proverb

R/VX™

Not all iron is the same! Blood "iron" is called **"heme"** iron as in **hem**oglobin. "Elemental" iron is different. Iron is an oxidizer—meaning it loses electrons when exposed to "oxygen." Rust is oxidized iron. In the body, **elemental** iron provides a "substrate" that pathogenic bacteria need to multiply. Deprive them of elemental iron and they can't do much damage.

R/VX™ is an elemental iron "scavenger!" It helps prevent the outbreak of iron-based infections by "binding" elemental iron and removing it from the body. Iron removal boosts immune system function and keeps the terrain healthy.

The body **"makes"** heme iron! Heme iron is **not** something you eat. Hemoglobin transports oxygen to the cells and carries carbon dioxide out of the body via the lungs. [People who are "anemic" benefit from taking racemized™ liver and algae plus Cobo-12 creme. See pages 291 and 383.]

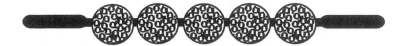

Biogenic™ Lymph Roller
• Breaks-up "cellulite"on hips and thighs •
• Tones the skin for a youthful look •

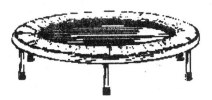

Rebounder or Mini Trampoline
Available from most discount stores.

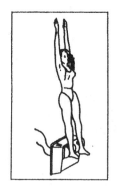
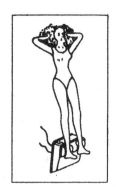
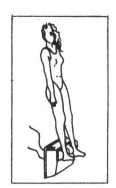

The L/CSF™ Machine
(See page 381 and Source Page400)

The Way It Is!

Meat Eater vs. Vegetarian/Vegan

"The savvy person is neither a heavy meat eater nor radical vegetarian. Balance is the key!"

Deep within the heart of the health movement is the **dogma** that "vegetarians" are *smarter* and *healthier* than meat eaters, and that "vegans" are smarter than **BOTH!** When sick, aging, meat eaters go "vegetarian" their health improves and they soon look and feel better—for awhile!

Question: Why do meat eaters enjoy improved health when they include fresh vegetables in their diet? **Answer"** Because they lacked **"balance"** in their diet. They suffer for what they **fail to eat, NOT** for the meat they do eat!

Having been on **both** sides of the fence, first a heavy meat eater and then a radical vegetarian, your author **returned to his senses** many years ago, mellower and smarter. Here is what I learned first hand!

Food imposes stress on the body—and it's the "terrain" that dictates how we digest the food we eat and how the body deals with acid waste left behind.

Bacteria are living "creatures" just like animals—and you cannot eat food without eating them, period! Plants have eyes and ears and blood and parasites just like animals and people. They are every bit as much alive as flesh and blood "animals!" Harvesting a plant or cutting its branches and leaves is **NO** different than *slaughtering* an animal!

If you have "spiritual" or "religious" hang-ups about eating meat, remember this: **Every living thing eats other living things.** It's the way it is; use it to your advantage!

The "terrain" and the liver control health and longevity. Health is **NOT** a meat vs. vegetarian issue. **In fact, the less food we eat, the longer we live!** Fresh "live" food and vegetable juices produce miracles because of the **"pigments"** they contain. [See Chapter 35.]

Vegetarians generaly **enjoy** better health and maintain their appearance longer than heavy meat eaters. But, vegetarians **do** experience secondary health problems with their connective tissues because of their diet. "Vegans" and macrobiotic folks deteriorate worst of all! **A few tips:** Eat only "healthy" meat. Red meat is better than chicken. Fish is in between. *Racemized*™ liver is a ZERO stress, super healthy food that is **predigested.** It is your author's **"meat"** of choice. R/BHCl™ and DiSorb Aid II™ should **always** accompany meals with animal or egg proteins to get good absorption.

The body cannibalizes itself every day of our lives—so everyone is a **"meat eater!"** Self-digestion of body proteins is unavoidable and the process accelerates as we grow older!

The U.C.C. Connection

Throughout this book your author has alluded to and pointed out that our legal system is in serious trouble. The problem is that we have two **"parallel"** systems operating side by side—one constitutional, the other unconstitutional—the latter being the source of most of the troubles we labor under every day of our lives—as well as the social injustice emanating from the attorney-controlled courts of "corporate" America.

Perhaps you are wondering why your author would raise this subject in a book about health and aging reversal? Because when **TRUTH** is cast aside, societies become corrupt and the people suffer "unnecessarily"—and in vain!

Citizens labor under layers of mistruths and half truths relating to law, health, medicine and politics—and the fastest way to expose a lie is to tell the truth!

If you would like to learn how the system "really" works and how your life is subservient to the Uniform Commercial Code, order the "UCC" Connection and the Yellow Fringed Flag 12-hour cassette series. The only way to dispel ignorance is with knowledge. The story will astound you and settle the confusion going on all around you! [See Source Page 400.]

P.S. Why do Americans salute the "flag" when they recite the pledge of allegiance? Want to better understand the events of September 11, 2001? Do you wonder why the "flag of peace" is on the cover of this book instead of the "flag" you know?

Chocolat

One of the best movies of year "2000" was *Chocolat*. The movie dealt with the human obsession for chocolate! Women have a particular obsession for chocolate, especially prior to the onset of their menstrual period. Chocolate is also considered to be a "love" food. What is overlooked in the chocolate story is the fact that good chocolate is very high in fat—and fat is "critical" to hormone production—especially in females. Women need lots of dietary fat to make their hormones. That is why "low fat" diets are so harmful to women.

Good fats [not to be confused with all the HDL and LDL and VLDL baloney] are loaded with essential fatty acids. Fats do **NOT** make you fat, but they sure improve body physiology and function. Use olive oil, butter and virgin coconut oil. R/ EFA's™ are racemized™ essential fatty acids in capsule form that insure proper intake of "essential" fats! The reader might be surprised to know that ADD and ADHD children need "fat to "nourish" their brain! That is why they are called "essential" [See page 84, 94, 124, 161, 182, 267 and 311.]

Germs, Disease & Aging

Your author totally **rejects** the Germ Theory of Disease—but he is in total **agreement** with the medical folks about germs, pathogenic microbes and parasites waging war against us. The real question is *"Why do they wage war against us?"*

When the body's "terrain" is burdened with acid waste, pathogenic microbes proliferate and cause us to suffer and die. So is it the "germs" or is it the "terrain" that dictates who wins and who loses this silent war going on in our bodies? The **TERRAIN** "controls!" But germs and parasites know how to "read" their environment. They communicate with each other—and when conditions are just right, they "explode" onto the scene with **devastating** consequences! In small numbers, germs can't accomplish much and they don't try. But create the right conditions, and their numbers exponentially multiply—and the war is on!

Modern medicine since the time of Pasteur, and especially since Lister and the advent of antibiotics, has attempted to kill the microbes when the real war has always been the "terrain." When you clear the body of acid waste, you change the terrain and deny the microbes a comfortable environment in which to live. Always remember that you don't catch disease! You develop **SIGNS** and symptoms that manifest as disease because of conditions of **EXCESS** in your body's "terrain!"

"Excess" stresses the system and diminishes vital organ function. **Excess** provides the perfect environment for illness and dis-ease to manifest. **Excess** causes loss of control of our lives—and it causes us to suffer. **Excess** cause us to age, grow old and die. We lose control of our "terrain" because of conditions of **"EXCESS"—NOT because of "deficiencies!"**

Human beings have free will. God gave us the right of choice. When we **choose** the path of ignorance or bullheadedness, we must pay the price. When we make correct choices, we "change" the **outcome** and the **direction** of our lives. We have **CHOICE!** Learn to exercise it!

10 Year Window

It has been your author's experience and personal observation that between ages 35-45, everyone enters a 10 year "test" and "training" period of crises like divorce, death, health, finance and career. These things **"seem"** to descend upon us out of nowhere. The test period lasts about 10 years. When it is over, we get our "wisdom" and life becomes rosey again. It is during this **"test"** period that we "grow" and "find" ourselves.

Ignorance is temporary. Stupidity is forever!

ATP-body's primary energy molecule; product of Crebs Cycle and burning of glucose in mitochondria.

Acetylcholine-a nerve impulse transmission chemical.

Acetylcholinease-an enzyme that splits acetylcholine.

Acid-any substance that liberates hydrogen ions; ion donor.

Acid reflux-regurgitation of stomach acids into esophagus; a bowel, liver & gut disorder.

Acid stomach-describes upset stomach/poor digestion; related to HCl, poor bowel & liver activity.

Acne-confirmation of poorly functioning liver and highly acid condition of body terrain.

Acupuncture-alternative manipulation of body energy fields with pins or their electrical equivalent.

Adenovirus-a virus associated with upper respiratory infections, associated with AIDS/HIV.

Adhesion-water's tendency to coat the surface of things.

Adrenals-glands located on each kidney; make cortisol and adrenaline; key to stress management.

Aerobes-bacteria that require an oxygen rich environment.

Aerobic-with air.

Aerobic exercise-exercise that produces a high oxygen state.

Aging process-begins at anabolic peak and ends with death; a cumulative and reversible process.

A/G ratio-ratio between albumin & globulins in blood, range 1.0-2.4; the higher the number the better.

Agglutination-clumping of the red blood corpuscles.

AIDS-Acquired Immune Deficiency Syndrome.

Albumin-a blood protein; elevated urine levels mean kidney trouble and catabolic tissue activity.

Alcohol-end product of fermentation; anaerobic process

Algae-lowest of plants; some edible (klamath, spirulina, chlorella)

Alkaline-above pH 7.0.

Alkaloid-physiologically active chemical compounds in plants.

Allopathic medicine-conventional cut, burn, and drug medicine.

Alum-double sulfate of aluminum; toxic; food additive; pickles.

Aluminum-a metal that releases toxic ions into food and water; involved in Alzheimers.

Alzheimer's -atrophy of brain tissue; invasion of brain by amyloid plaques; dementia, violence.

Amalgam-toxic metals used to fill teeth; up to 40% mercury; erroneously referred to as "silver" fillings.

Amenorrhea-absence or suppression of menstruation.

American Dental Association-mouthpiece of conventional dentistry; pharmaceutical surrogate.

Amyloid fluid-acidic, soluble, intracellular tissue waste not picked-up by lymphatic system; stagnant.

Amyloid plaque- non-soluble amyloid structural waste; forms scar tissue; cannot circulate.

Anabolic, anabolism-generation/regeneration of tissues; growth; repair; youth side of anabolic peak.

Anabolic Peak-high point of anabolism, growth and repair; opposite of catabolism/catabolic peak.

Anaerobes-bacteria that can live in the absence of oxygen.

Anaerobic-without air; oxygen deficient.

Analog-a molecule that is similar to another in it reactive and/or functional characteristics; a synthetic molecule; "-R" group location dictates analogous personality profile.

Andropause-male menopause; end of middle years; reversal of puberty; decline of sex drive; aging.

Angina pectoris-chest pain due to lack of oxygen in muscles.

Anemia-low number of circulating red blood corpuscles; low blood hemoglobin levels.

Anion-the smallest form of (+) energy released during a reaction; opposite of cation.

Antegenic Protein-protein with regenerative qualities; needed for regrowth of aged/damaged tissue.

Antibiotic-drug; useful for life threatening infections; major side effects on terrain and gut wall.

Appendix-organ distended from cecum; surrounded by Peyer's Patch; toxic energy release organ.

Arthritis-deterioration/inflammation of the connective tissues and joints.

Arteriosclerosis-hardening of arteries; see atherosclerosis

Antenna-device that receives a radio (energy) signal.

Antibody-immunity related blood immunoglobulin; product of a previous infection.

Applied kenesiology-hocus-pocus version of muscle testing; see muscle testing.

Aspartate-salt form of aspartic acid; aspartame; artificial sweetner; toxic.

Atherosclerosis-plaque formation/deterioration of arteries.

ATP-(adenosine triphosphate)-energy carrying molecule of body; product of mitochondrial oxidation of glucose; produced with and without oxygen; Crebs Cycle and glocolysis (lactic acid conversion to ATP).

Atrophy-deterioration and death of body tissue/gland/organ; loss of function.

Avogadro's Number-number of atoms in 12 grams of carbon-12; noted as [N].

Autonomic Nervous System-involuntary system controlling vital organs and activities.

Autodigestion-cannibalization of body's own tissues to meet its needs; autoimmune; aging/illness.

Aura-mirrow of bio-electric body; invisible body; life force; Fourth Dimension concept.

Axon-nerve fiber; includes synapses; involved in nerve signal transfer; Schwanns Cell activity.

Bacteria-microorganisms; microbes; may be aerobic, anaerobic or faciculate.

Bactericidal-a non-selective killer of bacteria, antiseptic.

Balding-loss of hair; hair follicle dormancy; not genetic; thyroid, liver, terrain and sex hormone issue.

Basal metabolism-minimum requirement for maintenance of vital body functions when at rest.

Basement membrane(s)-support tissue structure beneath the skin; soluble waste storage storage.

B-12 (vitamin B-12)-critical to body metabolism; female issue after age 35; aging related; cobalt.

BAT-brown adipose tissue high concentrations of mitochondria; seen in healthy, younger poeple.

Bent molecule-the water molecule; a polar molecule; hydrophilic substance.

B-vitamins-vitamins B-1 through B-17 vitamin complex; critical for good health; mineaal cofactors.

BFRV™-Biologically Friendly Racemized™ Vincent; trademark for Young Again Protocol™ water.

Bile-liver waste product; fat emulsifier; digestive related; primary waste product; controls bowels.

Biogenic-stimulation of body to produce new, healthy tissue and heal self.

Bio-dynamic-agricultural manipulation of energy for production of biologically live food.

Bio-electric age-true age based on health of the vital organs.

Bio-electric body-the physical and energy body's combined.

Bio-junk diet-dietary filler; unhealthy; unable to support life; causes accelerated aging.

Biological alchemy-transformation of the elements in liver, gut and soil via bacteria; fusion reactions.

Biologically friendly water-two hydrogens and one oxygen only; all contaminants (mineral or chemical) removed; erasure of memory of contaminants; bond angle adjustment.

Biological Theory of Ionization-release of ion energy by breaking of ionic mineral bonds.

Bio-magnetics-the use of therapeutic magnets for promotion health of bio-electric body.

Bio-magnetic Irrigator-dental hygiene appliance for oral hygiene and healthy teeth/gums.

Bladder-the urine storage organ in mamals; urinary system; down line from kidneys.

Blood-one of three "fluid" body fluids; protein communication system; lymphatic and cerebral spinal fluids are other two systems.

Body odor (BO)-odoriferous product of microbial oxidizing of skin waste; tissue waste exit portal.

Bond-energy "link" between elemental atoms and within molecules; energy release site when broken.

Bone spur-abnormal mineral deposit in/on joints and bones.

Bowel-colon or large intestine; final six feet of intestine; toxicity and cancer zone; controlled by bile flow.

Brain fog- inability to think clearly or to recall information; related to thyroid and hormonal issues.

Brix-a unit of measure of the sucrose sugars in plant juices; measured with a brix meter.
Brown fat-see BAT.
Bulimia-mental condition; forced vomiting of food after meals; related to anorexia.
Calcification-soft tissue invasion by alkaline mineral salts; precipitation of mineral salts.
Calcium-elemental alkaline metal; salt crystal when bonded with halogen gas; 229 known forms of.
Calculus-dental plaque; tartar.
Cancer-systemic collapse of terrain; 1 of 4 major diseases; other 3 are: arthritis, heart/stroke, diabetes..
Cannibalism (auto-digestion)-self consumption of one's own body tissues and muscle mass when body's needs not met; especially prevalent after age 35, and particularly in female vegetarians and vegans; occurs in all elderly people who are wasting away for lack of ability to regenerate due to loss of control of their terrain.
Canola oil-rape oil; toxic; mustard family; industrial oil; unfit for human consumption.
Capillaries-smallest blood vessels; can be venous or arterial; also lymphatic.
Carbohydrate-sugars, starches, dextrins; 1 of 3 classes of foods; other are protein and fats.
Carbon-essential element to all living things; atomic element #12; basis of "organic" poisons.
Carbon cycle-path of carbon: atmosphere through bacteria, soil, plant, animal, ocean and return.
Carbon dioxide- atmospheric gas; cellular waste; CO_2; exchanged for oxygen by hemoglobin.
Carcinogenic-poisonous.
Cardiovascular disease-dis-eases of the blood circulatory system and brain.
Carpal Tunnel Syndrome-occlusion/deterioration of nerve & nerve path in bones of wrist; aging.
Carrion-spoiled animal flesh.
Cartilage-one of seven connective tissues (bone, muscle, tendon, ligament, skin and gums).
Casts-albumin/amyloid proteins and mineral salts deposited in kidney's tubules; aging.
Catalyst-substance causing a chemical reaction that would not occur if substance not present.
Cataract-clouding of lens of the eye; waste accumulation; poor blood/lymph flow; amyloid waste.
Cation-smallest form of (-) energy ion released during a reaction; opposite of anion.
Catabolic, catabolism-degeneration of body; aging of tissues and organs; opposite of anabolism.
Cavities-rotting away of teeth; decay; confirmation of an acidic terrain; degerative; aging.
Cecum-junction of small/large intestine; gut/colon (bowel).
Cellulite-abnormal, waste filled, body fat; hips and thighs on females; aging issue; acid terrain.
Chemotherapy-treatment of dis-ease w/negative energy drugs; cancer treatment modality.
Chi energy-life force energy of the invisible, Fourth Dimension bio-electric body.
Chloroform-toxic substance from reaction of chlorinated water with organic molecules (chloramine).
Chlorine-a halogen gas; used to chlorinate drinking water; chemically unstable; terrain toxic.
Chloride-a salt form of chlorine i.e. sodium/pot./alum chlorides.
Chiropractic-modality for correction of spinal alignment and improvment of nerve/ vital organ function.
Chiropractic (Network)-multi-dimensional form of chiropractic.
Chloramine-highly toxic organic molecule; product of chlorinated water with organic molicules.
Chlorinated water-water treated with chlorine; toxic; source of leaky gut.
Chocolate pudding-highly acid wasted released during colon hydrotherapy; stored in cecum.
Cholesterol-chole=bile; sterol=chemically active fat; made by liver; not cause of cardiovascular disease.
Cilia-hair like projections in small intestine/respiratory tract; move waste; produce enzymes.
Cirrhosis-hardening/yellowing of liver; inflammation of liver; aging sign, not cause of disease.
Clinical Disease-a "diagnosed" medical condition based on recognized signs.
Cloak(ed)-under cover; hidden; non-detectable; subclinical condition; occult stage.
Cobalt-mineral element; intrinsic factor needed for absorption; critical to hemoglobin production (blood iron) and high metabolic rate; a very big female health issue; anemia.
Co-enzyme-necessary for the function of another enzyme.
Cohesion-water's tendency to stick together; hydrogen bond and electrical charge issue.
Colloid-a substance in suspension; refers to particle size not activity level; non-ionic mineral form.
Colon-large intestine; bowel; bottom 6 feet of intestine; begins at cecum.
Colonic (colon hydrotherapy)-water stimulation of colon nerves feeding vital organs from colon wall; accelerates bile flow and acid waste release; washing of colon; controls terrain; High Enema Therapy.
Collagen-basis of connective tissue (bone, cartilag/muscle/tendon/ligament/gums).
Comfrey-garden plant grown for spinach like leaves; a food; requires use of vinegar or lemon.
Congestive Heart Failure-heart overload; poor circulation; excess tissue fluid; edema; drowning.
Constipation-less than 2-3 bowel movements per day; byproduct of insufficient bile flow and water.
Cortisol-hormone produced by adrenal glands; produced when under stress; puts body in overdrive.
Cravings-desire for foods; sign of hunger and nutritional insufficiency; toxic terrain; poor bile flow.
Crowns (dental)-cap overlay on teeth; never use metal; always use ceramic materials.
Crypts of Lieberkuhn-where food nutrients are absorbed in gut; located between intestinal villi.
Crystal-a salt; combination of halogen gas and a metal ion.
Currency, electrical-energy money; mineral ions.
Cyanide-active component in rape seed and rape oil; from which canola oil is derived.
Cyanocobalamin-cobalt atom combined with an amine; Vitamin B-12 component.
Cytoplasm-intercellular fluid.
DMSO-dimethylsulfoxide; effective carrier solvent; stinks; promotes healing; basis of SOC.™
DNA-genetic code; deoxyribonucleic acid; defective genes product of terrain; genes don't cause disease.
Deacidification-removal of environmental and metabolic wastes from body tissues and fluids.
Defecate-a bowel movement; should have 3-5/day; controlled by bile flow; squat position best.
Deficiencies-imaginary, causative factors behind disease; invalid theory; result of excess in system.
Degenerative dis-ease-systemic acidification of the terrain; confirmed loss of control of the tettain.
Denature-alteration in form, function and/or shape of food enzymes/proteins.
Holistic dentistry-biologically friendly dentistry; no use of mercury amalgams, implants or root canals.
De-energize-neutralization of energy footprint; synchronization of chemical energy reaction.
Deodorant-a cover used to mask BO; confirmation of acidification of the terrain; toxic body.
Dermis-the true skin; beneath the epidermis (outer skin).
Detoxify-removal of waste from the body; deacidification of tissues.
Devitalized food-so-called food without life force and vitality; bio-junk diets.
Diabetes-dis-ease of pancreas; related to blood serum levels of insulin; loss of organ function; closely related to liver, adrenal and thyroid function; adult onset diabetes called Type-II; Type-I id childhood diabetes; Type-I linked to vaccinations; often occurs during puberty related stress.
Digestion-breakdown/conversion of food nutrients into energy (ATP) by mitochondria in Krebs cycle.
Dilution-technique and concept used in creation of homeopathic remedies.
Dirt-unproductive, dead, no or poor bacterial activity; unbalanced growth media for plants.
Dis-ease-lack of health; a left-spin condition; aging condition; loss of vital organ function; liver issue.
Diuretic-agent that forces excretion of body's extracellular fluids.
Dogma-established authoritative opinion.
Dowager's hump-hunchback condition; loss of bone density and discs; degenerative; very acid terrain.

Dowsing-tool for measuring/interpreting energy, choice of direction or sourcing answers to questions.
Drugs-chemical substances that cause a physiologic effect; toxic anti-life chemical molecules.
Ductless glands-glands that do not secrete into a lumen or duct.
Dynamic Reflex Analysis-kinesthetics; muscle testing; subjective testing methodology.
E. coli-un/friendly bacteria of the gut; critical for health; deadly in pathogenic form.
Eczema-inflammation of the cutaneous layers of the skin (dermis); dermatitis; toxicity related.
Edema-excess fluid retention; waste overload/poor lymph activity; potassium loss; acidic condition.
Enema-a swallow, partial cleansing of the lower colon; stimulates bile flow; deacidification of terrain.
Electrolytes-mineral ions capable of electrical conductivity; necessary for nerve signal transmission
    along nerve axon; minimize Rouleau effect in blood; critical for preventing/addressing heart attack.
Electron flow-movement of electrons along nerve fibers, metal wires or through a solution.
Endocrine system-system for production and distribution of hormones/messages via the blood.
Energy-electrical phenomenon.
Energy field-a field of electrical influence; signature may be left/right spin; signature; footprint.
Energy imbalance-bio-electric stress; dis-ease.
Energy manipulation-alteration of signature and frequency of an energy field.
Energy meridian-an energy highway or path in body; chakra; energy flow.
Energy (scrambled)-destructive, unpredictable skew of healthy energy; radiation/irradiation/food
    additives/halogens/; free radical production; enzyme destructive; skewing of proteins.
Enzymes-biological catalysts; all body functions require them; see catalyst.
Esoteric-unseen,; mysterious; beyond Third Dimension; Fourth Dimensional.
Estrogens-group of female horones (estrone, estradiol, estratriol, etc.); also part of male physiology.
Exit portal-waste removal avenue(s) in bio-electric body.
Excesses-causative condition behind manifestation of all diseases; opposite of deficiencies.
Exocrine glands-glands which secrete enzymes into lumens or hollow organs like the stomach or gut.
Extracellular fluid-fluid between (outside) cells; interstitial.
Exercise-physical activity for aerobic effect and circulation of body/lymphatic fluids; deacidification.
Fabale-a family of plants; parent family of the soy bean.
Facultative anaerobes-bacteria that can function with or without the presence of oxygen.
Fats (lipids)-dietary food category; critical for good health; source of 40% of energy production when
    terrain in balance; solid at room temperature; butter, lard and coconut oils; healthful.
Fat-body tissue; ideally 20% of total weight; adipose tissue; brown fat; excess=obesity.
Fatty acids-critical for health; essential; brain matter=80%; energy source for 40% of ATP production.
Fever (febrile reaction)-elevated body temperature due to infection/toxins/sepsis.
Floaters-yeast and waste debris in the eye; poor blood and lymphatic activity; acidic terrain.
Fission-splitting of atoms/molecules; catabolic; nuclear; metabolic process in a healthy terrain.
Fluorine-a halogen gas; toxic; a wildcat.
Fluoride-a salt form of fluorine gas combined with a metal ion.
Fluorosis-fluoride toxicity in teeth and bones.
Food-nutrient energy in form of fat, protein and carbohydrates; energy footprint may be lert/right.
Footprint-descriptive term indicating spin direction, intensity and depth.
Fourth Dimension-invisible/intangible energy dimension beyond the Third Dimension; esoteric.
Free radical-negative electron scavenger, very reactive; acceleration of aging; catabolic.
Functional cells-healthy cells of the vital organs; parenchyma cells; vitality producing; anabolic.
Fusion-transmutation/formation of molecules; anabolism; goes with a healthy terrain.
Gallbladder-holding vessel for liver produced bile; dumps into gut; gallstones; critical to food digestion.
Gall stones-precipitates from liver/bile; mineral/cholesterol based; called nails in liver's biliary ducts.
Gas-a state of energy; foul byproduct of incomplete digestion in an acid/anaerobic GI tract.
Gastric-related to stomach.
Genetically engineered-manipulated life forms; synthetic.
Germ Theory of Disease-allopathic medical theory; invalid; ignores terrain; single factor analysis.
GI tract-gastrointestinal tract; begins in mouth and goes to anus.
Glaucoma-eye dis-ease; atrophy of retina; supposedly due to eye pressure; blood, lymph, terrain issue.
Glycogen-form in which glucose is stored in muscle and in liver.
Glucose-blood sugar; product of liver and digestion; stored in liver and muscles as glycogen; fuel for
    production of ATP by mitochondria in the electron transport chain of the Krebs Cycle; glycololysis.
Glycerol-glycerin with alcohol(s) attached; present in fats.
Glycine-a nonessential amino acid; sweet; glycine max.
Glycocide-inhibit muscle enzymes; soy/canola contain them.
Glycolysis-splitting & oxidation of glucose; Krebs cycle; formation of ATP by mitochondria; health.
Glands-body organs with special functions and purpose; specialized cells and tissues.
Goiter-swollen thyroid gland; linked to stressed ovaries, pancreas, liver and adrenals; trophy; inability
    of thyroid gland to produce hormone; not related to iodine insufficiency.
Gout-uric acid toxicity in blood and joints; degenerative; acid terrain; degenerative if ignored.
Gua Sha-acupuncture without needles; manipulation of trauma memory via blood and lymph technique.
Greens-collards, broccoli leaves, spinach, cabbage, chard, etc.
Gut-small intestine (includes duodenum, jejunum, ileum; stomach to cecum; source of leaky gut.
HCL-(hydrochloric acid); stomach acid; breaks peptide bonds joining amino acids; critical for health and
    protein metabolism; kills incoming parasites and eggs by digesting their proteins.
hGh™-human growth hormone precursor in racemized™ form; use with Skin & Body Toner.
HIV-Human immunodeficiency virus; precursor virus to AIDS.
Halogen-an chemically unstable, acidic gas; a wildcat; toxic; combines with alkaline earth mineral ions.
Harmonic-a healthy frequency; causes body to resonate health/vitality.
Heart attack-insufficient oxygen to heart muscle; also result of skewing of calcium : magnesium ratio;
    insufficent mineral ion electrolytes in blood; sodium overload; potassium shortfall.
Heat stoke (exhaustion)-lack of circulating blood electrolytes; can occur when fully hydrated.
Herbicides-man made organic plant poisons.
Hemorrhoids-swollen, congested, displaced veins in the anus; bile, liver and water issue; constipation.
Hepatitis-inflammation of the liver (hepatocytes); invasion of liver by viruses; serious terrain issue.
Hepatocytes-functional cells of the liver; critical for good health; death of translates as aging.
Herpes-group of viral conditions; sexual/non- sexual; fever blister, genital blisters; liver terrain issue.
Hiatel hernia-deterioration in diaphragm near esopogus allowing stomach to infringe on lung cavity.
High blood pressure-hypertension; sign of systemic cardiovascular issues; amyloid plaque; acid terrain.
High Enema THeherapy™-manipulation and management protocol of colon; stimulation of bile flow and
    stimulation of nerve plexus from colon wall to vital organs; deacidification; critical to long term health.
Hologram-a multidimensional energy message; illusionary 3-D effect; beyond Third Dimension.
Homeopathic medicine-the medicine of similars; uses remedies; exact opposite of allopathic medicine.
Homeovitic-extension of homeopathy remedies; mixed multiple frequencies; esoteric.
Hormone-chemical messenger; powerful energy field; product of vital organs and glands.

Hormone Cycle-female cycle; not same as menstrual cycle; occurs monthly from puberty until death in all females; can be resurrected, measured and mapped; critical to all women.
Howdy Doody Lines-Facial lines from corners of mouth to sides of chin; sign of aging, toxicity, parasites.
Hyaline-albuminoid, involved in amyloid plaque formation; in healthy form part of hyaluronic acid.
Hyalinization-infusion of hyaline into cells or tissue; formation of amyloid plaque.
Hybrid food-food produced from genetically weak seed.
Hydration-the water level in tissues of the body.
Hydrochloric acid-produced by stomach wall; breaks peptide bonds linking amino acids into proteins.
Hydrogen-an element; high energy; bonds easily; bioactive; acidic.
Hydrogen peroxide-H_2O_2; therapeutic; antiseptic; oxidizer; kills all pathogenic organisms.
Hype-unrealistic thinking; mind over matter; bio-junk diet induced stress.
Hyperspace-Fourth Dimension energy space; beyond Third Dimension.
Hypertrophy-increased/abnormal change in organ function and size; i.e. goiter, prostate.
Hyper-exaggerated; enlarged
Hypo-diminished; smaller
Hypoglycemia-low blood sugar.
Hypotrophy-decline; abnormal change in organ function; diminished organ size; atrophy.
Hypovolemia-low blood fluid volume (also lymph0; low water levels in body/tissues.
Ileum-final section of small intestine; joins colon at cecum.
Ileocecal valve-gatekeeper of gut/colon flow rate; between small intestine and cecum.
Immune system-auto defense system; also offensive functions.
Immunization-bogus introduction of foreign microbial protiens into body; does not produce immunity.
Impotence-inability of male to get an erection; female clitoris non responsive, impotent.
In-camera-consideration of all body systems as a whole; not isolated.
Inflammation-redness; swelling; generates pain; body response to immobilize limb, part.
Indols-toxic whole molecules produced/absorbed via a leaky gut wall.
Insulin-blood protein, shuttles glucose transfer across cell membrane; diabetes related; magnesium and and leaky gut origin; autoimmune condition; one of four major disease of aging.
Integument-the skin (subcutaneous, dermis, epidermis); one of seven body connective tissues.
Intercellular substance-fluids, waste, protein matrix between cells; amyloid.
Interstitial fluid-fluid between the cells; extracellular fluid.
Intestine-small intestine (gut); large intestines (colon); approx. 20 feet long.
Intima-innermost layer of the artery blood vessel wall interfacing blood.
Intoxication-alcohol saturation of tissues beyond liver's ability to degrade and kidneys to excrete.
Intracellular fluid-fluid inside the cells.
Intrinsic factor-secreted by stomach; a Vitamin B-12 shuttle; production diminishes after age 30.
Intuition-instinct; Fourth Dimensional concept; esoteric; gut instinct.
Invisible-not seen; ; Fourth Dimensional; esoteric; positive/negative thought; prayer; magic.
Iodine-an element; needed for health; related to thyroid goiter formation; toxic in wrong form or quantity.
Ion-an atom that has gained or lost electrons.
Ionic bond-bond between two mineral ions.
Ionic minerals-minerals that have gained/lost electrons; unstable; seeing to bond; sea water.
Ionization-exchange of energy and electrons; anions/cations.
Irradiation-destruction/scrambling of food molecules; negative energy manipulation; anti-life.
Iridology-reading/interpretation of body health using iris of the eye.
Irritable Bowel Syndrome-collection of bowel disorders; leaky gut/liver related; stress/nervous effect.
Ischemia-reduced oxygen supply to heart muscle.
Isotope-an atom with same number of protons, but different number of neutrons.
Jaundice-effect of toxic liver; bilirubin buildup in blood; yellowing of eye sclera; toxic.
Juice/juicing-extraction of food plant juices for drinking; vegetable juices best; deacidification.
Kombucha tea-dynamic home preparaton used for rejuvenation.
Kidney-primary excretory organ of the body; exit portal.
Kidney stones-mineral/fat/waste precipitates in the kidneys.
Kinesiology-study of body movement.
Kinesthetics-muscle sense testing; kinesiology.
Krebs Cycle-cycle for production of energy molecule ATP; glycolysis part of; includes electron transport chain; mitochondria controlled process; anabolic; aka citric acid cycle.
Leaky gut-porous wall of small intestine; liver issue; drives all autoimmune disease; not age related.
Lactate-salt form of lactic acid.
Lactic acid-product of anaerobic fermentation; incomplete oxidation of glucose; acid waste; produces muscle soreness; liver recycles and clears body of.
Laying on of hands-healing through energy transfer; similar to chi gong and therapeutic touch.
L/CSF™-device for increased circulation of lymphatic and cerebral spinal fluids; very effective.
Lecithin-emulsifier and component of oils/fats/bile; soy derived but not a health issue when isolated.
Left-spin-negative energy; catabolic; anti life;
Lice-creatures that live on filth and negative energy in body hair; head, axillary and pubic unique.
Life expectancy-length of time one can expect to live.
Lightning, cellular-energy produced by the mitochondria in form of ATP.
Limb regeneration-regrowth of bone, nerve, tissues and limbs.
Live blood cell analysis-dark field microscopy used for diagnostic purposes; interesting but not reliable.
Liver-primary chemical/fusion/detox organ of the body; can regenerate; central to all body functions.
Liver breath-bad breath resulting from stress liver; smells like onions and/or metallic.
Liver stones (nails)-mineral precipitation from bile; clogs biliary ducts; slows bile flow; accelerates aging.
Load-bearing work-work involving movement and weight; improves circulation; builds muscle.
Localized condition-a condition that is not systemic.
Lungs-organs of external breathing.
Lye soap-saponification of fats/oils with lye (sodium hydroxide).
Lymph-lymphatic fluids in lymph vessels; intracellular plasma protein drained by lymphatic system.
Lymphocyte-immune system cell; B-cell; part of lymphatic system.
Lymphotrophic-change in lymph fluid; T-cell.
Lymph roller-mechanical device for degrading cellulite; moving toxic tissue waste; crushing of blood capillaries in tissues beneath the skin; detoxification.
Lyse-to split, cleave or break apart; to divide.
Macrophage-non circulating immune system 'attack' cell;T killer cell; defensive.
Macular degeneration-deterioration of macula of eye and loss of vision; aging issue for women; amyloid waste,oxygen and hormone driven condition; closely related to loss of hearing & osteoporosis.
Magic bullets-medical science's hype; false hope; drugs; cut, burn and poison.
Magnesium-an element; alkaline earth mineral; critical for heart muscle; must be in ratio to calcium.
Magnetism-the effect of a magnetic field; polarity; (+) (-) fields; therapeutic side of magnet is (-) side.

Magneto hydro dynamics-dental appliance modality for dental plaque management and gum health.
Malnutrition-insufficient absorption of right-spin food energy; digestion; inability to digest food; bile.
Manganese- trace mineral; builds serum iron via bioalchemy.
Mastication-chewing of food; critical to saliva secretion; beginning of digestion process.
Mass-energy exporting tissue growth; generally cancerous; opposite of a tumor; offensive in nature.
Matter-condensed energy.
Matriarchal society-blood line follows the woman.
Matrix-collagen framework for deposition of minerals/formation of bone; basis of all connective tissue.
Meat-animal tissue; may be right/left spin energy.
Menopause-negative shift in hormonal change; the change; opposite of puberty.
Menstruation-monthly shedding of endometrial lining of uterus in women from puberty until menopause; not same as female "hormone cycle; but should parallel menstrual cycle; female health.
Mental age-how old a person thinks.
Mercury-most toxic element on earth; quicksilver; evaporates; composes 40% of amalgam fillings.
Mercuric acid-extremely toxic heavy metal agent for treatment of water during warm months.
Metabolic rate-rate of metabolic activity in a living system; thyroid, waste, liver and hemoglobin related..
Metabolism-summary of all body functions and rate of operation; slow, sluggish, fast, hyper, etc.
Metabolite-end product of metabolism; synchronization.
Metaphysics-beyond normal physics of length, width, height; Fourth Dimension; esoteric.
Microbe-microscopic life forms; bacteria, viruses, molds and fungus; parasites.
Microwave oven-a negative energy cooking device.
Medical Grade Ionized Water™-reduced/oxidized water with very high ORP pH in both acid and alkaline forms; therapeutic water; made from BFRV™ water and racemized™ liquid mineral ions to supply needed electrons; used in Japan to address issues like diabetes, cancer, arthritis and cardiovascular disease; acid form destroys viruses, bacteria, fungi and yeast; water BEYOND conception point.
Mitochondria-bacteria within all cells that produce the ATP energy molecule; 10,000/cell; Krebs Cycle.
Modality-a methodology of therapy.
Molds-lowest life forms; toxic in most forms.
Molecular (intermolecular) bond-bond between molecules; not same as ionic bonds, hydrogen bonds.
Mononucleosis-viral condition of liver; inflamed lymph nodes/liver; severe immune system stress.
Monosodium glutamate (MSG)-a salt of sodium, glutamine and cytoic acid.
Morbid-related to dis-ease, death; life insurance morbidity tables.
Multiple sclerosis-inflammation of central nervous system; myelin sheath deterioration of nerve fibers.
Muscle tone-resistance of muscles to elongation or stretch; healthy musculature; buffed.
Mustard gas-chemical agent of war; made from rape seed oil.
Muscle testing-subjective/unreliable form of dowsing; not for diagnosis or treatment of disease.
Myocardial infarction-see heart attack.
Myelin-protective nerve fiber sheath; neurilemma; pH affected; progesterone related; important.
Myelinoma-deterioration of the nerve sheath/neurilemma.
Myxedema-low thyroid function/metabolic rate; thyroid atrophy; low BMR; hypothyroid.
Nano scale-one between 1 billionth and 1 trillionth of a meter; highly absorbable and active.
Nattokinase-product of correct fermentation of soy; must conatain Vitamin-K2 or unsafe.
Naturopathic-alternative methodology to allopathic medicine; uses multiple healing modalities.
Necrotic flesh-dead, non-gangrenous tissue.
Negative energy-left-spin energy; catabolic; toxic; acidic.
Nephron-kidney blood filter; critical to detoxification.
Nerve gas-toxic agent of war; blocks enzyme function.
Neti pot™-device used with Clear Head™ to purge sinus cavities of infection and mucous.
Neurolema-the outer sheath of nerve fibers; includes Schwann's cells; myelin sheath; synapse.
Neuropathy-nerve fiber deterioration in extremities; pH and hormone related; highly acid terrain.
Neutralize-denature; detoxify; prevent damage by toxic energy, substance or condition.
Niacin/niacinamide-names for synthetic vitamin B-3.
Nicotine-an alkaloid; not toxic in small amounts in natural form; synthesized form extremely toxic.
Nicotinic acid-acid form of nicotine; natural source is dry tobacco.
Nitrogen-elemental gas; critical for formation of protein in food molecules; 3 forms: ammonia, nitrate (metallic) and urea.
Node-part of lymphatic system; toxic energy storage sites; critical to health,y fluid, tissue protein communication system; tonisls.
Nonfunctional cells-cell that do not perform critical functions; covering of vital organs.
Nonshivering thermogenesis-heat produced w/o shivering.
Nourishment-positive food energy that fuels anabolism.
Obesity-slowdown in metabolic & vital organ function; excess weight; huge aging factor.
Old age-dis-ease; loss of vitality; acidification/breakdown of conective tissues; atrophy of vital organs.
Open pollinated seed-seeds that produce true to type; non hybrid; non freak; not genetically engineered.
Opportunistic-condition where microbes proliferate; low tissue vitality; catabolic; acidic.
Organic-a term used in reference to food that is supposed to be healthier than food produced by normal commercial agricultural practices; any molecule containing carbon; bogus, government hijacked term.
Organic poisons-poisons built on a carbon skeleton.
ORP-Oxidation/reduction potential; measure of life force (electrons) in Medical Grade Ionized Water™; symbol (+) means water is in oxidized state and electron positive; and exact opposite (-) for reduced water; high pH plus high ORP; rejuvenatory to body; electrons fuel mitochondrial production of ATP.
Osteoarthritis-calcification of joints and connective tissues; opposite of rheumatoid arthirtis where the joints dissolve and eventually kill the sufferer; both reversible conditions; very acid terrains.
Osteopenia- the rate of bone building as opposed to the rate of degredation.
Osteoporosis-loss of bone density; acidification of tissues and fluids; aging; driven by acidity, low hormonal activity and inability to lay down collagen faster than it is being destroyed.
Ovaries-glands that produce female reproductive cells called ova (eggs); female equivalent of testicles.
Oxidation-aging factor; health building process; can be either negative or positive; involved in free radical production; Krebs Cycle and glycolysis; conversion of glucose (sugars) molecule to ATP; chemistry term indicating loss of electrons (in need of electrons) as indicated by symbol (+).
Oxygen-a gas element; oxidizer; aerobic; anabolism.
Ozone-O_3; therapeutic if in medical grade form; kills pathogenic organisms of all types.
PACs-racemized™ formulation of proanthrocyanidins; very useful for free radical management and minimization of damage to healthy tissues during Young Again Tissue & Liver Protocol™.
pH-measure of acidity or alkalinity of a substance based on hydrogen donor ability; 7.0 is neutral.
PHG-phytohemaglutinin; a vegetable protein glue; heavy in soybeans.
P-P Factor-pellagra preventive agent; known as vitamin B-3 (niacin); commercial sources are synthetic.
Palliation-relief of signs/symptoms without cure of cause.
Pallor-skin color; abnormal or healthy pallor.

Pancreas-vital digestive organ; both duct and ductless; stress linked to liver; diabetes related.

Paradigm-a new model along side an older model.

Paralysis-loss of muscle function and tone; degenerative.

Parasite(s)-foreign life forms in the body living on toxic waste; burden/destroy vital organ function.

Parasympathetic nervous system-involuntary nervous; no control; part of autonomic system.

Parathyroid-four tiny glands on both sides of the thyroid; ductless glands.

Parenchyma cells-functional cells of a gland or organ.

Pathogenic-pertaining to dis-ease; dis-ease causing; degenerative condition of the terrain.

Patriarchal society-blood line follows the male.

Peer review-submission to review by conventional thinking; following the protocols of "legitimate" medical science; control of independent thought; public display of intimate details of discovery.

Pellagra-dis-ease related to unbalanced dietary intake; B-vitamin related; known by other names today.

Pellets-small waste vehicles produced by the liver from waste filtered from blood; if lodged in liver and calcified called nails; if in gall bladder called stones; body normally produces dozens of them each day.

Pendulum-an antenna; a tuning device; a transmitter; a tool.

Peristalsis-intestinal wave-like motions that move food/waste.

Pesticide-organic poison; man-made; attached to carbon atom.

Peyer's Patch-area surrounding appendix that is densely populated by lymph nodes designed to detoxify/neutralize waste energy; appendicitis is confirmation of waste energy overload and toxicity.

pH scale-normally from 1-14; 7 is neutral; ea. # increases 10x.

Phagocyte-a cell that eats invading cells/life forms/antigens.

Phenols-toxic whole molecules produced/absorbed via a leaky gut wall.

Phosphorous-mineral element; alkaline metal; critical to bone formation; calcium : phosphorous ratio.

Phytates-substance that interferes with digestion; heaviest in soy.

Phytohemaglutinin-see PHG.

Plants-nature's antennas; mediate cosmic energy; build soil; produce solar based food energy.

Pituitary-important ductless gland; linked to all other glands.

Plaque-waste deposits in vital organs, tissues and fluid vessels of body.

Plicae circularis-undulating folds in the walls of the small intestine (gut).

Plasma protein-fluid serum proteins; seep into cell spaces for delivery of oxygen and nutrients; approx. 10% loss of blood fluid volume seep into tissues; recirculates via lymphatic system (85-90% drainage); stagnant, residual tissue fluids left in tissues called amyloid fluid; highly acidic.

Polar molecule-a bent molecule like water; highly magnetic electrical charge.

Pollen-reproductive male sperm equivalent in plants.

Polycystic ovary-cysts on ovary(s);"incomplete" ovulation (non emergence of egg from wall of ovary.

Poly/pleo morphic-bacteria capable of morphing into a different specie according to the terrain.

Polluted-toxic; loaded with poisonous waste; raw city water.

Positive energy-right-spin; anabolic.

Positive thinking-mind over matter; helpful if realistic and without hype.

Post mortem-after death; examination after death.

Potassium-alkaline metallic element; (+) charge; sodium's twin; lines inside of cell menbranes.

Precipitate-formation of a solid by settling out of solution.

Precursor-a substance that precedes another; i.e. beta carotene/vitamin A.

Proof-something medical science demands, but can't deliver; a demand to cover lack of knowledge.

Prostate-sperm production and storage site; male ejaculatory organ; surrounds urinary tube.

Portal-an exit point or avenue or system for waste disposal from body

Portal hypertension-high blood pressure in the portal vein.

Portal vein-nutrient laden venous blood vein from gut to liver; 50% of blood is arterial; caries food molecules to liver; pathway to liver for all lipids.

Protein-one of three food nutrient forms; also fats and carbohydrates.

Proanthocyanidins (PAC)-plant derived, extremely active antioxidants; free radical scavengers.

Puberty-onset of reproductive ability; secondary sex charistics (breasts/body hair/body odor).

Pulmonary system-blood circulation from heart to lungs and return.

Pulse-beats per minute by heart muscle.

Pure (biologically friendly) water-two hydrogens and one oxygen only; all comtaminants (mineral or chemical) removed; erasure of memory of contaminants; bond angle adjustment.

Purine-a nitrogenous protein waste from incomplete digestion of animal tissue or self digestion of body muscle mass; catabolic; adenine, guanine; nucleic acid end product; gout factor.

Pyridine ring-a synthetic organic molecule used to make artificial B-vitamins; left-spin; will not support life; toxic to body; synthetic B vitamin molecule.

"-R"-group-a chemical group that gives an organic molecule its characteristic(s).

RNA-Ribonucleic acid; nucleic acid; genetic template material.

Racemize™-process that increases spin rate and energy field to boost biological availability and usefulness to body by a factor of 10x.

Radiation-energy radiating from a source (nuclear/solar); left/right spin)

Radionics-broadcasting of energy frequencies in agriculture.

Radiomimetic-ability of a substance alter body frequency to left/toxic state.

Rape oil-canola oil; toxic; not a food; radiomimetic.

Rebounder-a mini trampoline used to circulate lymphatic fluid.

Reduced-opposite of oxidized, oxidation. A high energy state.

Refractometer-brix meter;measures sugars in plant juices as an indicator of mineral load/plant health.

Rejuvenate-to rebuild; start anew; anabolism; opposite of aging; health.

Remedies-homeovitic, homeopathic substances for neutralizing negative energy and restoring health.

Replication-multiplication; reproduction.

Repolarization-stimulation and restoration of cellular matrix and organelles (mitochondria) to normal ize cellular function; healing through increased production of ATP.

Resiliency-return to previous condition; ability to bounce back.

Respiration, external-O_2/CO_2 exchange in the lungs.

Respiration, internal-O_2/CO_2 exchange in the cells.

Retrovirus-a virus capable of using a reverse enzyme to access the host; HIV virus is a retrovirus.

Right-spin energy-anabolic; positive; aerobic; health giving.

Royal Jelly-hormonal food fed to a bee to create a queen capable of living 5 years vs. 28 days; highly hormonal effects on humans; restoration of sexual peak; good for both sexes,

Rouleau effect-blood borne waste that produces clumping of blood corpuscles slowing movement of waste through blood capillary beds slowing production of bile by liver; goes with toxic terrain; aging.

Root canal-removal of nerve tissue in inflamed tooth; retention of dead tooth; cavitation; antigen antibody response; C Reactive Protein factor associated with non febrile terrain response; involved in degeneration of the heart muscle; alternative is to pull tooth; burr out tooth socket and bridge using ceramic material; cannot be checked by x-ray once crowned; requires "cavatat" for determination of

decay in months and years following canal; avoid.
Rotenone-a toxic poison derived from the soybean.
Roten-Japanese for derris: plant family to which the soybean belongs.
Rhythm (rhymicity)-scheduled, rhythmic, regular habits and lifestyle.
Saliva-secretion of the salivary glands; digestive juice; pH sensitive; beginning of the digestive system.
Salt-combination of halogen and metal ions.
Satiety-fullness beyond desire; nutritionally full.
Saponification-soap making; the hydrolysis or splitting of fat by an alkali; hydrolysis of an ester; (*sapo*-soap;*facere*-to make).
Sauerkraut-controlled fermentation of vegetables; nutritious; loaded with friendly microbes;avoid pasteurized forms; easy to make at home with cabbage, green beans and tomatoes (red or green), etc.
Scar tissue-non functional tissue; end product of formation of structural amyloid plaque; negative energy field; negative memory of tissue trauma, non soluble waste tissue; must be digested and circulated out of body via the lymphatic system; collagen formation critical to replacement of scar tissue.
Scientific Method-medical sciences official system of information gathering; anecdotal facts gathered to prove a pet theory rather than observation of the creator's handiwork; no vision involved.
Schwann's Cells-cells residing at the synapses of nerve axons; necessary for nerve signal transmission.
Sea water-naturally balanced mineral ion water; right-spin.
Sedentary lifestyle-lack of exercise and load bearing work.
Self digestion (cannibalism; auto-digestion)-consumption of one's own body tissues and muscle mass when body's needs not met; especially prevalent after age 35, and particularly in female vegetarians and vegans; occurs in all elderly people who are wasting away for lack of ability to regenerate due to loss of control of their terrain.
Senility-loss of mental faculties; Alzheimers; invasion of brain by amyloid plaque; greatly affected by loss of hormonal production in female after age 40; occurs in highly acid terrains.
Sepsis-infection of tissue or blood; usually fever producing; blood poisoning; pathogenic state
Signature (energy)-energy footprint; related to spin and intensity; Fourth Dimension energy factor.
Signs-visable and measurable conditions that support diagnosis and disease.
Silica-mineral element; body transmutes to calcium; of critical importance in soil.
Silicone-thixotrophic substance used in breast implants; highly toxic; destroys immune system.
Similar(s)-homeopathic principle; cancellation of one energy field by another of similar frequency.
Single factor analysis-a form of scientific myopia; head in the sand; one cause for each disease.
Silver dental fillings-not silver; mercury; dental misnomer to hide truth from public; deadly.
Sixth sense-intuition; Fourth Dimension; extension of mind.
Skatols-toxic whole molecules produced/absorbed via the gut.
Skin-our outer tube; a connective tissue; halographic; an organ and an exit portal; very first organ to form upon conception; organ from which tissue differentiation into other organs and tissues follows.
Sleep cycle-period of rest, detoxification and rejuvenation; ATP utilization; repair; deacidification.
Smoking-oxidation of dried tobacco via flame; cigars not a problem; cigarettes very bad.
Sodium-an element; a metal; alkaline; always involved in cancer; displaces potassium.
Soft drink-acid forming; electrolyte robbing; accelerates aging; toxic; heavy metals; avoid.
Soil-biologically live dirt; product of healthy practices, microbial activity, and balancing of medium.
Solar energy-anionic energy; right spin; anabolic; life giving.
Soluble waste-waste that is not in structural form; waste that will flow if given the opportunity; waste body stores in fatty tissue beneath the skin; opposite of structural waste.
Solvent-a substance that dissolves solids creating a solution; Yucca Blend,™ DMOS, alcohol,
Soybean-toxic plant of Derris family.
Soybean oil-degenerative left spinning energy from soybeans; industrial oil; avoid as food.
Space-extension of the mind; related to Time.
Sperm-male reproductive cells.
Spin-direction of energy flow of a substance or thought.
Spinach-an alkaloid; Goosefoot family; eat with vinegar/lemon.
Spirulina-a complete algae protein; good nutrient energy.
Sprouts-sprouted seeds eaten as food.
Spur-mineral/body waste deposits in joints/on bones.
Squat position-correct position for defecation; native position; use short stool or box; squat on toilet.
Stagnant waste-soluble waste that cannot or will not flow; amyloid fluid; intracellular tissue fluids.
Standard-a defined reference point; a known yardstick, measure by which all other things are compared.
Stannous-a tin containing compound.
Stannous fluoride-a toxic fluoride/tin containing compound used in tooth paste and rinses.
Static-standing still; not changing; no motion; synchronized.
Steroids-broad class of hormonal compounds including bile, vitamins and glucosides.
Stomach-digestive organ of GI tract prior to small intestine; holding/mixing reservoir.
Stones-waste vehicles produced by liver from waste filtered from blood; if lodged in liver and calcified called nails; if in gall bladder called stones; abnormal; slow bile flow; unhealthy.
Stool-forms bowel movement; should be very soft or loose; hard=constipation; should have 3-5/day.
Stress-bad energy; antagonistic to adrenal; increases cortisol levels; disrupts female hormonal balance.
Stroma cells-nonfunctional structional cells of the organs and glands; outer covering of vital organs.
Subatomic-below atom size; fusion; transmutation; alchemy; nano scale.
Subclinical-not diagnosable; symptoms only, conditions prior to appearance of clinical signs.
Subcutaneous-below the dermis or dermal layer of skin; shallow or deep facia; basement membranes; fatty tissue layer beneath skin.
Sugar-carbon containing sweet molecule; glucose in blood sugar; may be right/left-spin; glycolysis; conversion to ATP energy molecule by mitochondria in electron transport chain of Kerbs Cycle..
Sun-source of anionic energy; life giver; causes Earth to spin.
Supplement-vitamin, mineral, misc. factors added to routine, daily diet for improved health.
Sweat-a waste product; transport for water abased toxic molecules; good sigh; heat regulator.
Swiss chard-an alkaloid; Goosefoot family; eat with vinegar/lemon.
Symbiotic-one life form helping the other; buddy system; mutual beneficial relationship.
Sympathetic nervous system-under our conscious control; voluntary.
Symptoms-subclinical; undiagnosable; early stages of dis-ease; Fourth Dimensional; energy related.
Synapse-juncture points along nerve fibers where nerve signal is bolstered and transfered from one side of gap to the next; where Schwann's cells are located; receptor sites along nerve axon.
Synchronization-temporary neutralization of energy (electron) transference or reaction; energy stall.
Synergy-the coming together of two or more energy forces that produce outcome different than inputs.
Systemic-affecting the entire body; i.e. fever or infection or constipation or poor bile flow.
Synthesis-energy forces coming together to form a new substance.
Synthetic-artificially prepared; man-made analogous molecule; not real thing; isomer; mirror image.
T-cells-killer cells; defense cells of the immune/lymphatic systems.

Tartar-calculus; dental plaque; product of oral bacteria in an acid terrain.

Terrain-the TOTAL energy state of the bio-electric body physically and esoterically; both Third and Fourth Dimensional state of being; affected by and affects spiritual/mental state.

Testes-glands that produce male reproductive cells (sperm) and female cells (ova).

Testicles-male equivalent of ovaries; reproductive generating organs.

Therapeutic-having healing qualities; promoting health; not derived form cut, burn and poison tactics.

Therapeutic touch-healing through energy transfer or management; chi gong; laying on of hands.

Thermodynamics-study of energy creation and movement; three laws of.

Thermogenic hyperphagia-production of heat by metabolic conversion of food energy or body WAT (fat) and through oxidation of glucose by mitochondrial brown fat.

Thixotrophic-substance that when disturbed turns to liquid state and then reverts to a gel state when left undisturbed; silicone (breast implants).

Thymus-gland of the immune system systems; above heart; critical to good health.

Thyroid-controls metabolic rate; serious female issue; goiter/iodine; critical to good health.

Time-extension of mind; related to Space; Fourth Dimension.

Time & aging-passing of Time defines speed of aging; aging mirrors passing of Time.

Time made visible-signs of aging in the mirror or noted by the doctor for diagnosis of clinical condition.

Tin-mineral element; stannous; component of stannous fluoride as used in toothpaste.

Tissue-cells of the body; grouped by type, function, and organ; physical; palpable; or liquid.

Tobacco-richest source of natural, complete B-vitamin complex in the world; up to 30%; alkaloid when green; acid when dry; a good food; must be food grade tobacco; must be eaten with lemon or vinegar.

Tofu-soybean curd; unhealthy; loaded with phytohemoglutinins; damps thyroid function; influences and skews hormonal activity in male and females and children and the unborn.

Tone-resistance of muscles to elongation or stretch; that state in which body functions/parts are healthy and normal; retention of muscular shape, strength.

Tonsils-lymphatic nodes in the upper throat; swell when infection; toxic energy holding site.

Toxemia-blood poisoning; sepsis; waste overload; fever producing condition; febrile.

Toxic-poisonous; acidic; causes tissues to age; poor health.

Toxins-poisonous; negative energy fields; acidic; product of infection or waste accumulation; acids.

Trace minerals-mineral ions needed in minute amounts; electrolytes.

Transmutation-conversion of one mineral ion (energy field) into another in the gut or liver of animals, or in soil by bacteria.

Trophy-abnormal change in tissue structure or function; driven by conditions of excess in the terrain.

TRUTH-something that can be ignored, but not denied; something that is.

Tumor-abnormal, condensed, energy importing tissue field in the body; cancerous or benign; body either calcifies and walls-off tumors or dissolves them; not same as a mass.

TVP-textured vegetable protein; avoid; usually soy derived.

Ulcer-open sore on skin or mucous membranes of throat, intestine or lungs; degenerative; serious.

Unopposed estrogen dominance-female condition where progesterone is lacking or receptor sites are "blocked" by hormone analogs; estrogens lack opposing/offsetting hormonal influence; symptoms associated with menstrual troubles or menopausal complaints.

Uric acid-a waste product of nitrogen tissue breakdown; gout factor.

Urine-waste product of the body; therapeutic if drank fresh AM daily; contains carbamide; important.

Vaccine-live or attenuated microbes in animal protein serum; toxic; does not produce immunity.

Valence-property of an atom or group of atoms causing them to combine in definite proportion with other atoms or groups of atoms; valence may be as high as 8 and is determined by the number of electrons in the outer orbital shell of each atom; electrical charge; energy state.

Vascularization-blood vessel invasion into tissue or bone for purpose of building or degredation.

Vibrational medicine-manipulation of energy for healing; body friendly; opposite of allopathic medicine.

Villi-finger-like projections of the gut wall.

Vinegar-acidic substance of natural fermentation; good for body; causes bile and tissue acids wastes to flow; does NOT cause body to become acidic; causes body terrain to less acid not more alkaline.

Virulent-disease producing; pathogenic.

Virus-a non-life form; parasitic; steals/converts body's energy; proliferate when terrain is supportive; opportunistic; has ability to take control of DNA and cellular production of ATP; pathogenic.

Viscera-abdominal organs (stomach, pancreas, liver, intestine, ovaries, uterus; spleen and gallbladder).

Visible-tangible; Third Dimensional (length, width, and height); condensed energy.

Vital organs-ductless glands; necessary for survival and health.

Vital force-production of ATP energy; effect generated by vital organ activity; reflection of overall condition of energy state of body, mind and spirit.

Vitamins-co-factors; important to health and vitality; use only food derived.

Vorago™ Effect-condition of non aging and regeneration in females or males as a result of intake of massive amounts of plant pigments via diet or transdermally by the skin.

Waste-acid byproducts of metabolism; may be soluble or nonsoluble, structural or non structural; acidic; drives aging and loss of control of the body terrain, disease and early death.

Water-2 hydrogens + 1 oxygen; food; energy source; primary solvent in body; polar; bent molecule.

Water substitutes-soft drinks, beer, milk, etc.; not acceptable.

Weeds-negative energy antenna; detoxify the air/soil; part of natures garbage crew.

White blood cells-part of the immune defense system; defensive in nature; elevated=infection.

Wildcats-name given to the halogen gases (fluorine, chlorine, bromine, etc.).

Wrinkles-confirmation of the passing of Time; sign of aging in the vital organs; toxicity buildup in the dermal/subcutaneous tissues of the skin; acidification of the shallow fascia; poor thyroid function; sign of inability to lay down collagen faster than it is breaking down; cross linking of collagen.

Yucca Herbal Blend™-biological solvent for removing acid wastes from tisues and boosting bile flow.

Young Again Protocol™- program designed to restore good health and take control of the body terrain.

Yellow Fringed Flag-any flag of government where a yellow fringe, ball or spear is used to subordinate a flag of peace of any nation for the purpose of establishing a foreign "state" or condition repugnant to the constitution and vested rights of a nation's people; bogus; criminal; contempt for the constitution, perjury of oath, constructive treason; may also involve overt substitution of a nation's war flag to trick or obscure the state or condition of the hearing or court ritual under the pretense that the preceding is constitutional, fair, and designed to seek truth; a condition before the "bar;" activity by the bar association and attorneys, barristers, court officers and judges to subvert un-alien-able, constitutional rights of free citizens of a nation/state; a sham; a mockery; a Kabuchi dance!

Zeno (estrogen)-hormone analog; not real; synthetic/similar molecular structure; capable of grid-locking receptor sites in body; confuses body; stresses liver; skews hormonal balance; causes body to become a prisoner unto itself; loss of control over the terrain; aging issues.

"You want the truth? You can't handle the truth!
Jack Nicholson (from *A Few Good Men*)

Hot & Cold Therapy
For Chest & Head Congestion

1. Cover chest area (above breasts) with two double folded towels (four layers of toweling over chest area).
2. Bring large pan of water to a boil; remove pan and place near area where you will do procedure.
3. Fill another small pan with cold water and ice cubes and place near pan with hot water.
4. Using tongs, dip one double folded towel into hot water; lift out; drain excess water; and place towel over the four layers of toweling covering chest. Note: "open" hot wet towel so it covers entire chest area protected by four layers of dry towels.
5. Use two additional dry towels to cover the hot towel. Leave the entire "bunch" of towels on chest UNTIL it becomes too "hot" for person being treated. When that time comes, FLIP "all" towels over onto belly area to "uncover" chest.
6. QUICKLY take wet, ice-cold hand towel from ice water and slop it onto the chest area; rub down chest.
7. Begin again by FLIPPING all towels onto the chest. Re-dip the HOT towel in the hot water and REPEAT procedure.
8. Do HOT, cold, HOT, cold; **always** ending with "HOT!"
9. If possible, place person's feet in a plastic foot basin of HOT water during procedure; refill as needed.
10. Also, place cold, wet wash cloth filled with ice cubes over person's nose and forehead (breaks up head congestion).
11. Procedure is very effective for "breaking up" mucous congestion and "grid-locked" areas by **speeding** and **slowing** blood and lymphatic flow into and out of congestion zone(s).
12. If available, lightly rub down chest with Hysoppus Balm before procedure. Balm causes chest to "release!" **AVOID eyes!**

NOTE: Be very careful with pan of hot water. Be **very careful** to NOT "drip" hot water onto person when applying the wet, hot towel. Do procedure 2-3 times/day until congestion and breathing eases. The above procedure involves MECHANICAL intervention to dislodge chest and head congestion. Procedure works equally well on babies and seniors. When finished, see that the person gets into a warm bed to avoid "drafts!" Make sure the person has plenty of water and sea minerals in them **before** doing procedure or waste cannot flow and congestion is denied a "transport" vehicle. Keep bowels open with enemas 1-2 times a day. [Use High Enema Therapy™ for adults only!]

"They pretend they are telling us the truth and we pretend that we believe it!"

Russian proverb

Source Page

**For More Information
Request The**

Young Again
"Source Packet"

1-800-659-1882
Or Write

Young Again
P.O. Box 1240 Mead WA 99021-1240
(509) 465-4154 fax (509) 466-8103

➥ Free Books

Want to share the *Young Again* message with
friends? If you will pay the s&h, books will
be given at no cost. Books must go to
one address. To order books, call
(509) 465-4154, leave address,
and phone number; someone
will call you and confirm
shipping charges and
arrange payment.
32 books/case
6th edition

(Publisher reserves the right of limitation or cancellation of offer.)

Book Purchases
Wholesale & Resale
Author Interviews

Plexus Press
(509) 465-4154

(No email or web access)

P. O. Box 1240
Mead, WA 99021

Ph. (509) 465-4154 Fax: (509) 466-8103

Books Make Great Gifts!